VISUAL OPTICS

(Volume II)

VISUAL OPTICS

VOLUME II

PHYSIOLOGY OF VISION

BY

H. H. EMSLEY, B.Sc.

LATE HEAD OF APPLIED OPTICS DEPARTMENT,
NORTHAMPTON POLYTECHNIC, LONDON

FIFTH EDITION

BUTTERWORTHS

LONDON - BOSTON

Sydney - Wellington - Durban - Toronto

The Butterworth Group

United Kingdom	Butterworth & Co (Publishers) Ltd London: 88 Kingsway, WC2B 6AB
Australia	Butterworths Pty Ltd Sydney: 586 Pacific Highway, Chatswood, NSW 2067 Also at Melbourne, Brisbane, Adelaide and Perth
Canada	Butterworth & Co (Canada) Ltd Toronto: 2265 Midland Avenue, Scarborough, Ontario, M1P 4S1
New Zealand	Butterworths of New Zealand Ltd Wellington: 26–28 Waring Taylor Street, 1
South Africa	Butterworth & Co (South Africa) (Pty) Ltd Durban: 152–154 Gale Street
USA	Butterworths (Publishers) Inc Boston: 19 Cummings Park, Woburn, Mass. 01801

Originally published by The Hatton Press Ltd, which is now part of IPC Business Press Ltd. It is now reprinted by Butterworths in association with IPC Business Press Ltd, and the journal *The Optician.*

First Published 1936
Second Edition 1939
Third Edition 1942
Fourth Edition 1946
Reprinted 1948
Reprinted 1950
Fifth Edition 1952
Reprinted 1955
Reprinted 1963
Reprinted 1969
Reprinted 1971
Reprinted 1972
Reprinted 1973
Reprinted 1974
Reprinted 1976
Reprinted 1977

ISBN: 0 407 93414 6

Printed in Great Britain by Billings and Sons Ltd., Guildford and London

PREFACE

The kind reception accorded to my text on Visual Optics in various countries has encouraged me, in preparing this fifth edition, to accede to requests that I should extend the text by the addition of chapters devoted to the physiology of vision. In consequence of this extension the book is now subdivided into two volumes.

Volume I, being substantially the same as previous editions except for the transference to the second volume of the chapters on Binocular Vision and its Anomalies, thus deals with what may be called the optics of vision. Volume II, containing the transferred chapters and the new matter, is concerned with the physiology of vision.

The book is intended as a class book for students who are already familiar with the elements of ocular anatomy and physiology, optics and spectacle lenses. It has been found satisfactory for teaching purposes to commence the study of Chapters I and XVII simultaneously and then to proceed through the two volumes in parallel. Matter appearing in small (8 point) type may be omitted on a first reading.

The opportunity has been taken to carry out a systematic revision. Visual optics is concerned with events arising from the interaction of radiation and living organisms in the retina and nervous system and from the contemporaneous interplay of consciousness. Investigation into these events calls for the employment of the analytical methods of physics in association with the broader biological methods necessary when considering sensation and perception. Because of the difficulties involved in this association the progress of visual optics has been retarded. There has, however, been considerable research into the physiology of vision during the last twenty-five years, not only on account of the need to broaden the foundations on which rest the techniques of eye examination, particularly in relation to binocular vision, but also because of the need of physicists and illuminating engineers to know more about vision. The whole subject is consequently in a state of flux and some controversy. Controversial matters would be out of place in a class book of this kind, but the main trends of recent work have been incorporated in the simple outline here presented.

I have abstained from giving details of instruments; these are best obtained in the laboratory and from the manufacturers' literature. The exercises marked (S.M.C.) and (B.O.A.) have been taken from the examination papers of the Worshipful Company of Spectacle Makers and the British Optical Association respectively.

During the original writing of the book I received much help from discussions with my former colleagues at the Northampton Polytechnic, London. I am indebted to them and particularly to Mr. J. Adamson, M.Sc., who collaborated with me in the preparation of Chapters XII to XVI. It is a pleasure also to accord my thanks to Dr. W. D. Wright and Mr. E. F. Fincham for helpful criticism of many parts of my manuscript of Chapters XVII to XXIII. Naturally the great works of Helmholtz and Donders have provided inspiration and I am conscious of help received from the Report on the *Discussion on Vision* and other publications by the Physical Society and from the writings of my friend, Mr. W. Swaine.

In tracing the biographical details to be found here and there in the text and in the Appendix I was kindly assisted by the late Dr. M. von Rohr, Mr. Chas. Goulden and Professor A. K. Noyons of Utrecht; to whom and to those firms who have provided blocks and illustrations I tender my thanks.

H. H. EMSLEY.

EVESHAM,

January, 1952.

CONTENTS OF VOLUME II

VISUAL OPTICS

VOLUME II

BINOCULAR VISION AND ITS ANOMALIES

CHAPTER XII

BINOCULAR VISION

12.1. Conditions for Binocular Vision.

BINOCULAR vision may be defined as the use of two eyes in such a co-ordinated manner as to produce a single mental impression of external space. A complete retinal image of the objects in the field is formed in *each* eye, the two images being transmitted separately to the cortex. Our final mental percept is the result of the blending or fusing of the two neural representations in the higher levels of the brain—the third, psychological, stage of the visual act.* Thus binocular vision is essentially a perceptual process.

The outstanding advantage of binocular over monocular vision is the great superiority of the former in estimating the relative disposition of objects in space and in appreciating their depth and solidity. This is made evident at once by observing a garden or landscape, first with one eye occluded and then with both eyes. Whereas with one eye it is not easy to decide, for example, which of several trees or bushes in the middle distance is furthest away, they all immediately fall into their correct relative positions when the other eye is opened.

When both eyes are in use, we at once introduce the new element of convergence. To see singly objects at different distances it is necessary to exert varying amounts of convergence effort. It has, however, been established by DOVE (1841) and later experimenters that the effect of convergence, like accommodation, is feeble; for objects illuminated by a flash of one thousandth of a second, or less, are seen in relief. This period is less than the reaction time of muscle and less, consequently, than the time required to carry out changes in convergence. Nevertheless, although feeble, this factor of convergence is always present and is utilised when possible to strengthen the binocular perception of depth.

* §§ 1.7 and 1.8.

In the normal individual binocular vision is so greatly superior to monocular vision in this matter of depth perception that there must be some other new and potent factor in operation. We shall see that this lies in a certain kind of correspondence between the right and left retinal images. The eyes assume the rôle of observing stations, as it were, at the extremities of a base line—the interocular base line—a principle adopted in the measurement of

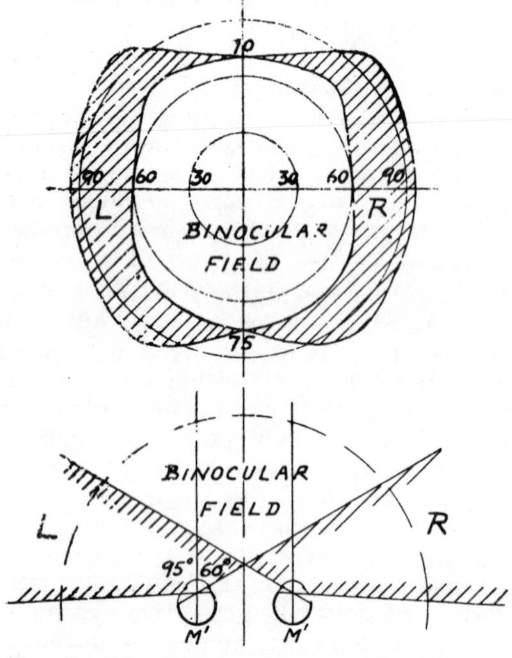

FIG. 12.1—THE COMMON BINOCULAR VISUAL FIELD. EYES LOOKING INTO DISTANCE.

distances by triangulation in surveying. The plane of triangulation, or plane of fixation, determined by the two eyes and the object fixed, is normally horizontal, or swings about the interocular base line as a horizontal axis. Because of this, incidentally, our judgment as to the relative distances of *horizontal* lines, lying in or parallel to the plane of fixation, is much more difficult than is the case with vertical lines, which are normal to that plane.

Granted the possession of two forward-looking eyes, we are thereby provided with two separate and slightly dissimilar uniocular views of objects lying within that portion of space where the monocular visual fields overlap —the binocular visual field. In order that these two views may be brought into association in the cortex so that there emerges out of them a single mental perception, with objects taking up their correct relative disposition in space, further conditions must be satisfied. If the eyes and their connections with the cortex were quite independent of one another, even although each eye possess an orderly arrangement of receptors around its fovea together with the innate faculty of local sign* and consequently a correct monocular sense of direction, the brain would have to contend with two uniocular presentations bearing no relation to one another. Diplopia and a conflicting sense of direction would result. It is clearly necessary that there shall be an orderly spatial correspondence between the *two* retinæ ; a means of bringing their impressions into a corresponding association in the cortex ; and a brain properly equipped by heredity and acquired experience to fuse these uniocular impressions into a single binocular picture. And again, the movements of the eyes necessary to shift fixation over various portions of the field, and from distant to near objects, must be linked together or co-ordinated in order to preserve this correspondence.

We may summarise these requirements for binocular vision thus :

1. The two monocular fields must overlap so as to include an appreciable extent of binocular field within which objects may be imaged on *both* retinæ, each of which contains a pre-eminent central area, the fovea.

2. The retino-cerebral pathways must be such as to convey the two (right and left) impressions of each object to associated regions of the cortex.

3. The eyes must be capable of co-ordinated movements so that the visual axes may be directed to bring corresponding areas of the two retinæ, particularly the foveæ, to bear successively upon chosen objects in the binocular field.

4. The brain must possess the capacity to fuse the two impressions and co-ordinate them into a single binocular percept.

---

* § 2.5.

We have seen, in Chapter I, that the visual mechanism of man and the primates has arrived at a stage of evolutionary development in which the anatomical basis necessary to meet these conditions is provided. The visual fields of the two frontally directed eyes overlap considerably. The visual pathways are such that the two retinal impressions of an object, e.g. Q in Fig. 1.2, are converged to adjacent, or at least associated cell stations in the *one* lobe of the cortex, which is not only convenient for mental fusion but, equally important, introduces the impressions received to a common efferent motor path.* And the system of eye muscles with their motor nerves is arranged to provide the required co-ordinated movements of the eyes.

What we know concerning the manner in which this visual apparatus functions in satisfying the stated conditions necessary for binocular vision, will be outlined in the following pages. Binocular vision of the kind described is enjoyed only by the higher animals.

THE FIRST CONDITION FOR BINOCULAR VISION

12.2. The Binocular Visual Field.

With the eyes looking straight ahead at a distant object, the two monocular fields overlap as indicated in Fig. 12.1, enclosing a considerable region, the common or BINOCULAR VISUAL FIELD, within which each object is imaged on both retinæ. The total field extends over a region exceeding 180° horizontally, but within the portions marked L and R vision is only monocular, R being invisible to the left eye, because of the nose, and L invisible to the right eye. The binocular field of 120° or so is therefore about two thirds of the total extent; this is much larger than the field obtainable with artificial optical instruments. The usefulness of this wide extent of field has already been mentioned.† The upper part of the figure illustrates the projection of the field upon a hemispherical surface such as that indicated by the curved dotted line in the lower diagram; were the field projected upon a plane surface, the monocular portions L and R would extend to infinity in each direction since the temporal side of the monocular field exceeds 90°.

Large as the total field is in any one fixed direction of the gaze, it is still further increased by the movements of

---

* § 12.18. † § 2.5.

the eyes and head as the gaze is continually shifted from one point of attention to another.*

THE SECOND AND FOURTH CONDITIONS FOR BINOCULAR VISION

12.3. Binocular Projection. Physiological Diplopia.

It is important for the student to realise that each eye always receives its own view of the external field and that both views are transmitted and separately presented to the brain; and that it is not until the nervous impulses have reached the brain that the two presentations, in so far as they are suitable, are fused into a single perception.

Experiment. Hold up a pencil ten inches or so before the eyes and look, not at the pencil, but at the wall beyond it or at the sky. Two "images" or projections† of the pencil will be seen; and by closing each eye in turn and noting which image disappears it will be observed that the left image belongs to the right eye and the right image to the left eye. The images have a shadowy or semi-transparent appearance since the portion of the wall hidden by the pencil from one eye is seen by the other eye, giving the impression that the wall is seen through the pencil. The images may be described as "phantom" images.

Hold up the forefinger before the eyes and the pencil further away and a little higher than the finger. Fixing the gaze steadily on the finger, two projections of the pencil appear, the left projection belonging to the left eye and the right projection to the right eye. As the pencil is slowly approached towards the finger, the extent of the doubling or diplopia of the pencil is observed to decrease until when the pencil is approximately at the same distance as the finger it appears single. When the pencil is approached still more, until it lies between the eyes and the finger, the doubling again appears, but now the right eye projection is to the left and the left eye projection to the right, as in the first experiment. The projections are now crossed or heteronymous whereas with the pencil beyond the finger, which is the fixation point, they were uncrossed or homonymous.

We conclude that when we look directly at an object, such as the finger in the experiment, we see it singly; we obtain BINOCULAR SINGLE VISION of that object; and that objects further away or nearer are seen double. This PHYSIOLOGICAL DIPLOPIA of objects seen by indirect vision does not arise in consciousness in ordinary vision: we apparently see only one view of the external world as if we possessed only one centrally placed eye. Nevertheless, the dual nature of the view, and the diplopia, are always present and are of great importance. In drowsiness we

* §12.11. † §13.4.

see double because we are not directing both eyes at the object of attention.

Referring to Fig. 12.2, suppose the eyes rotate and accommodate to fix binocularly an object point O, in the median plane. This point is imaged on the two foveæ M'_L and M'_R and, for reasons already stated, it stands out with greater emphasis and more clearly than any other point in the binocular field. It occupies the centre of the field in both monocular presentations and is perceived as a single point in space situated at the intersection O of the visual axes M'_LN_L and M'_RN_R, N_L and N_R being the nodal points. A nearer object B is imaged at b′ in the temporal retina of the left eye and at b″ in the temporal retina of the right eye. The former stimulation is transmitted to the left occipital lobe and is projected into the right half of the visual field along the direction line $b'N_L$. The latter stimulation is transmitted to the right occipital lobe and projected into the left half of the visual field. There is conflict, as it were, between the two monocular directions; when the mind's attention is directed to the object B, the two cortical impressions are not fused into a single united percept and the object B appears as two objects projected along the directions b′B and b″B respectively. The diplopia may be represented on the diagram by marking the points M_L and M_R along the visual axis in, or about, the frontal plane containing B; it is then given by the distance M_L M_R and is at once seen to be crossed since the projection B is to the right of the left fovea projection M_L and to left of the right fovea projection M_R. *In the frontal plane containing the object, the diplopia is equal to the separation of the two foveal projections.*

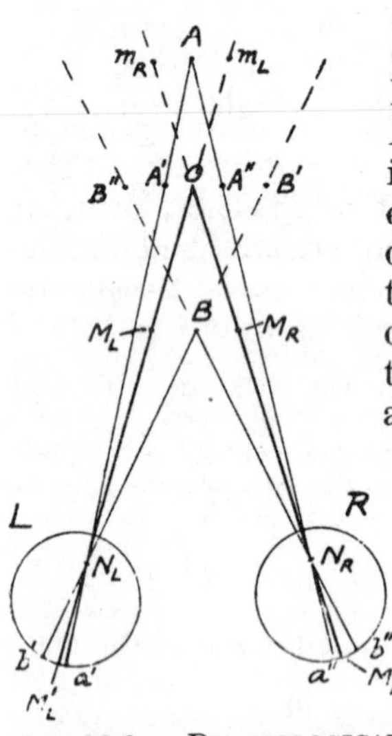

FIG. 12.2 — PHYSIOLOGICAL DIPLOPIA OF A AND B—EYES FIXING O.

An object A more distant than the point of fixation O is similarly seen double. The images a′ and a″ are formed on the nasal portions of the retinæ and the condition is UNCROSSED OR HOMONYMOUS DIPLOPIA. The extent of the diplopia is represented by $m_L\ m_R$, the diagram revealing its uncrossed nature since the projection A is to the right of the right fovea projection m_R and to the left of the left fovea projection m_L.

This physiological diplopia of all objects except the one fixed is constantly present in everyday vision. We do not ordinarily appreciate it as diplopia, however, because the fusion faculty builds out of it a mental picture in which the diplopia is interpreted as nearness or distance relative to the point fixed, according as it is crossed or uncrossed. And further confirmation of the depth impression thus obtained may be derived by varying the convergence to fix different objects O, A, B, etc., in succession. This ranging of the eyes from one object to another, bringing with it the " feel " of changes in convergence and accommodation, is the more needful the greater is the *lateral* separation of the objects. It is only within a limited lateral distance from the point fixed that the relative distances of objects stand out clearly. To confirm the relative distance of objects further removed laterally, the gaze has to be shifted back and forth between them and the original fixation point.

Consider now a point Q, Fig. 12.3, lying upon a circle passing through O and the two nodal points, the eyes still fixing the point O. The retinal images of Q are q′ and q″. The direction lines q′Q and q″Q make equal angles θ with the visual axes M'_LO and M'_RO (from the properties of the circle); hence also

$$M'_Lq' = M'_Rq'' = f_e\theta$$

where f_e is the anterior focal length of the eye $= M'_LN_L$ or M'_RN_R. The nervous impulses from q′ and q″ both travel to the right occipital lobe; both presentations are projected to the left visual field and, because of the above equality, by *equal displacements* θ from the centre of the field O. Thus they possess a common " local sign " and Q is perceived as a single point in space.

On account of the fusion of the two uniocular impressions into a single mental percept, we are unconscious of the fact that two foveæ and retinæ are in operation. Our projection into space takes place without conscious awareness of the dual mechanism. *The projections of the two foveæ are conceived as one point in space.* Estimates of direction when both eyes are used together in binocular vision are mentally referred to an imaginary origin lying between the eyes, as if the latter were acting as one eye, the so-called CYCLOPEAN EYE or binoculus, situated midway between but somewhat further back than the actual eyes.

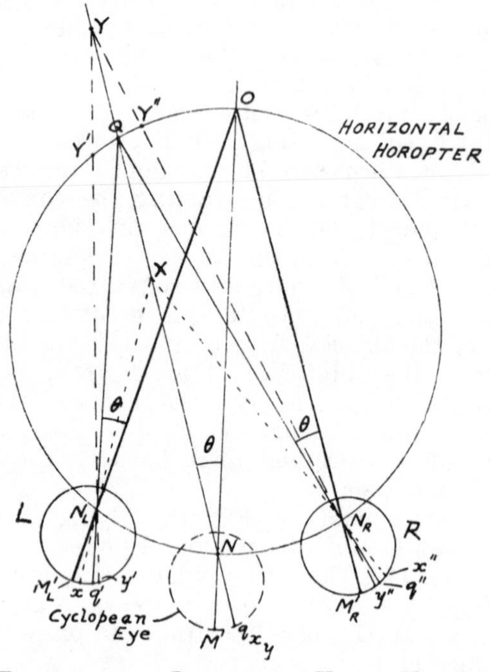

FIG. 12.3—PHYSIOLOGICAL DIPLOPIA OF X AND Y—EYES FIXING O. HOROPTER.

It will be seen from the diagram that the visual axis NO of this imaginary centrally situated eye and the direction line NQ of the point Q with respect to it, are also inclined to one another at the angle θ.

An object at Y, lying in the same general direction as Q, but beyond it, will be imaged at y′ and y″, the impulses from which both travel to the right occipital lobe so that Y is projected to the left of O, by an angular amount θ. (It will also be seen from the geometry of the diagram that $\frac{1}{2}(M'_L\, y' + M'_R\, y'') = M'_L\, q' = M'_R\, q'' = f_e\theta$). Although Q and Y are thus judged to lie along the same direction, there is a significant difference between their respective retinal representations. Whereas the images q′ and q″ are equi-distant from the fovea, the images y′ and y″ are removed from the fovea by appreciably unequal amounts, that is

$$M'_L y' > M'_R y''$$

The object Y is seen double, along the respective directions y′Y and y″Y, the diplopia being homonymous. The diplopia as such is ordinarily ignored, however, and interpreted in terms of greater distance, the retinal images y′ and y″ being binocularly projected along $y'N_L$ and $y''N_R$ to the point Y.

In a similar manner the object X suffers from heteronymous diplopia and is judged to lie nearer than Q, but along the same direction θ.

The diplopia of the point Y may be conveniently represented on the diagram by the distance Y′Y″, which depends upon the amount QY = *dl*, say, by which the distance of Y exceeds that of Q, which we will call *l*. It is made evident to the brain by the difference between the retinal distances $M'_L y'$ and $M'_R y''$, this quantity $(M'_L y' - M'_R y'')$ being a measure of the relative distances of the object Y and the object fixed. Representing the interocular distance $N_L N_R$ by *p*, which is small in comparison with the distance of O or Q, we obtain from the diagram:

$$\begin{aligned} M'_L y' - M'_R y'' &= \frac{f_e}{l}(OY' - OY'') \\ &= \frac{f_e}{l} Y'Y'' \\ &= \frac{f_e}{l}\frac{dl \, . \, p}{l + dl} \\ &= f \, . \, \frac{p \, . \, dl}{l^2} \qquad (12.1) \end{aligned}$$

if *dl* is small in comparison with *l*.

When an object is observed from two stations, the angle included between the two sighting lines to the object is called the angle of parallax. In the case of the observation of an object, such as O, in binocular vision the angle, $N_L O N_R$, is referred to as the BINOCULAR PARALLAX of the object O. The difference between the parallax of O or Q and of Y is thus given by

$$\frac{p}{l} - \frac{p}{l + dl} = p \, . \, \frac{dl}{l^2} \qquad \text{when } dl \text{ is small.} \qquad (12.2)$$

Hence the retinal difference $(M'_L y' - M'_R y'')$ is equal to the product of the eye's focal length and the relative binocular parallax of the two objects.

12.4. Retinal Correspondence. The Horopter.

The above discussion indicates that binocular projection and the perception of depth are closely linked with, and largely depend upon, the faculty of monocular projection described in §2.5. When the two foveæ are stimulated, the mental interpretation is that of a single object at the intersection of the visual axes ; when two retinal points,

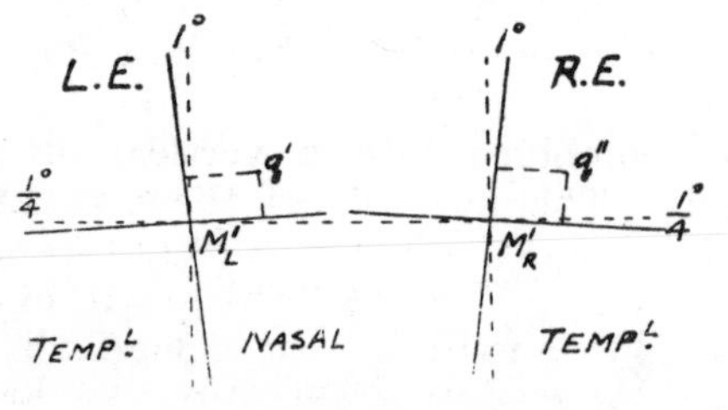

Fig. 12.4—Apparently Vertical and Horizontal Retinal Meridians.

such as q′ and q″ in Fig. 12.3, in corresponding halves of the retinæ and at equal distances from the foveæ are stimulated, the interpretation is again that of a single object at the intersection of their direction lines. Those pairs of retinal points which when stimulated give the impression of a single object point, we may conveniently call identical or CORRESPONDING POINTS. All other pairs of retinal points, which when stimulated give diplopia—ordinarily interpreted in terms of an object beyond or within the point fixed—we may call non-corresponding or DISPARATE POINTS. The two foveæ are the outstanding corresponding points.

From Fig. 12.1 it will be seen that points in the nasal periphery of each retina are projected outside the common binocular field and so can have no correspondence with points in the other retina ; but in all other portions of the retina each point is related physiologically to a corresponding point in the other retina.

We have used the term " corresponding halves " of the two retinæ. We have to define the dividing line between these halves. Experiments in which pairs of fine lines are presented as objects to the eyes, each eye seeing only one line of the pair, show that the meridians of the retinæ which, when projected into space unite to form a single vertical line, are not truly vertical.* They are inclined to one another at a average angle of about two degrees, diverging upwards, the eyes being in their primary position. That is, a line of one retina inclined one degree to the true vertical " corresponds " to a line inclined one degree to the vertical in the other retina. These two meridians may be called the *apparently* vertical meridians of the retinæ ; see Fig. 12.4.

* §12.13.

If they are stimulated, the sensation in the brain is that of a vertical line in space. Similarly the two retinal meridians which are projected to a common horizontal line in space are not quite horizontal, but are inclined usually downwards and temporalwards by about a quarter of a degree in each eye.* These may be called the *apparently* horizontal meridians of the retinæ.

We will, however, ignore these small departures from true verticality and horizontality and will assume that when, with the head erect, the eyes are in the primary position gazing at a distant point on the horizon, the truly vertical and horizontal meridians of the retinæ passing through the two foveæ are mentally combined into a vertical or a horizontal line, respectively. These we will call the PRIMARY VERTICAL MERIDIANS, and PRIMARY HORIZONTAL MERIDIANS of the retinæ. They divide each retina into four quadrants, and external space into four quadrants correspondingly. Corresponding points such as q′ and q″ of Fig. 12.3 are equidistant from these meridians.

Although there is evidence that corresponding areas of the two retinæ are physiologically connected to associated regions of the one lobe of the cortex, this does not necessarily mean that a given pair of corresponding points is anatomically connected rigidly together. The question as to whether this retinal correspondence and the faculty of depth perception resulting from it† are innate and inherited, or whether acquired by experience, has been much discussed. The former idea, the *natavistic theory* of perception, was formulated by the philosopher KANT and expounded by HERING ; the latter, the *empiristic theory*, received support from NAGEL and HELMHOLTZ. Probably both views are in part correct.

It is probable that retinal correspondence does not consist strictly of correspondence point for point, but between small *areas* of the two retinæ,‡ so that single vision would result from the stimulation of any point within such small area of one retina and any point within the corresponding small area of the other retina ; in which case it would be better to speak of corresponding areas rather than corresponding points.

When the eyes fix a single point in space, the two visual axes intersecting in that point, the direction lines from each

---

* There is much variation in different individuals here, however ; the inclination is sometimes in the opposite direction.

† See also the later paragraphs on stereoscopic vision.

‡ PANUM's areas.

pair of corresponding points intersect in some other point in space. The locus of all such points in space is called the HOROPTER,* for that pair of eyes and for the particular point fixed. All points on the horopter are seen single since their images fall on corresponding points. The horopter is a complex surface and many investigators have sought to determine its form experimentally and, by making certain assumptions, mathematically. Actually it will be a different surface for each pair of eyes. If we assume that the retinæ are truly spherical, that the nodal points and centres of rotation coincide, that there is true mathematical symmetry in the correspondence of the retinal points, and that no rotation of the globes around their visual axes takes place—none of which assumptions is true—then the horopter becomes simplified to a toroidal surface the intersection of which by a horizontal plane containing the nodal points is the circle N_LON_R in Fig. 12.3, the eyes fixing the point O. For, as we have already seen, M'_Lq' and M'_Rq'' are equal, or the images of any point Q on this circle fall on corresponding points. This is the horizontal horopter of MÜLLER. If the eyes change their convergence so as to fix some other point, then this horizontal horopter will become a new circle passing through the nodal points and the new point of fixation. There will be a different horopter for each point fixed. This simple horoptic circle will not coincide with the true horopter for a given pair of eyes, since it is based on so many assumptions, but it serves to illustrate the principle. Object points such as X and Y (Fig. 12.3) lying off the horopter, stimulate disparate retinal points and produce physiological diplopia, the extent of which depends upon the distance of such points from the horopter.

12.5. Binocular Projection with Two Objects.

Further illustration of the mental union of the two uniocular images is afforded by considering the binocular vision of two objects.

Experiments. Hold up the two forefingers or two similar pencils before the eyes a foot or so distant and rather more than two inches apart. With both eyes open look beyond the pencils at the wall or

* This term is due to FRANCOIS AGUILLON, whose work entitled *Opticorum* was published in Antwerp in 1613. He made extensive studies in binocular vision. Other investigators in this field have been HERING, HILLEBRAND and TSCHERMAK.

sky. At first four pencils will be seen; the middle ones being less substantial than the outer ones; but on adjusting the separation the two middle ones will coalesce into one, leaving three apparent pencils. The middle one will appear more substantial than the outer ones for the reason given in the first experiment of § 12.3. Since we are gazing beyond the objects, the diplopia of each is heteronymous. The middle pencil is formed by the right eye's right projection and the left eye's left projection, as will be seen by closing each eye in turn.

Repeat the experiment using as objects two similar coins, similarly placed on the table, or two small equal circles (or other geometrical figure) drawn on paper. When the two middle projections have been combined into one, place a sheet of cardboard (S, Fig. 12.5) in the median plane extending from the nose to the table. This screens the right object from the left eye and the left object from the right eye, and the two lateral shadowy projections then disappear.

Each experiment may be repeated by converging the eyes considerably (squinting) until their visual axes intersect at a point nearer than the two objects. The left eye can thus be made to look at the right object and the right eye at the left object. The diplopia of each will then be homonymous.

The conditions when the eyes fix a point beyond the objects are represented in Fig. 12.5. The objects are A and B. When the eyes are converged such an amount that their visual axes are directed respectively towards A and B, as indicated in the figure, the left eye receives an image of A on its fovea and an image of B to the temporal side of the fovea. Similarly in the right eye B is imaged centrally and A temporally. These images are projected, through the respective nodal points, along the directions $M'_L AA'$ and $b'BB'$ for the left eye and along $M'_R BB''$ and $a''AA''$ for the right eye. The projections from the foveæ coalesce at $A'B''$; A'' and B' appear to the left and right respectively. Ignoring for a moment the object B, the diplopia of A is seen to be heteronymous: the diplopia of B is similarly crossed. If the median screen or septum S be interposed, A is screened from the right eye and B from the left, in which case the view is limited to the combined middle object at $A'B''$. This will appear fused into a single

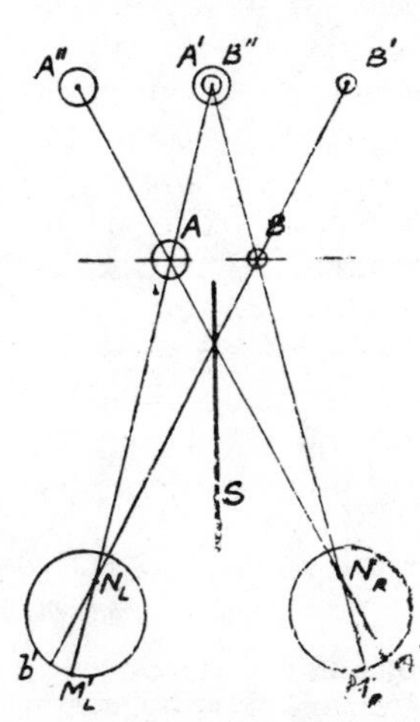

FIG. 12.5 — BINCCULAR VISION OF TWO OBJECTS A AND B WITHIN POINT OF FIXATION.

and apparently real object if A and B are similar, or nearly so ; but merely as two objects superimposed one on the other if the dissimilarity between A and B is marked.

Some students may at first experience a little difficulty in carrying out these binocular experiments. This may be partly due to their initial difficulty in distinguishing between what they *know* of the object or objects exposed and what they actually see. They must learn to examine carefully and analyse what they see as distinct from their conscious knowledge of the objects. Closing the eyes in turn helps.

In the above experiments, when the combined middle image has been obtained, it may appear indistinct and remain so, or it may presently clear up. This is due to the fact that since the eyes have converged on a point at A′B″ (Fig. 12.5), the accommodation will also be appropriate for that distance, whereas actually the objects are nearer. They will not appear distinct, as well as combined, until the accommodation has adjusted itself to the true distance of the objects without any corresponding change in convergence.*

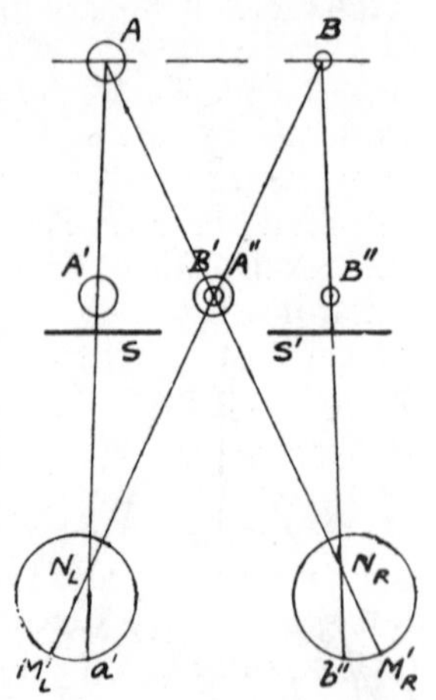

Fig. 12.6—Binocular Vision of two Objects A and B beyond point of fixation.

Fig. 12.6 represents the conditions when the eyes fix a point nearer than the object plane AB. To get rid of the lateral monocular images A′ and B″ in this case, screens are required at S and S′ as shown. These are preferably placed in the plane containing the combined image, since then they will themselves not be doubled.

There is an instrument, due to the Frenchman Remy, called the *diploscope*, based on these phenomena of binocular projection. It is used for examining subjects with anomalous binocular vision. Suppose, in Fig. 12.5, that in the plane containing A and B, about 25 cm. from the eyes, there is a metal plate containing two equal holes at A and B, each about 7 mm. in diameter and 15 mm. apart ; and that a white screen lies in the further plane A″ B′,

* § 5.3.

carrying three printed characters, say D at the position A″, O at the central position A′ B″ and G at position B′. The screen, which is about 33 cm. from the eyes, thus carries the word DOG. A person with normal binocular vision, who sees with both eyes and can direct his visual axes as shown in the diagram, with his attention on the letters on the screen, will see through the two apertures the letters D and O with his right eye, and the letters O and G with his left eye. The retinal images of O fall on the foveæ so that their projections are mentally fused, and the subject reads the word DOG correctly. If, on the other hand, the subject cannot direct his visual axes to pass through the apertures, but leaves them relatively divergent (e.g. divergent squint), then the images of O and G will both fall on the temporal side of the left fovea, and the images of D and O on the temporal side of the right fovea. The subject will then read DO OG, the space separating the two letters O depending upon the extent of the divergence of the two eyes. The instrument can be used to check the relative positioning of the eyes and the subject's binocular vision ; and to provide a certain amount of exercise for an anomalous subject. The diploscope is supplied in various models with additional apertures, but the essential principle is the same in all.

From the above considerations we see that the mental percept of a single object lying at a certain position in space may be the result of the fusion of the impulses from the retinal images of two separate objects. It is necessary to remember that what is seen is the projection outwards of the mental percept ;* in ordinary circumstances this will be a true symbol or token of the actual object or objects, but may in special circumstances be untrue or illusive.

The subject of this paragraph will be continued later.†

12.6. Fusion.

We have seen how the arrangement of the nerve connections from corresponding regions of the retinæ provides an anatomical basis for fusion. It has been advanced that there is a definite " centre " in the brain responsible for fusion, as in the case of the centres for speech, etc. ; and certain kinds of squint have been attributed to failure of development of this centre. There is, however, no anatomical

---

* § 1.4. † § 12.19 *et seq.*

evidence of its existence or of the existence of an innate fusion sense. The probability is that the function is rather the result of operations in the brain as a whole, through the agency of its association pathways. Nevertheless, it is convenient to refer to the function as the fusion sense or impulse.

Momentary fixation is present at birth, or at any rate in earliest infancy, indicating the innate dominance of the fovea. The action is purely reflex and fixation cannot be maintained. At two or three weeks the power of monocular fixation for longer periods develops. Binocular fixation follows and can be maintained at the age of six months or so; until then the eye movements are uncertain in the horizontal plane but they appear always to move together in a co-ordinated manner in vertical movements. During this early period the child learns to correlate the positions of things as seen with their positions as experienced by feeling them; out of the ensuing system of reflexes in the brain, the faculty of fusing the two monocular presentations into a unitary binocular perception gradually gains strength and precision.

The final binocular percept is created in the brain out of the two separately elaborated monocular neural images. If these two images appear alike under introspection, the fused binocular impression is the same as either monocular component. SHERRINGTON suggests that it is contemporaneity in time that leads the mind to "see" just one percept; the mind cannot help but see singly. The two monocular sensations may differ from one another, however. Even when a single object is under observation, the two retinal images may differ in distinctness because of anisometropia or unequal visual acuities in the two eyes; or they may differ in size or shape in corrected anisometropia, a particular case arising when one eye is aphakic; or the images may differ in luminosity.

When different objects are presented to the eyes as in the experiment of § 12.5 or in some kind of stereoscopic device,* or if, viewing a single object, differently tinted glasses are interposed before the eyes, the retinal images may differ in brightness or in colour.

If the brain finds the monocular sensations so widely different as to prevent fusion, there arises a state of

---

* § 12.20.

antagonism or RIVALRY between them. They may co-exist for a while superimposed one on the other; first one and then the other may assume preponderance in the mind.* To overcome the disturbing effects of such retinal rivalry, one or the other may be mentally suppressed, the attention being concentrated on one to the exclusion of the other. The trained microscopist, for example, learns to suppress what he sees with the eye that is not looking into the instrument, which eye he keeps open for comfort. Clearly, if the two impressions are unequal in potency, the stronger one will occupy the attention and the weaker will be suppressed. Such suppressions may be entirely psychological, the attention being focused upon either of the two sensations if they are not widely different. This state of affairs exists in cases of alternating squint.† In other cases of squint, which are non-alternating, where the image in one eye is definitely inferior in quality, the continual suppression of this image results in disuse of the retino-cerebral and higher nervous pathways of the poorer eye, the visual efficiency of which degenerates, perhaps approaching near to blindness. This condition, known as *amblyopia ex anopsia* (amblyopia due to disuse) will be mentioned later when dealing with squint. We shall see that at a certain stage of squint treatment it is necessary to investigate the fusion powers of the subject (§§ 14.5 and 14.12).

An interesting and useful phenomenon due to unequal illumination intensities of the two retinal images of a given object is the PULFRICH phenomenon, discovered by PULFRICH (1922) when experimenting with stereo-comparators. The effect may be obtained by viewing a simple pendulum with both eyes, a dark glass being interposed before one eye. The pendulum, although swinging actually in a vertical plane, appears to be describing a horizontal ellipse. When the dark glass is before the left eye so that the left retinal image is reduced in brightness, the direction of the apparent elliptical path is clockwise as observed from above. The effect is noticeable when the difference between the amounts of light entering the two eyes is about twelve per cent. If the difference be increased beyond a certain ratio, the illusion of the elliptical path ceases, as the feebler image is suppressed and binocular vision ceases.

---

* § 12.5. † § 14.3.

The explanation lies in the fact that the time required for a retinal stimulation to appear as a perception increases as the illumination is reduced. Thus suppose the eyes to be fixed, at a given moment, on the pendulum bob as it passes its mid-position O in the direction of the arrow, Fig. 12.7. The retinal images are on the foveæ M'_L and M'_R. A moment later the bob is actually at A. At the moment when the image a″ of this in the right eye is perceived, the left eye image a′ of the bob when it passed through the position a has just been perceived. The reaction time is longer in the relatively dark-adapted left eye. Thus the retinal distance $M'_R a''$ exceeds $M'_L a'$ and the object momentarily appears to lie at the intersection A′ of the direction lines $a'N_L$ and $a''N_R$; and A′ is further away than the line of swing OA. Thus the bob appears to move along the elliptical path indicated by the dotted line.

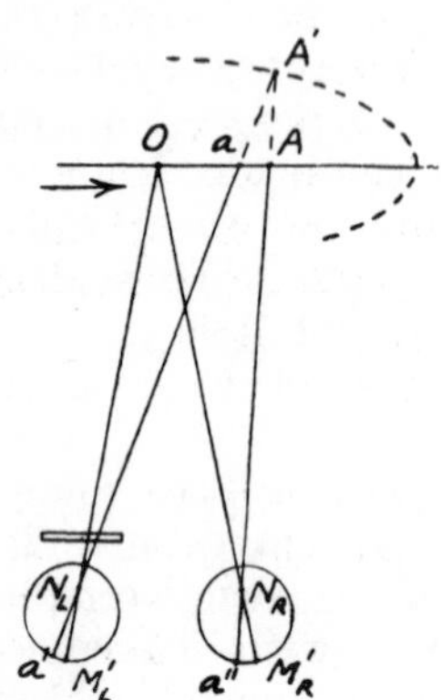

FIG. 12.7—APPARENTLY ELLIPTICAL PATH OF A SIMPLE PENDULUM WHEN RETINAL IMAGES ARE OF UNEQUAL INTENSITY.

This is a striking example of the manner in which depth perception can be falsified by an inequality between the two eyes. It was sought to adapt this phenomenon as a method for comparing the luminosities of two light sources (*photometry*), but it appears not to be accurate. It has been proposed that since it will operate in the case of a pair of eyes in which one eye has a relatively diminished light sense, it has some clinical importance for people who experience difficulty in games, such as tennis. For its effect can be eliminated by putting a smoked glass before the better eye, conducing to more correct judgment of position and movement.

Just how the physiological actions that take place in the nerve cells of the cortex finally emerge into a fused picture in consciousness and is projected outwards when the nerve impulses arrive there, we do not know, and perhaps never will know. It is probably beyond the power of our mind to probe the nature of its own actions. This does not prevent us from investigating the causes and results of such actions and formulating rules concerning them, much of which can be done, in the normal case, from purely physical and geometrical considerations; nor from designing binocular instruments of great service to vision. We do not know the precise nature of light or of electricity or of matter, but we can nevertheless discover laws governing their effects and harness them to useful ends.

To sum up: to obtain binocular single vision of an object, (*a*) there must be foveal vision in both eyes; (*b*) both visual axes must be directed so as to intersect at that object; and (*c*) the neural images resulting from the two retinal images of it must be brought together, projected into space and fused in the cortex. If, for some reason, the visual axis do not intersect at the object of attention, the object will be seen in diplopia; this is *simultaneous vision*, but not binocular vision.

12.7. Dominance of One Eye.

In many individuals one eye seems to assume a state of dominance and is relied upon more than the other; it is from this eye that sighting (pointing, reaching, grasping) takes place. There is disagreement as to the significance of ocular dominance and its bearing on binocular vision. It would seem that any theory concerning the nature of binocular vision must explain the need for a dominant eye for sighting purposes as well as the co-operation of the two eyes in giving us our appreciation of spatial relief. By some who have specially studied this subject* the following conclusions have been stated, though they are by no means universally accepted; indeed the subject is a very controversial one:

(*a*) There is a relation between ocular dominance and general sidedness (eye, hand, foot). The important motor

* E.g. W. H. Fink, "The Dominant Eye"; *Arch. of Ophthal.*, April 1938; F. S. Lavery, "Ocular Dominance", *Trans. Ophthal. Soc.*, LXIII, 1943.

and sensory co-ordination centres should be grouped together in one cerebral hemisphere—the left for right-sided persons—and the dominance of one side of the brain should be complete.

(*b*) Ocular dominance is established early in life, probably about the age of three, and remains stable thereafter.

(*c*) Ocular dominance promotes mental stability and better co-ordination.

Training aimed at making a left-handed child right-handed stimulates the development of previously dormant " centres " in the non-dominant cerebral hemisphere and produces conflict which may manifest itself in many ways including stuttering and difficulty in learning, particularly in subjects involving the use of symbols—reading, writing, etc.—and, even in adults, in hesitation and slowness in making decisions.

(*d*) Ocular dominance is independent of visual acuity and facial asymmetry and does not shift as vision changes from distance to near.

Of the many tests that have been proposed for the recognition of the dominant eye, a good one is the Remy separator test. In the holder of the instrument are two transparent slides, one carrying a black star and the other a black circle. The subject, seeing them first widely separated, is asked to gaze through them at a distant object ; they then come together and he is asked to state whether it is the star or circle which appears to move. That which moves is in front of the non-dominant eye. The dominant eye is master and moves little ; it is the other which has to follow.

As stated above, such conclusions are to be accepted with much caution. The methods used by experimenters to determine which is the dominant eye, or even to define clearly in what sense it is dominant, are of doubtful value ; it is not clear what is being measured.

THE THIRD CONDITION FOR BINOCULAR VISION

EYE MOVEMENTS. MONOCULAR

It is necessary to enquire into the means provided in the visual apparatus for moving the eyes in such a way as to satisfy the third requirement for binocular vision stated in § 12.1; into the nature of these movements and the rôles played by the various extra-ocular muscles and their nervous connections in producing them. The efficiency of the visual apparatus depends largely on the speed and precision with which these movements are executed. They may be initiated in two ways: *voluntarily*, the gaze being consciously directed from one place to another as, for example, in reading: or *involuntarily*, as when the eyes turn without conscious volition to examine some object that has appeared in the field of view, or when the eyes follow a moving object—the *fixation reflex*, to which further reference will be made.* The eyes have to be moved in such a way that not only in their primary position, but also when looking sideways, up or down or obliquely, or when converged in near vision, objects shall be seen in their proper positions and orientations, so that the two uniocular images shall be fusible into a single perception in three dimensions.

12.8. Planes and Axes of Reference.

We may consider the head as symmetrically divided into two lateral halves by a vertical plane called the MEDIAN PLANE. Vertical planes parallel to this are sagittal sections and vertical planes perpendicular to it, frontal sections. Horizontal planes are sometimes called transversal sections. The lines formed by the intersection of such planes are: sagittal lines running from front to back; transversal lines running from left to right; and vertical lines. Since we are concerned with forward-looking eyes with their entrances (pupils) lying on the front-to-back axis of the globe, it is convenient to refer eye movements to the rectangular system of co-ordinates formed by those sagittal, transversal and vertical lines that pass through the centre of projection of the globe. These three co-ordinate axes are fixed in the head and will be termed the *sagittal*, *transversal* and *vertical* axes of rotation.

By various ligaments and elastic fascia the globe of the eye is held in its bed of orbital fat in such a way that, except for extreme rotations, its normal movements are practically limited to pure rotations around a fixed point which we have called the centre of rotation and which we take to lie about 15 mm. back from the cornea and nearly

* § 12.18.

on the optic axis.* The means of moving it being provided, such a globe has theoretically the same freedom of movement i.e. three degrees of freedom, as a ball-and-socket joint. All its movements can be resolved into rotations around the three co-ordinate axes.

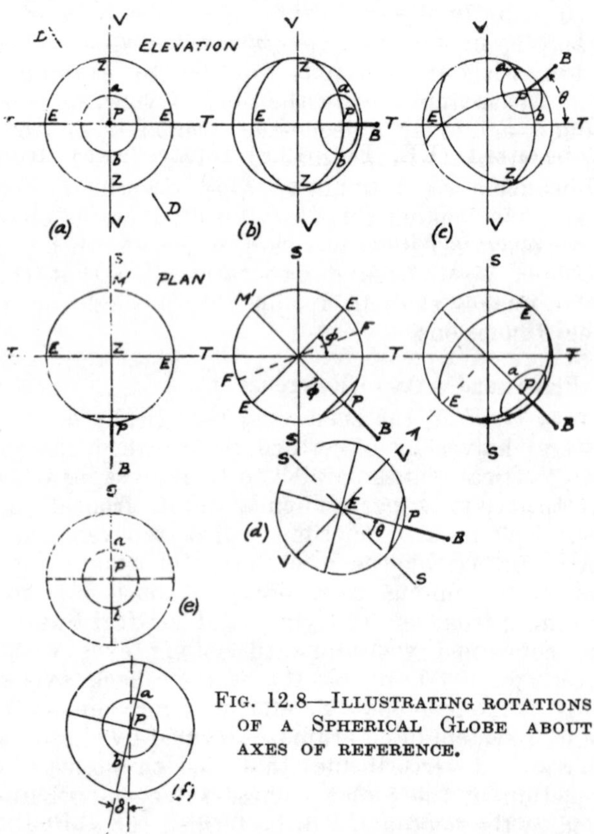

FIG. 12.8—ILLUSTRATING ROTATIONS OF A SPHERICAL GLOBE ABOUT AXES OF REFERENCE.

When, with the head erect, the eye is looking straight ahead along the sagittal axis and with the primary vertical meridian of the retina lying vertical, it is said to be in its zero or PRIMARY POSITION. If both eyes occupy their primary positions, the plane of fixation is horizontal. In this primary position of each eye the visual axis coincides

* See § 10.7.

(CO in Fig. 5.2) with the sagittal axis. If, from the primary position, the globe rotates sideways about the vertical axis, or up and down (elevation and depression) about the transversal axis, such motions are termed CARDINAL ROTATIONS, the eye having moved from the primary to a SECONDARY POSITION. In cardinal movements the direction of gaze of the globe sweeps over a horizontal plane or over a vertical plane; and the primary vertical meridian of the retina remains vertical. In a horizontal cardinal rotation as when the left eye turns to observe an object to the left (Fig. 12.8 b), the horizontal equatorial diameter of the globe itself (EE, Fig. 12.8) rotates away from the transversal axis TT which is fixed in the head, its nasal extremity advancing forwards. The visual axis has described an angle of *azimuth* ϕ. If the eye look upward from the primary position, a vertical cardinal rotation, it has described an angle of altitude.

Should the globe move so that the fixation line does not lie in a horizontal plane or a vertical plane, but in some oblique position between them (left eye looking out and up, for example) the globe is said to be in a TERTIARY POSITION. Whether or not the primary vertical meridian remains vertical will depend upon the manner in which the globe arrives into this position.

12.9. The Rotation of a Spherical Globe.

Consider Fig. 12.8 (a) showing a plan and front view of a spherical ball which may be taken to represent the left eye in its primary position. Although in this paragraph we shall use terms applicable to the eye, we are here discussing the movements, not of the eye, but of any spherical globe. The co-ordinate axes are SS, sagittal; TT, transversal; and VV, vertical. The equatorial plane EZEZ of the globe itself lies in the frontal plane. Suppose the globe to rotate around the vertical axis VV into the new position (b). It has executed a horizontal cardinal rotation through an angle of azimuth ϕ into a secondary position; its horizontal equatorial diameter EE is inclined at this angle to the frontal plane TT. The primary vertical meridian is still vertical, passing through M′, which may be taken to represent the fovea. M′PB represents the fixation line.

Now suppose the globe to rotate upwards around its own horizontal equatorial diameter EE, describing an angle of elevation θ in the vertical plane containing the fixation line. It is now in an oblique or tertiary position represented by diagram (c). (Diagram (d) shows a view of the globe in this position, looking along the direction EE, as indicated by the arrow.) The primary vertical meridian still remains vertical since this second movement was a pure rotation around EE and has not involved any rotation around the globe's front-to-back axis BPM′. The view to an observer looking on the globe from position B along BP would be as shown in diagram (e), the vertical meridian ab of the cornea and the primary vertical meridian of the retina lying in a vertical plane. It will be clear from the diagram that if the second rotation were to be performed about any axis other than EE, about TT for example, the primary vertical meridian through M′ would be tilted out of the vertical.

The student should construct a simple model or " ophthalmophore " from an ordinary rubber ball, drawing three great circles round it in the three co-ordinate planes and a small circle ab to represent the cornea. Or a circular disc of cardboard will suffice. Holding the ball or disc at the points ZZ for the horizontal rotation and then at EE for the elevation, the effects can be seen easily. A pin might be stuck into the model at P along the direction of the front-to-back axis to represent the fixation line.

The globe could move from the primary position to the tertiary position by means of *one* rotation about an oblique axis DD lying in the frontal plane, DD being perpendicular to the plane containing the original primary position of the fixation line and its final oblique position. If this movement be carefully executed on the model, it will be found that the vertical corneal meridian ab, and hence the primary vertical meridian of the retina, are no longer vertical but are tilted over clockwise (to the observer in front) as indicated in diagram (f). To restore these meridians to verticality would require a counter-clockwise rotation of the globe around its front-to-back axis. Such rotations around the front-to-back axis, i.e. around the sagittal axis when the globe is in the primary position, we will call CYCLO-ROTATIONS OF TORSIONS.

Thus rotation about an oblique axis DD not only shifts the fixation line to an out-and-up position, but at the same time rolls the globe over so that the primary vertical meridian is tilted, *as if* the globe had suffered a torsion.

A tilted position of the primary vertical meridian arrived at in this way, by a rolling of the globe around an oblique axis in the frontal plane, we will call a FALSE TORSION, to distinguish it from a condition in which a tilted position has been obtained by an actual or true torsion. (True torsions, we shall see, are executed by the eye only to compensate the subsidiary actions of the recti muscles.)

The position and false torsion attained by the single rotation about an oblique axis DD from the primary position could be attained by two rotations: such as a horizontal cardinal rotation to the secondary position shown in (b), followed by an elevation around an appropriate axis lying in the horizontal plane. It can be shown that the axis around which this second rotation must be executed is FF, lying midway between the transversal axis TT and the new position EE of the globe's horizontal equatorial diameter.

Thus if the globe be initially in a secondary position such as (b), then to arrive at a tertiary position with the same amount of false torsion as would result by one rotation about an oblique axis DD in the frontal plane, the rotation must be executed around an axis *not* lying in the frontal plane.

12.10. The Rotation of the Eye.

The combination of two rotations, first about the axis VV and then about the globe's own equatorial diameter EE (represented in Fig. 12.8 (a), (b) and (c)), which leaves the primary vertical meridian vertical, could be executed by means of two pairs of muscles, provided their point of origin moved round with the globe, remaining always on the fixation line produced backwards; one pair to rotate the globe about its vertical diameter ZZ and the other pair about its horizontal diameter EE. The anatomical arrangement of the eyes and sockets in the head does not allow of such movement, however; and each eye is, in fact, provided with three pairs of muscles with which the student is familiar.

Under the action of these six muscles, which we will examine in the next paragraph, the eye executes its *cardinal* movements in such a way that the primary vertical meridian remains vertical. In movements from the primary position to an oblique or tertiary position, the primary vertical meridian is tilted as if the movement had been one of pure rotation about an oblique axis DD lying in the frontal plane and perpendicular to the plane containing the initial and final directions of the line of fixation. It does not matter how the eye does actually arrive at the final position it may have moved out and then up, or up and then out, or in some other manner; whatever the actual sequence of movements, the false torsion will finally be the same. The state of tension of the muscles will also be the same.

The immediately preceding statements sum up the laws enunciated by DONDERS (1847) and LISTING (1854). Other prominent investigators in this field were HELMHOLTZ, HERING and MEISSNER.

DONDER'S LAW states: *When the position of the line of fixation is given with respect to the head, the angle of false torsion will invariably have a perfectly definite value for that particular adjustment*; which is independent not only of the volition of the observer but of the way in which the line of fixation arrived in the position in question.

The subject was carried a stage further in LISTING'S LAW, which states: *When the line of fixation is brought from the primary position to any other position, the angle of false torsion of the eye in this second position will be the same as if the eye had arrived at this position by turning about a fixed axis perpendicular to the initial and final positions of the line of fixation.*

The vertical and horizontal axes about which cardinal rotations are executed and the oblique axes (such as DD) about which rotations to tertiary positions are attained from the primary position all lie in the frontal plane containing the centre of rotation of the globe. It is fixed in relation to the head and is sometimes called LISTING'S PLANE.

Since, for a given direction of the gaze, the eye always takes up a definite position of false torsion, the orientation of the globe is sufficiently defined by stating the direction of the line of fixation.

The angle of false torsion, δ in Fig. 12.8 (f), is the angle between the plane containing the tilted primary vertical meridian of the retina and the vertical plane containing the line of fixation. For a tertiary position of which the angle of azimuth is ϕ and the angle of elevation θ, the false torsion is given by the expression*

$$\cos\delta = \frac{\cos\theta + \cos\phi}{1 + \cos\theta . \cos\phi} \qquad (12.3).$$

* J. ADAMSON: *A Study of the Cyclo-rotational powers of the Eyes*; Trans. Opt. Soc. XXXIII, No. 5, 1931–32.

The fact that the eye suffers no false torsion when making cardinal rotations supplies a physiological definition for the primary position : namely, as that position of the eye from which pure vertical and horizontal rotations result in no false torsion being produced.

That the eye does move in the manner described above may be demonstrated in various ways, of which the subjective method of after-images is accurate and instructive. A bright object in the form of a cross A, Fig. 12.9, with its limbs disposed vertically and horizontally is placed

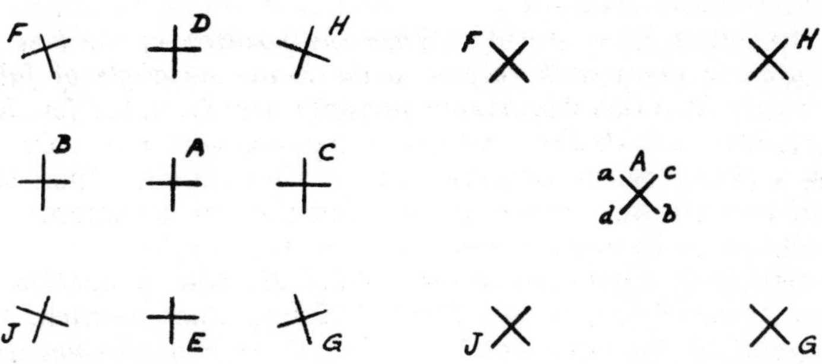

Fig. 12.9—Demonstration of Eye Movements by After-Images.

Fig. 12.10—Demonstration of Eye Movements by After-Images.

on a wall opposite the eye in its primary position. After fixing the centre of the cross steadily for some time and then shifting the gaze to some other part of the wall, an after-image is observed. Since this is the projection of the fatigued area of the retina, it follows the eye accurately in all its movements. If the eye rotate horizontally to fix position B or C situated on a horizontal line through A, the after-image will be observed with its limbs still vertical and horizontal, as indicated in the diagram. If, starting from position A, the gaze is moved to positions D and E on the vertical line through A, again the limbs of the after-image are vertical and horizontal. This demonstrates that for horizontal and vertical cardinal rotations the primary vertical meridian of the retina has remained vertical, the rotations having been executed about the vertical and transverse axes respectively and no torsion having taken place.

If, however, starting from position A, the point of fixation is shifted to oblique positions such as F, G, H, J, the limbs of the after image no longer remain vertical and horizontal. If the line of fixation is directed up and to the left to position F, the upper end of the " vertical " limb appears tilted to the left, as shown. (The diagram indicates the appearances to the subject.) With the gaze directed down and to the right towards G, the lower end of the " vertical " limb appears turned to the right, and so on. If the surface upon which the after image is projected in these tertiary positions is held so as to be always normal to the line of fixation, a condition that would be satisfied if, for example, the surface were spherical with the eye as centre, the " horizontal " limb of the after image will in every case be perpendicular to the " vertical " limb; the cross will still remain rectangular, although tilted. These appearances demonstrate that the primary vertical meridian of the retina is no longer vertical in tertiary positions of fixation.

That this tilted position is not due to a true torsion about the globe's front-to-back axis, but is the result of rotation of the eye about an oblique axis in the frontal (Listing's) plane through the centre of rotation, is proved by repeating the experiment using as the object a cross A, Fig. 12.10, disposed obliquely. If, after a steady gaze at A, the fixation is changed so as to follow a prolongation of the arm ab of the cross to position F, the after image will be seen as a rectangular cross parallel to the cross A, as shown in the diagram. Similarly for positions G, H, and J. The results are similar to those obtained with the cross of Fig. 12.9 when the rotations carried the gaze to A, B, C and D. The retinal strips fatigued by the limb ab and cd (Fig. 12.10) remain parallel to themselves for rotations of the globe to fix F, G, H and J, showing that the rotation of the globe to change fixation from A to any of the tertiary positions is accomplished about an axis perpendicular to the plane containing the initial and final positions of the fixation line.

In the first experiment (Fig. 12·9), had the after-images been observed projected on a flat wall situated in a frontal plane and not therefore normal to the direction of gaze in the tertiary positions, the " horizontal " limb of the after-image would not have been perpendicular to the " vertical " limb. This is merely because the projection of the horizontal limb is distorted by perspective, which has nothing to do with the eye. For example, if the subject were surrounded by a spherical wire cage with the wires running in meridians and parallels, the projections, on a flat wall, of the meridians would be vertical lines, but the projections of the parallels would be hyperbolæ and not horizontal lines.

Because of the tilted position of the eye in a tertiary position, a vertical line object will be imaged on a row of retinal receptors which is inclined to the primary vertical meridian. The occipital lobes will therefore receive *via* the visual fibres the impression of a leaning object. The brain is, however, also receiving information—proprioceptive impulses—from the ocular muscles as to the oblique position of the globe and from the neck muscles and labyrinthe as to the posture of the head. The final verdict, on summing up these constituent messages into a complete mental picture, is that the line is vertical and that it lies to one side of and above, or below, the straight ahead direction.

The false torsion of the eye when it moves into a tertiary position has no special clinical significance. It, and the experiments on after-images, have been described merely to establish the kind of movement that the eye does execute. Having regard to the anatomical arrangement of the forward-looking eyes held in divergent orbits and operated by muscles with origins placed nearer to the median plane of the head, the various movements of the two eyes required to fix objects in differing situations in the visual field are executed in what is probably the most efficient manner and with the least expenditure of nervous energy.

12.11. Field of Fixation.

The extent of the excursions of the eye is naturally limited by its fastening in the orbit. With the head in a fixed position, the extent of external space over which direct foveal vision can be obtained is the FIELD OF FIXATION or the motor field. It may be measured on the perimeter. The limiting rotation of the globe in any direction may be measured as the angle between the sagittal axis and the line joining the centre of rotation to the limiting point that can be fixed by the fovea in that direction. The field varies for different individuals but is approximately as represented in Fig. 12.11, more rotation being possible downwards than upwards. The student should distinguish between the field of fixation, which concerns eye movements and direct vision and the field of vision,* which is the extent visible by indirect vision with the eye *stationary*. The field of fixation is usually smaller than normal in myopes, the greater length of the globe offering obstruction to rotation, particularly in the horizontal direction.

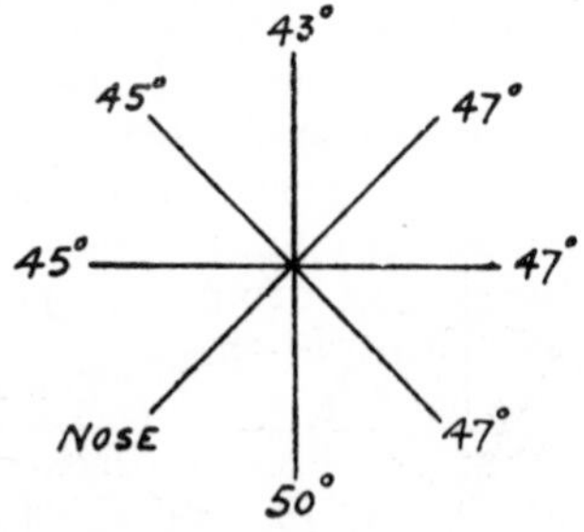

FIG. 12.11—FIELD OF FIXATION.

12.12. Action of Extra-Ocular Muscles.

Each of the six muscles plays its part in produ ng any of the possible rotations of the eye. Their arrangement is illustrated diagrammatically in Fig. 12.12, the lettering of which corresponds to that of Fig. 12.8. The place of origin of all the muscles is fixed in the head, all except the inferior oblique originating around the optic foramen at W which, it is important to note, is situated medially (nasally) with respect to the centre of rotation of the globe. Each muscle exerts a tangential force on the globe, rotating it about an axis passing through the centre of rotation. A plane through the centre of rotation and the direction of traction of a muscle is termed a MUSCLE PLANE. There are thus six muscle planes associated with the globe. A normal to a muscle plane through the centre of rotation will be the axis about which that particular muscle produces its rotation. The muscle pattern of the human eye is such that the six muscles are grouped into three distinct pairs; the medial and lateral recti, the superior and inferior recti, and the superior and inferior obliques. Measurements on the planes of attachment and directions of traction of the muscles show that the muscle planes of the two members of each of the above pairs, although not absolutely coincident, are so nearly so that we may regard them as

* §§ 2.4 and 12.2.

having a common axis of rotation, fixed in the head. The individual muscles of each pair thus rotate the globe in opposite senses, and are *antagonistic* to one another. The deviations from exact antagonism are only slight, being negligible in the case of the recti muscles and amounting to not more than about six degrees in the obliques.

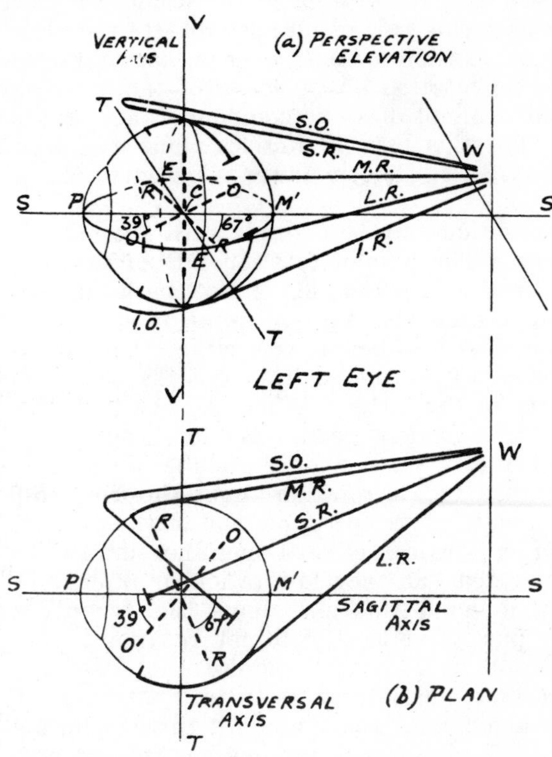

FIG. 12.12—LEFT EYE. AXES OF REFERENCE. EXTRA-OCULAR MUSCLES AND THEIR AXES OF ROTATION.

The common axis of rotation of the medial and lateral recti is vertical, coinciding with the vertical axis of reference VV, Figs. 12.8 and 12.12. The superior and inferior recti have a common axis of rotation RR (Fig. 12.12) which lies in a horizontal plane and makes an angle of about 67 degrees with the median plane, being forward on the nasal side. The obliques are regarded as having a common axis of rotation OO which lies also in a horizontal plane, making an angle of about 50 degrees with the median plane, and being forward temporally. These directions will be appreciated from Fig. 12.12, in which (a) represents a perspective view and (b) a plan, of the left eye in the primary position. From the fact that the axis of rotation of the medial and lateral recti is normal to the plane containing the axes of rotation of the other two pairs, it will be clear that this pair of muscles rotates the globe so that its line of fixation sweeps over a horizontal plane and produces no rotation about either of the other axes, since a rotation cannot have a component at right angles to itself. Thus this pair of muscles alone can produce only lateral rotations, directly inwards or outwards, about the vertical axis.

The conditions are less simple with the other two pairs of muscles. The axis of rotation RR of the superior and inferior recti, for example, is not perpendicular to the plane containing the axes of rotation of the other two pairs, nor does it coincide with either the transversal axis of reference TT or the sagittal axis SS but is inclined at 67 degrees to the latter. When the eye is in the primary position the vertical recti, therefore, not only produce elevation and depression of the globe about the axis TT, but also introduce a rotation about the front-to-back axis PM′ such as to move the upper end of the primary vertical meridian or vertical corneal meridian inwards when the eye is elevated—an *in*cyclo-rotation or *in*torsion; and, in addition, a small rotation about the vertical axis. To produce purely vertical cardinal rotations, the superior and inferior recti clearly require the assistance of the obliques and the lateral recti to neutralise this cyclo-rotation and lateral rotation. All three pairs are then in operation. Suppose now the eye has rotated outwards by 23 degrees until its line of fixation coincides with the direction of traction of the vertical recti. The action of the latter pair of muscles is then one of pure elevation and depression. If, on the other hand, the eye has rotated inwards to a position of appreciable convergence, then the action of the vertical recti muscles is predominantly one of torsion. Thus the action of the superior and inferior recti depends upon the position of the globe at the time their contraction commences. It will be seen from Fig. 12.12, however, that in the usual positions of the globe their action is mainly one of elevation and depression, which may therefore be conveniently looked upon as their *primary function*; torsion and rotations about the vertical axis are somewhat *subsidiary* effects of theirs.

Similarly with the oblique muscles: their effect varies from one predominantly torsional when the eye is turned outwards to one mainly of elevation and depression when the eye converges inwards. Which of these two functions is in the ascendency depends upon the position of the globe at the moment considered.

The following table may be useful as a guide to the primary and subsidiary functions of the various muscles, but it must be borne in mind that the medial situation of the origin of the muscles renders the subsidiary functions properties of the orientation of the globe.

PRIMARY AND SUBSIDIARY FUNCTIONS OF THE MUSCLES.

Muscle	Primary Function	Subsidiary Action(s)
Medial Rectus ..	Medial Rotation (in)	Nil.
Lateral Rectus..	Lateral Rotation (out) ..	Nil.
Superior Rectus	Upward Rotation or Elevation..	Medial Rotation Incyclo Rotation
Inferior Rectus..	Downward Rotation or Depression	Medial Rotation Excyclo Rotation
Superior Oblique	Incyclo-Rotation. Depression ..	Outward Rotation
Inferior Oblique	Excyclo-Rotation. Elevation ..	Outward Rotation

The actions described are easily understood by reference to Fig. 12.12 or to the model ophthalmophore. In considering them the student should also bear in mind that the muscles are not equal in weight and cross-section, the medial and lateral recti being the heaviest and thickest pair, followed by the vertical recti and obliques, in that order.

Even when the eyes are gazing passively forward into distance and the attention is not actively engaged, there is tone in all the muscles* and any movement, whether to

* §12.14.

a secondary or a tertiary position, will utilise the co-operative or SYNERGIC action of all three pairs. It is to be remembered that the coincidence of the axes of rotation of the two members of a pair is not absolute, and that in any movement where certain muscles are scarcely required for positive action, as in the case of the vertical recti and obliques when the movement is a lateral cardinal rotation, they are nevertheless of service (along with the check ligaments) in steadying the globe and preventing deviations from the movement desired. By the co-operative action of all three pairs of muscles all types of motion (within limits) possible to a body with three rotatory degrees of freedom are possible: but the muscles work together with such wonderful precision that only those movements required in the interests of co-ordinated binocular vision are executed and these—*vide* Listing's law—in the most efficient manner and with the least expenditure of nervous energy. The means whereby the innervations are supplied to the muscles will be referred to later.

The position of passive equilibrium just referred to, in which all the muscles are in a state of tonus and in which the brain is appreciative of the presence of light stimulus so that the eyes are ready to spring to attention, as it were, and move towards binocular fixation and fusion of any object that excites the individual's attention, is termed the position of FUNCTIONAL REST. This position is to be contrasted with that of anatomical rest.* The muscles are ready to respond instantly to RECIPROCAL INNERVATIONS, by which we refer to the fact that the contraction of a given muscle to execute a given movement of the globe is always accompanied by just the correct amount of inhibitory innervation, or relaxation, to its antagonistic muscle or group of muscles. The tonic contraction of the muscles when the eyes are in the passive condition of functional rest is only slight, however, compared with the contractions that occur when an active movement of the eyes is called for.

TORSION.

This movement is a rotation of the globe around its fixation line and places the primary vertical meridian of the retina in various meridians. It occurs in certain excursions of the eye as a compensatory movement. For

* §5.2.

example, to produce a pure cardinal rotation upwards from the primary position, the oblique muscles operate to compensate the torsional movement that would result from the action of the recti muscles alone. In one excursion of the eyes torsion of each globe occurs when it is not required in its usual compensatory capacity; this is when the eyes converge from a distant to a near object, a movement of extorsion of each globe taking place when the plane of fixation is elevated above a certain position. This will be referred to in §12.13.

EYE MOVEMENTS. BINOCULAR

12.13. Conjugate and Disjunctive Movements.

To preserve the retinal correspondence necessary for binocular single vision in all directions of the gaze, the two eyes must move together in a co-ordinated manner. It is common experience that they rotate together vertically, sideways and obliquely, keeping their fixation lines parallel, so as to view distant objects in various parts of the binocular motor field; and that, in any direction of the gaze, they can rotate in opposite directions in the plane of fixation in the act of convergence, to scrutinise nearer objects. These associated movements are executed with great facility and cannot voluntarily be dissociated in normal vision. It is not possible, for example, to turn one eye to the right or upwards without a corresponding movement of the other eye, except in special circumstances.* Which is evidence of the truth of the important basic principle that in all normal eye movements there is an equal distribution of nervous energy between the two eyes so that they rotate equally and symmetrically (HERING).

Following MADDOX, we shall find it convenient to divide the *possible* binocular movements into the two broad groups set out in the following table, namely:

(1) CONJUGATE MOVEMENTS OR VERSIONS, in which the fixation lines remain at a constant inclination to one another, parallel when viewing distant objects in various directions, and the primary vertical meridians remain parallel;

(2) DISJUNCTIVE MOVEMENTS OR VERGENCES, in which the fixation lines or the primary vertical meridians vary their inclination to one another, as they do in convergence

* E.g. see §§ 5.4 and 5.5.

or relaxation of convergence (divergence) when viewing objects successively at unequal distances.

Of these possible movements, those that may be described as necessary for binocular vision in ordinary circumstances, and which are normally executed, are the versions Nos. 1, 2, 3 and 4 and the vergences Nos. 7 and 8. These are the only movements that can be executed voluntarily in the normal visual apparatus; it is considered, by MADDOX for example, that definite subcortical "centres" for the first five of these movements have been established. Of the other movements in the table, which are involuntary or reflex, the cycloversions are called into play when the head is tilted to one side;* the supravergence and cyclovergence movements, Nos. 9 to 12, may be required in corrective movements during the complicated act of fusion. Cyclovergence may also take place, as we have seen, when the eyes are converged in near vision, depending upon the elevation (or depression) of the plane of fixation. A cyclomovement is a torsion; in the same direction in both eyes in the case of a version movement and in opposite directions in a vergence movement.

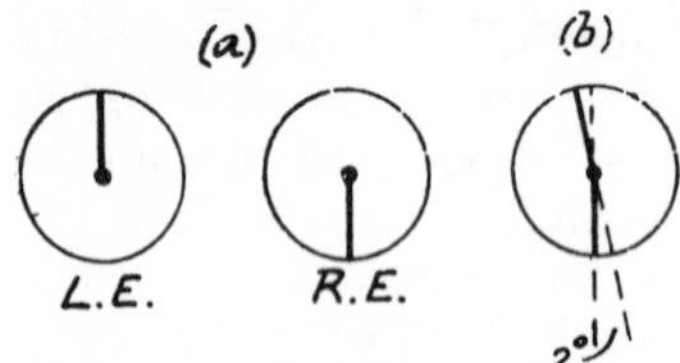

FIG. 12.13—ILLUSTRATING INCLINATION OF APPARENTLY VERTICAL RETINAL MERIDIANS–VOLKMANN'S DISCS.

It will be observed that the first four version movements are those carried out to place the eyes in different directions when dealing with two-dimensional space; and the first two vergence movements those executed when dealing with the third dimension, or depth.

In the conjugate movements each eye separately obeys Listing's law, except for extreme movements, the eyes rotating equally and symmetrically. The primary vertical meridians of the retinæ remain substantially parallel to one another as the eyes move over the visual field. If VOLKMANN's discs, Fig. 12.13, are presented at an appreciable distance, so that each eye is allowed to see only one disc, as in a stereoscope, when the two central spots are

* §12.18 and Fig. 12.16.

fused the two radii do not appear as an unbroken vertical diameter but inclined at about 2° as in (b); this inclination

CONJUGATE MOVEMENTS or VERSIONS.	DISJUNCTIVE MOVEMENTS or VERGENCES.
1* DEXTRO-	7* CON
2* LÆVO-	8 DI-
3* SUPRA- (or Elevation)	9 RIGHT SUPRA-
4* INFRA-(or Depression)	10 LEFT SUPRA-
5 DEXTRO CYCLO-	11 INCYCLO-
6 LÆVOCYCLO-	12 EXCYCLO-

TABLE. POSSIBLE BINOCULAR MOVEMENTS.
* Voluntary Movements.

remains constant with the gaze in various directions. We have already mentioned this inclination of the apparently vertical meridians.*

* §12.4.

If the eyes are made to converge, a disjunctive movement, the experiment with Volkmann's discs shows that the angle between the apparently vertical meridians, and hence also between the primary vertical meridians, gradually increases with increase of convergence, so long as the plane of fixation remains horizontal. The average angle seems to be about 6 to 8 degrees in extreme convergence and 4 degrees at the reading distance of one third metre. These extents of excyclovergence, or extorsion, decrease if the eyes are depressed below the horizontal plane as they converge, until at a certain angle of depression there is no extorsion. If the eyes are depressed more than this, there is a movement of *in*torsion as they converge. The special value of the depression angle at which there is no torsion is about the amount of depression ordinarily used in reading. It appears to be the case that the opposed torsion effects of the superior rectus and inferior oblique during elevation and convergence, and of the inferior rectus and superior oblique during depression and convergence,* neutralise one another at the particular value of depression referred to. The gradual change in the relative inclination of the retinal meridians with the plane of fixation in other positions is a true torsion of the globes around their fixation lines.

The co-ordinated movements of the two eyes are made possible by the fact that, in addition to the association of the muscles of each eye into a synergic whole, certain muscles of one eye share a common innervational control with certain muscles of the other eye. Such muscles are yoked in their action into a common team, as it were, and parallel movements are executed as if the two eyes were a single instrument. Thus the outward rotating muscle (lateral rectus) of the right eye is yoked to the inward rotating muscle (medial rectus) of the left eye, the two behaving, when required to do so, as a single right-handed mechanism. The muscles functionally concerned with one side are controlled by the cerebral hemisphere on the other side, as in the case of all limbs of the body.

Fig. 12.14 is intended to represent diagrammatically the muscles positively associated for the various conjugate rotations from the primary position. In looking upwards the right and left superior recti are mainly concerned, but the two inferior obliques are also associated in maintaining

---

* See below in this paragraph.

verticality of the primary vertical meridians. To look downwards the inferior recti are mainly required, the superior obliques acting with them in a minor capacity. To look to the right and upwards, positive action is required by six muscles, three for each eye; the dextroversion movement is produced by the right lateral rectus and the left medial rectus. During the first part of the excursion from the primary position, the elevation is brought about by the superior rectus and inferior oblique in each eye; as the movement proceeds, however, the left superior rectus and the right inferior oblique become gradually less effective in producing elevation, so that towards the limit of the movement this task is almost completely taken over by the left inferior oblique and the right superior rectus, only four muscles being concerned at this stage. This is indicated in Fig. 12.14; small letters are used for the four muscles which attend to elevation at first and capital letters for the two muscles, R.S.R. and L.I.O. which are responsible for elevation at the limit of the movement.

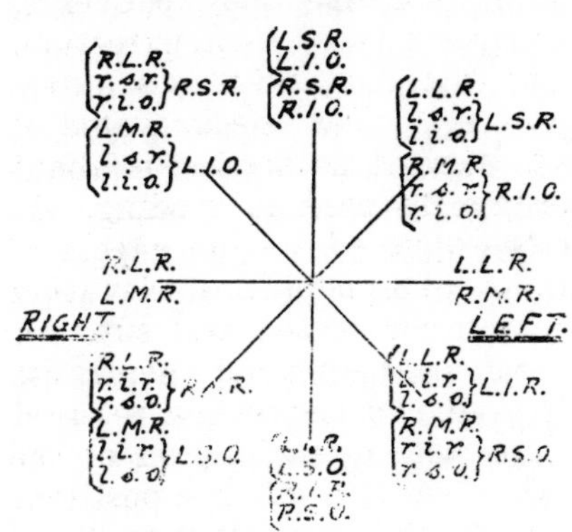

FIG. 12.14—ASSOCIATED MUSCLES FOR BINOCULAR CONJUGATE MOVEMENTS.

The other three oblique movements are lettered in a similar manner; the student should check the diagram, using Fig. 12.12 to assist him. Pure lateral rotations require the operation of only two muscles, the lateral and medial recti.

12.14. Functional Rest. Orthophoria.

If, the attention being directed towards a distant object on the median line, fusion is prevented, as by holding a card in front of one eye, the eyes will take up their position of functional rest, or as near that position (CP_D in Fig. 5.3) as we can practically attain. (We can never be sure of the extent to which other influences, such as the impulses from the neck muscles and labyrinthe and the factor of the individual's interest and attention, may

be tending to urge the eyes somewhat away from the rest position towards the fixation position.) Fusion being prevented, the eyes are freed from the controlling influence of the fusion impulse and the position (CP_p) they take up is the position of passive equilibrium of the oculo-motor system. This position *may* coincide with the desired fixation position, which in the case of a distant object is the primary position; in which event no further movement of the eyes is required to effect fusion of the uniocular images.

The balance of the oculo-motor system may not be so perfect as this, however. It may be that, in the passive position, the visual axes are convergent or divergent or supravergent; or that the primary vertical meridians of the retinæ are not vertical. In such a state of imperfect motor balance further movements of the eyes, under the direction of fusion, are necessary in order to place the eyes in the desired primary position and so effect fusion; extra fusional *effort* is required.

When the passive position of functional rest is also the primary position, such a perfectly balanced condition of the oculo-motor system is described as ORTHOPHORIA, *for* DISTANCE.*

When, for some reason, the passive position deviates from the primary position, we have a condition of HETEROPHORIA. Such deviations from the orthophoric condition may be remedied by corrective fusional movements of the eyes, when fusion is allowed. Upon completion of such movements binocular single vision, and depth perception, take place in a normal individual.

12.15. Composition and Speed of Eye Movements.

The actual composition of the movement from one fixation point to another is not as simple as might appear. If fixation is changed rapidly from one object to another, the point of fixation does not sweep smoothly over the straight line joining the objects, but usually describes an irregular curve between the two. The movement may carry fixation beyond the second object and so is followed by a short return movement, the to-and-fro process being repeated until fixation is achieved, the eyes then remaining at rest except for the fine tremor that always accompanies fixation. If the eyes are called upon to follow a slowly

* This definition will be somewhat amplified in the next chapter.

moving object, their more or less regular path includes a series of undulations. If such gliding movements are executed without the aid of a moving fixation object, the undulations become short jerking movements alternating with momentary pauses.

In reading, the eyes advance along the print in short rapid jerks, each jerk being followed by a fixation pause of a quarter of a second or so, this interval being probably sufficient to allow of interpretation of the retinal image. The eyes usually make four or five stops in the ordinary line of print, but this may vary according to the individual and the difficulty of the test.

The movements executed in changing fixation are very rapid ; they are quicker at the start and gradually decellerate as the point of fixation is approached. Lateral movements are the quickest and vertical movements the slowest. It is found that the movement is speeded up if the attention is concentrated upon the final fixation point.

The smallest voluntary conjugate rotations possible are of the order of 5 to 10 minutes of arc.

CONTROL OF OCULAR MOVEMENTS

12.16. The Oculo-Motor Nerves.

The wonderfully co-ordinated movements of the eyes, carried out mainly in the interests of binocular single vision, are governed by certain areas of the central nervous system which together constitute what we may describe as the oculo-motor system, consisting broadly of (*a*) the oculo-motor nerves which supply the innervation to the ocular muscles ; and (*b*) the cortical and sub-cortical areas of the brain which direct and co-ordinate the action of the nerves. The anatomy of the nerves and their connections with one another and with the brain, are matters of considerable complexity and their ramifications are by no means fully understood. Only an outline can be presented here.

Of the twelve cranial nerves, those concerned with eye movements are the third, fourth and sixth,* situated in the grey matter of the mid-brain.† These discharge the efferent impulses to the intra- and extra-ocular muscles.

---

* The seventh (facial) nerve controls the closing of the eyes.

† §1.4 and Figs. 1.1 and 1.2.

The disposition of the nuclei of these oculo-motor nerves is indicated *diagrammatically* in Fig. 12.15. Compare Fig. 1.2.

THE THIRD CRANIAL, OR OCULO-MOTOR NERVE, situated below the superior colliculus, supplies all the external

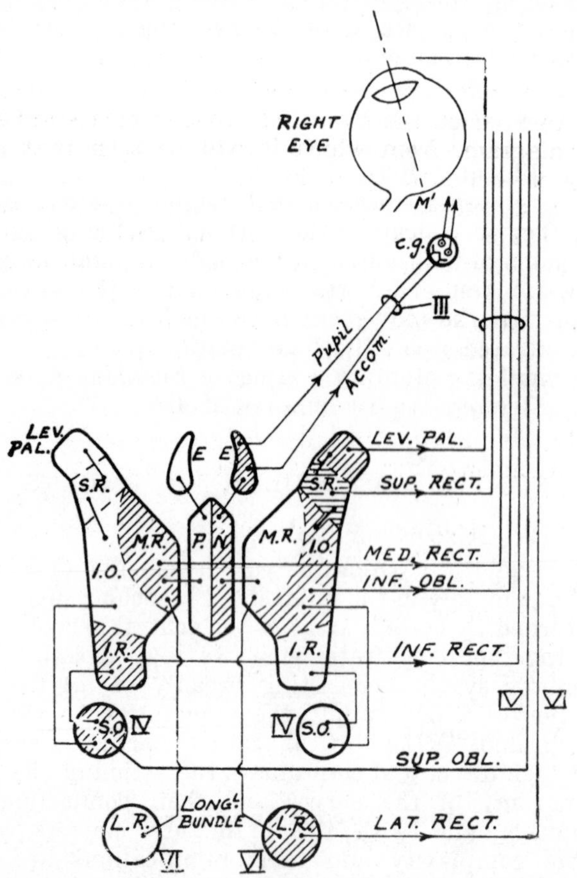

FIG. 12.15—THE THIRD, FOURTH AND SIXTH NUCLEI AND THEIR EFFERENT PATHS (DIAGRAMMATIC).

muscles of the eyes except the lateral recti and superior obliques. It also serves the sphincter of the iris, the ciliary muscle and the levator palpebræ. The constitution of its nucleus is as complex as its wide distribution would suggest. It consists of two large groups of cells disposed laterally round the median group known as Perlia's nucleus (P.N.). Anterior to the nucleus of Perlia are two smaller central groups forming the Edinger-Westphal nucleus (E). These two nuclei supply the intra-ocular muscles and Perlia's nucleus is considered mainly responsible for convergence. The remaining lateral groups of the third nerve, as well as nerves IV and VI, send efferent fibres to the various extra ocular muscles. The diagram indicates bundles of nerve fibres passing to the muscles of the right eye. The nuclei from which the indicated fibres originate are shaded in the diagram, from which it will be seen that all the muscles are supplied by nuclei on the same side except the medial and inferior recti (IIIrd nerve) and the superior oblique (IVth nerve). The various nuclei of all three nerves are inter-connected by means of bundles of association fibres. They are also connected with the superior colliculus, the cerebellum and the vestibular nerve (concerned with equilibrium) in the mid-brain; and with the frontal lobes and occipital lobes of the cerebrum. It is this intricate system of central connections that is responsible not only for initiating but also for co-ordinating the movements of the two eyes, but the manner of its operation has not yet been worked out. Thus the medial rectus of one eye may be required to operate in conjunction with the medial rectus of the other eye, to produce convergence; or it may be required to operate along with the external rectus of the other eye in order to produce a lateral version movement. In effect we may take it that the various nuclei of the three nerves are connected, either directly or indirectly through a network of paths in the mid-brain, in a manner partially suggested in the diagram, Fig. 12.15.

Thus the connection between the nuclei for the medial erctus (M.R.) of one side and the lateral rectus (L.R.) of the other side would account for the correlation of conjugate lateral movements. Similarly, connections between the nuclei of the superior rectus and levator palpebræ of the same eye permit of simultaneous upward rotation of the eyes and raising of the eyelids. The adjustments of convergence, accommodation and pupil contraction required for near vision are associated by the connections between the nuclei for (*a*) the sphincter-pupillæ (E); (*b*) ciliary muscles (P.N.); and (*c*) the medial recti (M.R.). The connection between the superior rectus (S.R.) and the inferior oblique (I.O.) of the same eye would permit of the balancing out of torsional movements when the eyes are raised. The superior recti of the two eyes are joined and also the inferior recti, allowing for conjugate elevation and depression. The scheme of association must also provide for conjugate innervation to such pairs of muscles as the right superior rectus and left inferior oblique when the eyes are to be moved to the right and up (see Fig. 12.14).

It is also supposed that there are connections between the nuclei of the various muscles and their antagonists to regulate the relaxation of one muscle as the other contracts under the influence of reciprocal innervations.*

THE FOURTH CRANIAL, OR TROCHLEAR, NERVE is the smallest cranial nerve and supplies the superior oblique muscle only. It is in close association with the third nerve, as already stated.

THE SIXTH CRANIAL, OR ABDUCENS (out-turning) nerve supplies the lateral rectus.

12.17. Cortical Control. Voluntary Movements.

The oculo-motor nerves just described are themselves stimulated and called into action in appropriate combinations by efferent impulses sent down to them from the " higher centres " of the cerebral cortex or from the " lower " or " secondary centres " of the sub-cortical areas. If the external conditions of the individual's environment are such that his conscious attention is definitely engaged and he decides to move his eyes to examine some chosen object in the field, the impulse for such voluntary movement originates in the motor area of the frontal lobe, in that part of this motor area that is concerned with the eyes (Fig. 1.1). The movements thus voluntarily initiated are Nos. 1, 2, 3, 4 and 7 of the table in §12.13.

These same movements and, in addition, the remaining movements listed in the table may, however, take place without the conscious intervention of the higher levels of the cortex. In that case they are reflex movements and are under the control of the *sub*-cortical regions of the oculomotor system embracing the superior colliculus, cerebellum, and other stations ; or, maybe, of the occipital lobes. We will postpone consideration of reflex movements to the next paragraph.

---

* §12.12.

The central nervous system is continuously receiving impulses from the peripheral receptors of the organs of special sense, informing it of the varying conditions in the individual's environment; and from the muscles of the body (the proprioceptive impulses) as to their state of contraction in meeting these conditions. It responds in such a way as to provide just the correct kind and amount of movement of the various limbs and organs to preserve the body's safety, equilibrium and comfort. The individual may decide to move his eyes, not only in response to some visual stimulus, but also in response to stimuli derived from the other senses. An unusual sound may be heard, the eyes and perhaps the head and body being moved in the appropriate direction to investigate; and the arm on that side of the body may be raised to ward off danger. Such simultaneous movements clearly involve association between those (sensory) areas of the brain concerned with the reception of stimuli from all the senses, as well as association between the motor areas, and between the motor areas and the sensory areas. And they require some kind of mechanism of co-ordination between all the areas involved in order to ensure that the proper combination of innervation is discharged to the muscles concerned, in the correct relative amounts.

It is supposed by some that the intermediary mid-brain region, lying between the cortex and the motor nerve nuclei, contains definite "centres" charged with this duty of co-ordination. According to this view there is a separate centre for each of the conjugate lateral and conjugate vertical movements (Nos. 1 to 4 of table, §12.13) and one for convergence (No. 7). They have not been determined anatomically, but are inferred from clinical observations. Whatever the actual mechanism of co-ordination may be, it is convenient to speak of centres for the various functions—the cortical regions as the higher centres and the sub-cortical regions as the secondary or lower centres; but it should be understood that all the visual functions (fusion, eye movements, etc.) require the co-operation of the whole central nervous system.

Illustration of eye movements in the absence of visual stimulus is afforded by the fact that the eyes can be moved in a dark room; convergence, however, is not easy of precise accomplishment in the absence of an object upon which to fix.

12.18. Involuntary or Reflex Movements. Cortical and Sub-Cortical Control.

In the course of our everyday visual tasks the globes are continuously moved about by reflex action. Sometimes the operation is purely reflex in character, being directed entirely by the sub-cortical regions of the brain without conscious intervention by the higher centres. Alternatively, there are movements which, although executed involuntarily, do to some extent, or perhaps on certain occasions, involve the operation of consciousness.*

In this group of partially-reflex movements, as we may perhaps call them, may be included the movements carried out during the process of fixation and the movements of adjustment executed during the final act of fusion. In both of these processes the visual stimulus is first appreciated by consciousness and it is thought that the efferent impulses originate in the occipital lobes which, for the purpose of these reflexes, are acting not only as sensory areas but as motor areas also, in response to visual stimuli only.

The Fixation Reflex

If, when the eyes are regarding some object B, Fig. 1.2, another object Q in the right visual field attracts the individual's attention, Q will at first be seen in diplopia. The afferent paths from the stimulated receptors at q′ and q″ lead to the left occipital lobe. Efferent impulses will be sent down from this lobe, through the mid-brain regions, to the motor nerve nuclei innervating the right-acting muscles; the right lateral rectus and left medial rectus will be chiefly concerned. The eyes will execute a version movement to the right, accompanied by convergence if Q is nearer than B.

Thus the conjugate (version) movements and convergence may be directed involuntarily from the occipital lobes or voluntarily from the frontal lobes. The impulses from the latter are the more intense, however, and will over-ride those from the occipital lobes if necessary.

Corrective Fusional Movements.

Under the action of the fixation reflex only, the eyes would take up their passive position in the neighbourhood of the point Q. If they are orthophoric for this point, no further adjustment will be necessary to fix Q binocularly

* See §1.4(c).

and fuse the impressions received from the retinal areas q′ and q″. If, however, they are heterophoric for the point Q, some corrective movement of the globes will be necessary to achieve binocular fixation and, maybe, some adjustment of accommodation. The corrective movement required may be one of horizontal, or vertical, or cyclo-vergence.* The impulses transmitted to the motor nerves to execute these final adjustments are directed to permit of fusion of the two uniocular impressions.

If the retinal images are markedly different from one another, or if they are made so artificially, the motive force for these fusional movements will be withheld; the eyes will settle into their passive position and the subject will experience diplopia unless one retinal image is suppressed.

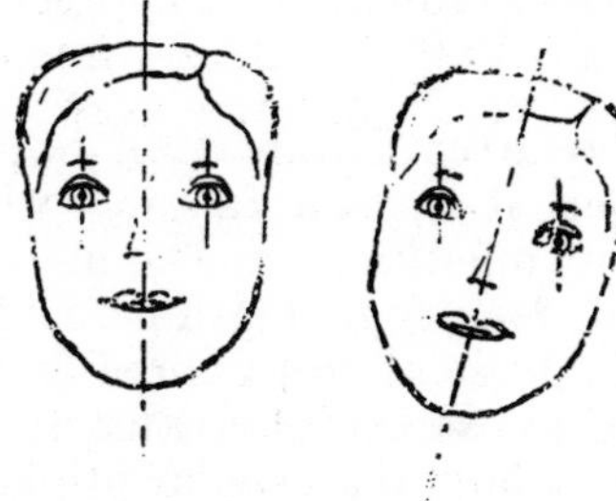

Fig. 12.16—Compensatory rotation of Eyes when Head is inclined.

When the conditions are at all favourable for fusion, however, great efforts will be made to achieve it. If the fixation lines are thrown out of alignment by a prism before one eye or the other, the eyes will move to place their fixation lines into the new position demanded and so regain single vision unless the prism is too strong.†

Postural Reflexes.

These are true reflex movements, controlled by the sub-cortical centres. If the head or body be tilted into some stationary abnormal position, the eyes are given a partial compensatory rotation (cycloversion) in the opposite direction in the attempt to maintain the visual field in its normal orientation, as suggested in Fig. 12.16. The reflex mechanism concerned in such movements, which are called *static reflexes*, includes the labyrinthe and neck muscles.

Again, to preserve the proper appreciation of space during movements of the head the eyes are moved reflexly, probably

* §5.6. † §5.4.

by means of stimuli from the semi-circular canals, in the attempt to maintain the eyes for some time in a constant position relative to the visual field. The eyes first move in the opposite direction to the head to maintain fixation and then rapidly jerk back to a new position, this latter movement being too quick to allow of a visual impression. The involuntary continuance of this to-and-fro movement of the eyes results in the visual field appearing stationary in spite of the sweeping of the gaze over it. Such are called *stato-kinetic reflexes*. They are called into action also, to serve the same purpose, when the eyes are rotated from one part of the field to another.

STEREOSCOPIC VISION

12.19. Stereoscopic Vision.

Although judgment of the relative distances of objects is possible in monocular vision if certain factors, which have been enumerated,* are in operation, and some one-eyed people acquire considerable facility in depth perception after long experience, the full appreciation of three dimensional space which we call STEREOSCOPY or STEREOSCOPIC VISION depends upon the blending of two uniocular presentations, which is possible only in binocular vision.

Suppose the object under binocular observation to be an arrow AB lying in the plane of fixation, i.e. the horizontal plane containing the nodal points N_L and N_R of the eyes, the arrow sloping away from the observer as indicated in plan in Fig. 12.17. Although the retinal images a′b′ and a″b″ possess only the two dimensional attributes of the retinal surfaces, the projected perceptual image is an arrow receding into the distance, the impression of depth being strengthened by moving the point of regard back and forth from one end of the object to the other. If the gaze be fixed steadily on the point O, careful attention (of the mind) on the extremities A and B will reveal that they are seen double—the images a′ and a″, as also b′ and b″, falling on disparate retinal points. Each eye receives its own perspective picture, the " centres of perspective " being N_L and N_R. Suppose further that the eyes are observing the object through a plane glass window WW.

* §2.6.

Projected on this plane the object appears as A′B′ to the left eye and A″B″ to the right eye; these lines could be drawn on the glass, closing one eye at a time. These two projections are slightly dissimilar because of the separation of the viewing stations or projection centres N_L and N_R. If now the original object be removed and the eyes presented with the horizontal arrows A′B′ and A″B″ before the left and right eyes respectively in the plane WW, and the visual axes directed towards O′ and O″, the retinal images will be identical in size and position with those obtained when viewing the original object. The resultant visual sensation will be that of an arrow occupying the position of the original object at AB.

Such stereoscopic or perspective pairs may be obtained by taking photographs a′b′ and a″b″ of the object with two cameras placed with the nodal points of their lenses at N_L and N_R, the focal lengths of the lenses being equal to the distance N_LO' or N_RO''. The photographs thus obtained, reversed and mounted correctly in the plane WW, would correspond to the arrows A′B′ and A″B″ and would form therefore a perspective pair which, viewed from the positions N_L and N_R, would fuse and give rise to the sense of stereoscopic relief.

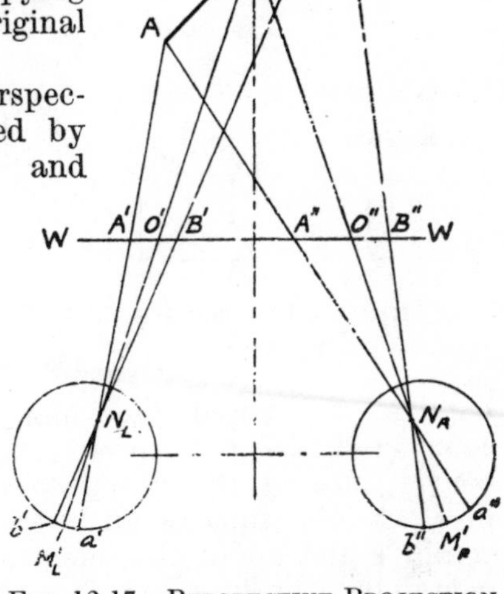

FIG. 12.17—PERSPECTIVE PROJECTION.

Fig. 12.18 illustrates a perspective pair corresponding to a truncated pyramid with the small end towards the observer. The student should fuse these as explained in §12.5, using a median screen so that each eye can see only its appropriate picture. The two figures will approach and presently unite and appear as a real skeleton pyramid of considerable height. The small end of the pyramid is to the right of the middle of the picture seen by the left eye and to the left of the middle as seen by the right eye.

The brain performs some process whereby both these small ends are individually *suppressed* and builds out of them a new picture of the small end of the pyramid in the middle of the united picture. Further, when the upper end of the line a, into which the lines a′ and a″ fuse, is steadily fixed the lower end of it is double, and vice versa. Those who find difficulty with such experiments will probably obtain assistance by using positive lenses of 2 or 3 dioptres before the eyes.

If a series of exactly similar and equally spaced objects, such as a tessellated pavement or papered wall of regular

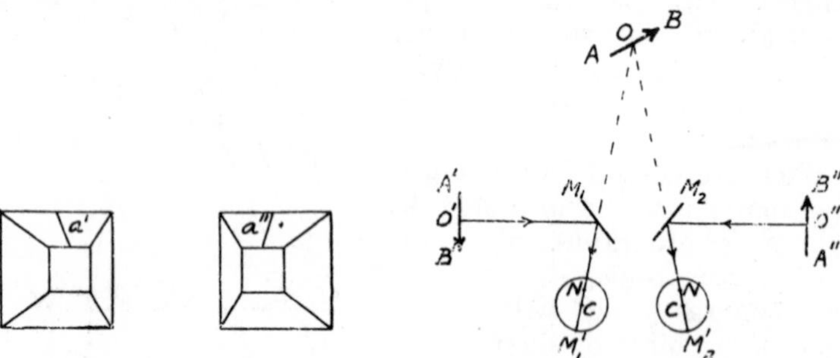

FIG. 12.18—A PERSPECTIVE PAIR.

FIG. 12.19—WHEATSTONE'S MIRROR STEREOSCOPE.

pattern, is viewed binocularly, and two neighbouring squares of the pattern are combined by increasing the convergence of the visual axes (squinting) as explained in §12.5, the squares all over the pattern will similarly combine and appear to come forward to the frontal plane containing the intersection of the visual axes (e.g. B′A″ in Fig. 12.6). If convergence is increased until a square and the next-but-one square are combined, again the whole combined pattern advances still further towards the observer. The forward advance of the pattern is accompanied by an apparent reduction in its size.* With practice this can be carried on by increasing the convergence until the pattern appears in miniature, but with an appearance of reality, only a few inches from the face.

12.20. The Stereoscope.

WHEATSTONE was one of the first who realised that the sensation of depth or relief should result from the

* §5.4.

presentation of two perspective pictures such as A′B′ and A″B″ above; and he first incorporated the principle in his reflecting STEREOSCOPE (1838). His instrument is represented in Fig. 12.19. M_1 and M_2 are plane mirrors in which the images of the pair of stereoscopic objects A′B′ and A″B″ are viewed by the left and right eyes respectively. The combined stereoscopic picture is seen in relief in the region AB. In later types of stereoscope the stereoscopic pair is placed directly in front of the eyes in the focal planes of two equal positive lenses L_1 and L_2, Fig. 12.20.*

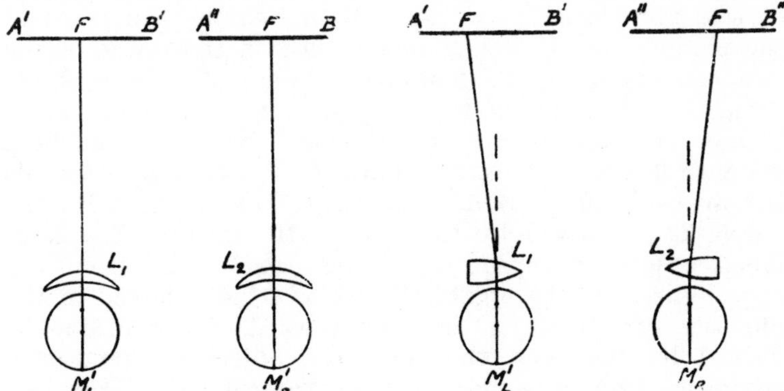

FIG. 12.20—LENS STEREOSCOPE.

FIG. 12.21—BREWSTER'S STEREOSCOPE.

In this case the pictures are seen at infinity, the two slightly dissimilar images being fused when the visual axes are parallel and accommodation relaxed. The size of the pictures is obviously limited by the inter-ocular distance in this case. Larger pictures, giving a larger field, can be viewed in the stereoscope introduced by BREWSTER (1843), which is still in fairly common use (Fig. 12.21). The positive lenses are decentred out—lens-prisms. It will be observed that the normal relationship between accommodation and convergence is not interfered with; more particularly, the points of the stereoscopic pictures the images of which are situated on the axes of the lenses will be fused with zero accommodation and zero convergence. Other pairs of points, appearing at different distances when fused, will require slight relative adjustments of accommodation and convergence.

* The lenses should be of the "verant" type designed by von Rohr.

In order that the correct angular perspective shall be obtained with these lens stereoscopes, the photographic pairs must be taken with lenses of the same focal length as those used for viewing in the stereoscope.

To provide the sensation of relief the pictures of a pair must be dissimilar in the same way that the views presented to the right and left eyes are dissimilar. If two exactly similar pictures, *not* a stereoscopic pair, be mounted in a stereoscope, for example with their centres at O′ and O″ in Wheatstone's stereoscope, Fig. 12.19, they appear as a single combined *flat* picture at O. Suppose two small objects are placed at O′ and O″ immediately in front of the pictures, so that their images fall on the foveæ of the two converging eyes. They will be fused into a single projection standing in the middle of the flat view at O. If now the objects, or one of them, be moved a short distance laterally across the slides A′B′ and B″A″, towards the arrow head in B″A″ and away from it in A′B′, i.e. outwards as viewed by the eyes in the mirrors, the combined object O appears to retreat backwards from the flat picture. If the object O′ and/or O″ are moved in the opposite direction, i.e. inwards towards the mid-line as viewed by the eyes, the combined object O apparently advances from the flat picture towards the observer. The approach and retreat into distance are most realistic, especially if the objects used represent some familiar figure such as a man or an animal. If the lateral movements are carried too far, the depth illusion suddenly ceases and two men appear in the plane of the flat picture, one on each side of the middle point. And if one of the objects (men) O′ or O″ be taken away, lateral movement of the remaining one merely produces a corresponding lateral movement in the plane of the combined picture.

This illustrates the necessity for two slightly dissimilar images in order to produce depth perception.

If two pictures are exactly alike over most of their extent but in one or two places there is a lack of the regular correspondence, the objects at these positions will stand away from the flat plane of the combined picture. This is utilised in many practical ways, as, for example, in detecting counterfeit banknotes, comparing patterns, etc. Slight variations between the two patterns reveal themselves as undulations in the combined picture.

PSEUDOSCOPIC VISION occurs when the left-hand picture of a stereoscopic pair is presented to the right eye and the right-hand picture to the left eye. The stereoscopic relief is then reversed, due to the reversal of binocular parallax, and near objects seem distant, convex bodies concave, etc. The effect may be obtained by cutting an ordinary stereoscopic slide and inserting the left-hand picture in the right side of the stereoscope, and vice versa. The effect can be conveniently demonstrated also, for slides or an object at a distance, with the aid of STRATTON'S pseudoscope (Fig. 12.22). The plane mirrors M_1 and M_2 are inclined at

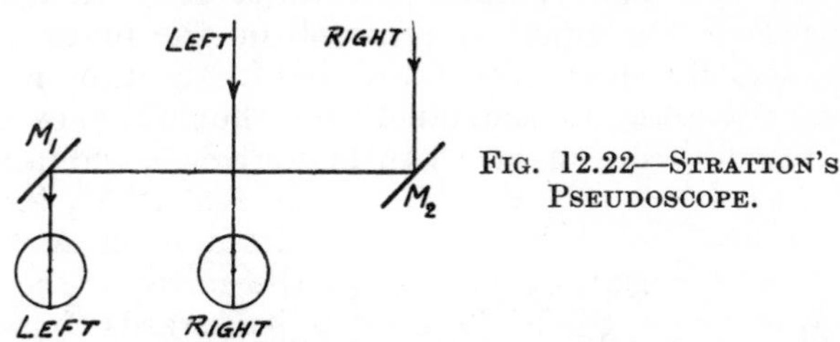

FIG. 12.22—STRATTON'S PSEUDOSCOPE.

45° to the direction of view and separated by twice the interocular distance. A near object is better seen in pseudoscopic relief by means of WHEATSTONE'S pseudoscope, in which each eye sees the object through a reflecting prism. The effect is most striking, a hollow hemisphere appearing like the outer surface of a sphere.

12.21. Stereoscopic Effects with Coloured Objects.

If two stereoscopic photographs are printed, one in red and the other green, and superposed one over the other on one piece of paper, then the picture is seen in stereoscopic relief if observed through a red and green glass, one in front of each eye (KOHLRAUSCH, 1871). To the eye with the green glass the background appears green, the green outlines of the picture are likewise green and hence invisible, and the outline of the red picture appear black, since red light will not pass through the green glass. Similarly the green picture is seen in black by the other eye; and the two are fused into a strikingly realistic stereoscopic impression. Such coloured picture-pairs have been called ANAGLYPHS. It is possible to buy picture books of this kind with an accompanying mask containing red and green celluloid peepholes. The green of the picture and the green glass or celluloid should reasonably correspond or fictitious results are obtained; likewise with the red.

When viewing a flat coloured picture, or when looking at the spectrum thrown on a screen during a lecture, it is frequently noticed that the parts coloured red stand out in front of the plane of the picture, or spectrum. To some observers it is the short wave length, blue or green, that appears to be the nearer. This effect is seen usually in binocular vision and is due probably to the chromatic aberration of the eye and the eccentricity of the pupil relative to the visual axis. It is the more marked the greater the spectral separation of the colours concerned. Assuming that the pupil is centred on the optical axis, the temporal situation of the fovea M′ (Fig. 2.3) relative to this axis results in the pupil being temporally eccentric relative to the visual axis. Thus, referring to Fig. 12.23,

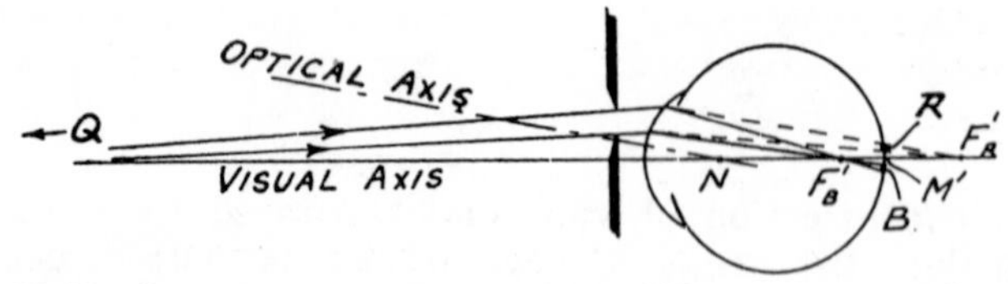

Fig. 12.23—Illustrating Stereoscope Effect with Coloured Objects.

in which this eccentricity is further exaggerated by means of a small artificial pupil placed in front of the eye, an object point Q is imaged in red light on a part of the retina R situated temporally in relation to the blue image B. The fusion of the images of a red object by the two eyes will result in that object appearing nearer than a blue object situated in the same object plane. If the centre of the pupil is on the nasal side of the visual axis (e.g. a person with a negative value of angle alpha), or if the artificial pupil is moved nasally across the pupil the blue images will be on the temporal side of the red and blue objects will appear to stand out in front of red objects.

This phenomenon is easily demonstrated by viewing binocularly through artificial pupils, or even through lenses, a red line and a blue line marked on a card, and moving the pupils or lenses across the eyes so as to vary their separation. When the pinholes are so placed that there is no stereoscopic effect between the red and blue lines, the red and blue images overlapping on the retina, the pinholes are situated on the visual axes. The inter-ocular distance can be accurately measured in this way.

Some individuals appear to see differently coloured objects at different distances even in monocular vision, and in the peripheral field; to what extent this may be due to variation of accommodation or other causes is not clear. The intensity of illumination of the objects seems to have some effect. Thus the localisation of coloured objects in space is dependent upon several factors, and errors in their depth perception might easily be made.

12.22. Stereoscopic Acuity.

Two objects, such as O and A of Fig. 12.2 or Q and Y of Fig. 12.3, must be separated by a certain distance before the greater distance of the one over the other can be appreciated. When two objects are just perceived as lying at unequal distances, i.e. in stereoscopic relief, their relative binocular parallax,* expressed in angular measure, measures the BINOCULAR OR STEREOSCOPIC ACUITY of the individual. Thus

$$\text{Stereoscopic acuity} = p \cdot \frac{dl}{l^2} \qquad (12.4)$$

where dl is the smallest resolvable difference in depth at the distance l by an observer with inter-ocular distance p. If the distances concerned in this relation are expressed in the same unit, the acuity is obtained in radians.

The stereoscopic acuity may be determined experimentally by presenting to the subject three vertical wires, the two outer ones being fixed in a frontal plane while the middle one is movable back and forth along the median plane. The positions are noted at which the subject can state with certainty, and correctly, that the middle wire is nearer or further than the fixed wires. To obtain accuracy care must be taken to shield the wires so that other factors, such as parallax with external objects, shadows, etc., and also alteration of size with distance, are eliminated. The results are found to vary considerably from one individual to another. Individuals with good visual acuity and training in binocular observations have stereoscopic acuity as precise as 5 seconds of arc, or even 2 seconds under favourable conditions. Others cannot detect parallax

* §12.3.

differences of whole minutes of angle, while in some the stereoscopic sense is lacking altogether. LANGLANDS showed (1926) that with practically instantaneous illumination the acuity falls to 10 seconds, rising to 5 seconds of arc when about 0·3 second exposure is allowed and to 2 seconds of arc under constant illumination. Thus, whereas depth perception is possible within a period of time so short that ocular movements could not have taken place, and also before the objects in the field are properly recognised, its accuracy is increased when time is allowed for such movements.*

Although the accuracy of the stereoscopic sense is so high (comparable with vernier acuity),† its *range* is comparatively limited. Thus to a person with stereoscopic acuity of say, 20 seconds, an object at a distance of 618 metres will not be separable from one at infinity; 618 metres being the distance at which the interocular base line, assumed to be 60 mm., subtends an angle of 20 seconds.

12.23. Accommodation and Convergence.

It will be of interest to obtain expressions giving the accommodative and convergence state of the eyes when viewing a stereoscopic pair with the aid of a stereoscope. By simple modifications or extensions the expressions will also serve to give useful information concerning the state of the eyes when observing objects through lenses generally.‡

In Fig. 12.24 the eyes are indicated looking at two objects Q, such as points on a pair of stereoscopic slides, through their centred correcting lenses at S and also through the lenses of the stereoscope, each of which is decentred a distance c cm. from the primary lines of the eyes. O, O are the optical centres of the stereoscope lenses. Consider the left eye. The object point Q is distant l metres from the stereoscope lens and is displaced laterally (inwards) by h cm. from the eye's primary line. If h is reckoned from the primary line and the lens decentration c is reckoned from the lens axis to the primary line, then the distance of the object from the lens axis is $(h + c)$ cm. The object Q is imaged at Q'_a by the stereoscope lens and this point is in turn imaged at Q'_b by the correcting lens. The light enters the eye along the direction Q'_b C, the eye having rotated through angle θ from its primary direction in order to receive the image on its fovea M'; and having at the same time accommodated for the image Q'_b.

The right eye is similarly affected and the stereoscopic objects Q are seen as a single projection at Q″.

Let F_a and F_b be the powers of the stereoscope and correcting lenses respectively. We find the distance (depth) CB′ of Q'_b and its lateral displacement $B'Q'_b$ from the primary line by successive applications of the conjugate foci and magnification formulæ to the two lenses in turn.

* §12.1. † §2.8. ‡ See, for example, §16.5.

To determine the Convergence of the Eyes :

First lens $L'_a = L + F_a$

Distance of Q'_a from axis of $F_a = (h + c)\dfrac{L}{L'_a} = \dfrac{(h + c) L}{L + F_a}$

" " " axis of $F_b = \dfrac{(h + c) L}{L + F_a} - c.$

Second Lens.

Object distance $l_b = l'_a - t$ or $L_b = \dfrac{L'_a}{1 - t L'_a} = \dfrac{L + F_a}{1 - t(L + F_a)}$

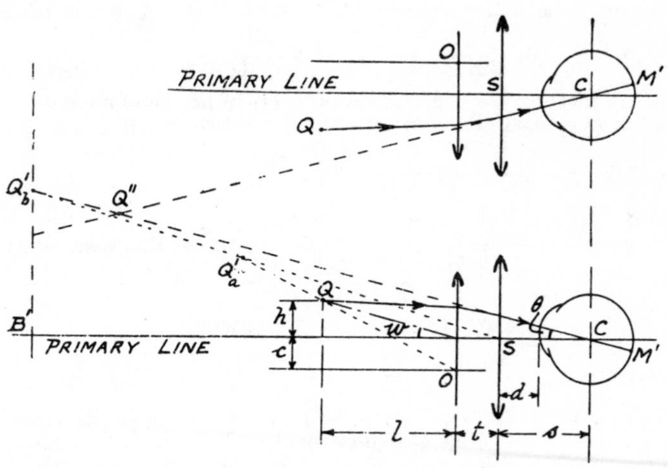

FIG. 12.24—ACCOMMODATION AND CONVERGENCE (θ) TO VIEW OBJECTS (Q) THROUGH LENSES.

We will neglect the separation of the two lenses and put $t = 0$ so that $L_b = L'_a = L + F_a$

Dioptral image distance $L'_b = L_b + F_b = L + F_a + F_b$

Distance of Q'_b from primary line $= \left\{ \dfrac{(h + c)L}{L + F_a} - c \right\} \dfrac{L + F_a}{L + F_a + F_b}$

$$\text{Hence } \theta = \frac{\left\{ \dfrac{(h + c) L}{L + F_a} - c \right\} \dfrac{L + F_a}{L + F_a + F_b}}{- \dfrac{1}{L + F_a + F_b} + s}$$

$$= - \frac{(h L - c F_a) S}{(S - L - F_a - F_b)} \qquad (12.5)$$

where s = distance from correcting lens to eye's centre of rotation and $S = \dfrac{1}{s}$ In the standard case $s = 27$ mm. and $S = 37$ D.

θ is given in prism dioptres if the lateral distances h and c are expressed in cm. and the remaining quantities in dioptres.

If the inter-ocular distance is p cm., the rotation of the eye in metre-angles is given by

$$\frac{\theta}{\frac{1}{2}p}$$

Accommodation. (Refer also to §6.1.)

In order to be sharply focused on the retina when the eye is relaxed light must reach it with a vergence K

$$\text{where } K = \frac{F_b}{1 - d\,F_b}$$

When observing object Q through the two lenses, the light leaves the correcting lens with vergence $L'_b = L + F_a + F_b$ which becomes

$$\frac{L'_b}{1 - d\,L'_b} = \frac{L + F_a + F_b}{1 - d\,(L + F_a + F_b)}$$

when it reaches the eye. Hence the eye must accommodate by an amount (reckoned at the eye itself)

$$A = \frac{F_b}{1 - dF_b} - \frac{L + F_a + F_b}{1 - d\,(L + F_a + F_b)}$$

$$= -\frac{L + F_a}{(1 - dF_b)\left\{1 - d\,(L + F_a + F_b)\right\}} \text{ dioptres} \qquad (12.6)$$

$$= -\frac{(L + F_a)\,D^2}{(D - F_b)\,(D - L - F_a - F_b)} \text{ dioptres} \qquad (12.6a)$$

where $D = \frac{1}{d} = \frac{1000}{14} = 71\cdot43$ dioptres in our standard case.

In a form of Brewster's stereoscope commonly used for laboratory purposes the lenses are approximately of + 6 D power (F_a) their optical centres being separated by 85 mm. For an individual with P.D. = 60 mm. the quantity $c = 4\cdot25 - 3\cdot0 = 1\cdot25$ cm. If the individual using the instrument is emmetropic, we have $F_b = 0$. Suppose the stereoscopic pictures to be viewed at a distance of 15 cm. from the lenses ($L = -6\cdot67$ D). Points situate 1 cm. inwards from the eyes' primary lines will require a rotation of each eye of

$$\theta = -\frac{(-6\cdot67 - 1\cdot25 \times 6) \times 37}{(37 + 6\cdot67 - 6)} = +13\cdot91\Delta \text{ or } 4\cdot64 \text{ M.A.}$$

the positive sign signifying convergence.

The accommodation exerted is given by

$$A = -\frac{(-6\cdot67 + 6)\,71\cdot4 \times 71\cdot4}{71\cdot4\,(71\cdot4 + 6\cdot67 - 6)} = 0\cdot66 \text{ D.}$$

An appreciable amount of convergence but very little accommodation are required to fuse two such points on the pictures.

Points situated 1 cm. *outwards* from the primary lines, ($h = -1$ cm.) will require an eye rotation of

$$\theta = -\frac{(6\cdot67 - 1\cdot25 \times 6)\,37}{(37 + 6\cdot67 - 6)} = +0\cdot82\Delta \text{ or } 0\cdot27 \text{ M.A.}$$

and the same accommodation as before.

In many problems dealing with the convergence and accommodation the eyes are called upon to make, only one lens before each eye has to be considered: e.g. in the case of an emmetrope using a stereoscope or a person wearing just his distance correction. Frequently such problems can be solved graphically, using a diagram similar to Fig. 12.24 with one of the two lenses before each eye omitted. If the result is sought by calculation, the method of this paragraph is applied, either F_a or F_b being omitted according to the nature of the problem. We shall meet with problems of this kind in Chapter XVI.

12.24. The Telestereoscope and Stereo-telescopes.

Other things being equal, the stereoscopic acuity and consequently the range of stereoscopic vision, will be increased by an increase in the inter-ocular separation, p. This may be done artificially by means of the TELESTEREOSCOPE, proposed by HELMHOLTZ (1857). As indicated in Fig. 12.25, the actual eye separation $N_L N_R$ is in effect increased to $n_L n_R$ by means of the system of plane mirrors. The relative parallax of two objects at distances l and $(l + dl)$ will now be given by

$$\frac{b \cdot dl}{l^2} = \frac{N \cdot p \cdot dl}{l^2}$$

where $b = N.p$ is the separation, or base, $n_L n_R$. The stereoscopic relief, or plastic relief as it is sometimes called, has been increased in the ratio N. The stereoscopic range is increased in the same proportion.

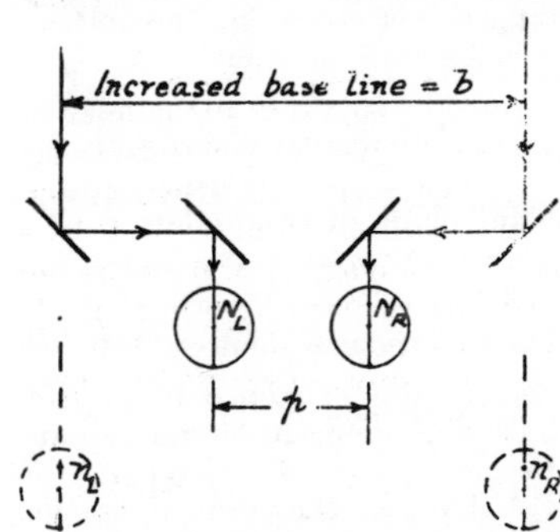

FIG. 12.25—SIMPLE TELESTEREOSCOPE.

If, in addition, a telescopic system magnifying M times is incorporated into the arrangement in front of each eye, all visual angles are magnified in the ratio M; or alternatively all objects in the field are brought, in effect, M times nearer. From these geometrical considerations, the relative parallax of the two objects would be

$$\frac{M \cdot b \cdot dl}{l^2} = M \cdot N \cdot p \cdot \frac{dl}{l^2} \tag{12.7}$$

i.e., if two objects at the mean distance l are viewed, the least separation dl that could be observed in unaided vision would be reduced to dl/MN. (In practice, however, the reduction is not thus proportional to 1/M.)

These principles are incorporated in prismatic binoculars; their magnification is 6 fold (M = 6) and the objectives are separated by a distance 1·5 times the eye-piece separation (N = 1·5) then the stereoscopic range to a person with stereoscopic acuity of 20 seconds will be 618 × 6 × 1·5 = 5560 metres, or about 3·5 miles. The stereoscopic effect is still greater in such instruments as the stereoscopic range finder in which the base length (b) may be one metre or more and the magnification 10 fold or more. Enormous increase in stereoscopic effect can be obtained by taking two photographs of the same scene from widely separated stations and viewing the two pictures, or stereograms, in a stereoscope. In this way the moon and the planets may be viewed in remarkable relief, the two photographs having been taken at different periods during which the viewing station has moved with the earth relative to the moon over a distance that provides a base length of the order of hundreds of thousands of miles.

EXERCISES. CHAPTER XII.

1. Write an account of the conditions to be satisfied by the visual apparatus in order to provide binocular vision; and indicate briefly the manner in which the anatomical basis necessary to meet these conditions is provided in the visual mechanism of man.

2. In what main respect is binocular vision superior to monocular vision? Explain how this superiority arises in binocular vision and why it is absent in the two-eyed vision of a bird.

Define the terms: plane of fixation and plane of triangulation.

3. Explain carefully the terms field of vision and field of fixation and give the average dimensions of each. Give a diagram illustrating the relation between the binocular visual field and the two monocular fields.

4. Describe simple experiments to reveal the existence of physiological diplopia. Explain, with the aid of a diagram, homonymous and heteronymous diplopia. Indicate clearly on the diagram the positions of the foveæ and nodal points of the eyes, the point of fixation and the projections of the foveæ. How is the extent of the diplopia represented on the diagram?

5. Explain, with an appropriate diagram, how the physiological diplopia of a given point in space is ordinarily interpreted in terms of the distance of that point relative to the distance of the point fixed. Indicate on your diagram the "cyclopean eye" and explain how the direction of the given spatial point is correctly estimated.

6. Explain what is meant by binocular parallax and show that the relative binocular parallax of two spatial points at distances l and $(l + dl)$ is given approximately by:

$$\text{relative binocular parallax} = \frac{p.dl}{l^2}$$

when the points are observed by a person whose inter-ocular distance is p.

Show also that, one of the two points being fixed, the distances of the retinal images of the other point from the respective foveæ differ by the quantity:

$$f_e p \cdot \frac{dl}{l^2}$$

f_e being the anterior focal length of the eye.

7. The binocular parallax of two objects A and B as observed by a person with an inter-ocular distance of 60 mm. are respectively 45 and 55 seconds of angle. Find the distances of the two objects.

If the objects lie in the median plane and the nearer one is fixed by the observer, what will be the positions of the right and left retinal images of the further object? Assume normal emmetropic eyes.

8. Explain carefully the meaning of retinal correspondence. In what way do the so-called corresponding points or areas correspond? What perceptual result follows from the stimulation of two corresponding retinal points or areas?

9. Explain the terms: apparently vertical and apparently horizontal meridians of the retina.

Explain also the meaning of the term horopter and, with a diagram, of the horizontal horopter of Müller.

10. Describe simple experiments, without a stereoscope, in which the mental percept of a single object in space is obtained by using two separate objects. Why may some difficulty be experienced in seeing the single combined "object" both clearly and singly? Give an explanatory diagram.

11. Explain what is meant by the fusion of the two presentations obtained of a single object in binocular vision; and describe the anatomical arrangement of the retino-cerebral connections providing a basis for such fusion. What conditions must be satisfied by the two retinal images for fusion to take place?

12. Describe the terms: retinal rivalry and suppression. Write a brief account of the development of monocular fixation, binocular fixation and fusion.

13. If a simple pendulum swinging in a vertical plane is observed binocularly in a direction perpendicular to this plane, a tinted or rather dark glass being placed before one eye, the end of the pendulum appears to take an elliptical course. Explain this effect carefully, with an explanatory diagram.

14. What constitutes binocular vision? On what anatomical conformations does it depend from the point of view of the shape of the skull and the visual centres of the brain, in contradistinction to the lower vertebrates having monocular vision only, although possessing two eyes? What conditions are necessary for perfect binocular vision in man? (B.O.A.)

15. With the aid of a clear diagram explain the following terms relating to eye movements: median plane; frontal section; sagittal section; transversal section; sagittal, transversal and vertical axes of rotation. Indicate on your diagram the eye's centre of rotation.

What is a cardinal rotation of the eye?

16. Explain the terms: primary vertical meridian of the retina; primary position of the eyes; secondary position; tertiary position.

If an eye has occupied a secondary position by means of rotation through an angle of azimuth from the primary position, indicate on a diagram around what axis, approximately, the eye will rotate in order to move from the secondary into a tertiary position. Give a brief explanation.

17. Explain the difference between cyclo-rotation or torsion of the eye and false torsion. Describe clearly how the condition of false torsion is brought about.

18. Distinguish between true voluntary torsion and incidental or false involuntary torsion; and describe how the latter may be experimentally measured in the living human eye. (S.M.C.)

19. Give a diagram showing in an approximate manner the course of the six extrinsic muscles from their origins to their insertions in the globe.

Explain what is meant by a muscle plane; and describe the situation of the axes around which the three pairs of muscles rotate the eye.

20. State the pre-eminent and subsidiary effects on the movements of the globe of each of the extrinsic ocular muscles and explain clearly how the subsidiary effects vary with the lateral and vertical binocular rotations. (S.M.C. Hons.)

21. State and explain carefully the law of Listing concerning the movements of the eye. What muscles are employed in each of the four cardinal movements of the eye? Explain how the effect of, say, the superior and inferior recti varies as the eye rotates outwards.

22. Give a description with diagrams of the extrinsic muscles of the eye, indicating the axes around which they severally rotate the globe. Explain the functions of the muscles that must be employed to rotate the eye upward and downward from its primary position.

23. Account for the torsional effects of the recti muscles and explain why torsion does not occur in the normal rotations of the eye.

24. Explain why it is necessary for more than one muscle to contract to produce a simple cardinal rotation of the eye in the vertical direction.

How would the action of the muscles be affected if the eye were turned (*a*) to the nasal, (*b*) to the temporal side before the vertical movement commenced?

25. Set out in tabular form the possible conjugate and disjunctive binocular movements of the eyes. State which of these are required for binocular vision in ordinary circumstances and describe briefly the conditions under which the others may be brought into play.

26. Distinguish between version movements and vergence movements of the eyes. In what circumstances may (*a*) cyclo-version and (*b*) cyclo-vergence movements of the eyes be required?

Describe briefly an experiment which indicates that a cyclo-vergence or torsional movement of the eyes is executed when they converge on a near object.

27. What is meant by conjugate action of the extra-ocular muscles and how many such conjugate actions are there?

Which muscles act in turning the eye from the horizontal medial plane down and out ? Name the muscles acting in both right and left eyes. (B.O.A.)

28. Explain the following statements and make clear the meanings of the terms used : In a person who is orthophoric for distance the passive position of functional rest coincides with the primary position of the eyes. In a heterophoric person the passive position deviates from the primary or distance fixation position, the eyes being convergent or divergent or supravergent or cyclovergent in the passive position.

29. What are the advantages of binocular vision ? Explain the innervations that produce conjugate movements of the eyes.

30. Give a diagrammatic sketch of the general arrangement of the nuclei of the nerves responsible for innervating the extraocular muscles. The medial rectus of one eye is sometimes required to operate in association with the medial rectus of the other eye and at other times in association with the external rectus of the other eye. Give a brief account of the means provided for meeting such different co-ordinations of the muscles.

31. Write a general account of the cortical and sub-cortical control of the ocular movements, differentiating between voluntary movements and involuntary or reflex movements.

Account for the movements of the eyes in response to stimuli other than visual stimuli.

32. Draw a diagram to show the course and the connections of nerve fibres from the retinæ to the visual centres of the brain. Describe briefly, in simple terms, what you consider would be the subjective and objective effects of disease conditions in the following situations :—

(*a*) the temporal side of the retina of the left eye,
(*b*) the left optic nerve,
(*c*) The left optic tract.

33. Describe the series of events that constitute the fixation reflex. If the person concerned be heterophoric what further reflex actions may be necessary before binocular fixation is finally achieved ?

Are the above true reflex movements ? If not, give a brief account of a true reflex movement.

34. Enumerate the factors that enable an appreciation of depth to be obtained in monocular vision and explain carefully what additional factor or factors are introduced when both eyes are used. What effect on our appreciation of depth has the length of time of exposure of the visual field ?

35. Give an account of the stereoscopic sense, mentioning the various factors upon which the monocular and binocular perception of depth depend. Describe the principle of any form of stereoscope.

36. Explain the principle of stereoscopic vision. Make drawings of a stereoscopic pair of some simple geometrical object and show how they are made to produce the impression of the single solid object.

How can it be shown that convergence is not an essential factor in stereoscopy ?

37. Explain how two photographs of a solid object may be obtained and mounted as a stereoscopic pair for use in a stereoscope.

Give a diagram of a simple stereoscopic pair in some form of stereoscope and discuss the relation between the convergence and accommodation of the observer when fusing selected portions of the pair.

38. With the aid of diagrams, describe the stereoscopes of Wheatstone and of Brewster. What condition must be satisfied when preparing the stereoscopic pair for the latter instrument in order that the proper angular perspective shall be obtained when using the instrument ?

Discuss briefly the adjustments of convergence in relation to accommodation as different portions of the pictures are successively observed.

39. Explain how the principle of stereoscopy may be utilised in the detection of spurious banknotes, in comparing patterns with a master pattern, etc.

When an object consisting of a regular pattern is observed binocularly under varying conditions of convergence of the observer, the pattern may appear on a reduced scale and nearer to the observer than its true position. Explain this.

40. Explain how it is that a stereoscopic appearance results from an " anaglyph," i.e. a picture in which red and green printings are superposed and viewed through red and green gelatine. (B.O.A. Hons.)

41. Explain carefully, with an explanatory diagram, why to many people the red portions of a flat multi-coloured object appear to stand out in front of the plane of the object. To some people the blue portions stand out in this manner ; explain this also.

How may this phenomenon be utilised to locate a subject's visual axes ?

42. Explain what is meant by stereoscopic acuity and derive an expression for this acuity for a person of inter-ocular distance p.

How would you proceed to measure the stereoscopic acuity of a person ? State the precautions to be observed.

43. A person with inter-ocular distance 65 mm. can detect the relative binocular parallax of two objects that are situated respectively 100 metres and 106·5 metres. Find the stereoscopic acuity and the stereoscopic range of this person.

Give a brief account of the effect on stereoscopic acuity of the length of time the test objects are exposed to the observer.

44. Find graphically the convergence and accommodation required when an emmetropic person with inter-ocular distance 60 mm. observes a pair of points through spheres of + 6 D the optical centres of which are separated by 80 mm., each point of the pair being situated one cm. inwards from the eye's primary line and 9 cm. from its corresponding lens. Assume the lenses are thin and placed 27 mm. in front of the centres of rotation ; distance of lenses from eye's principal points 14 mm.

Check by calculation.

(N.B. The diagram will be similar to Fig. 12.24 the second lens F. being omitted.)

45. A spectacle frame is glazed with centred lenses (+ 10 D spheres) and is fitted to a person with 60 mm. interpupillary distance (frame P.D. is also 60 mm.). A point 25 cm. in front of the left eye lens lies on its axis and is fixed by both eyes.

Draw a diagram to half scale to show the prismatic effect introduced by the right eye lens and measure the convergence in prism dioptres from your diagram. Assume the eyes are situated 20 mm. behind the lens plane. (S.M.C.)

46. Explain, with a careful diagram, the principle of the telestereoscope. Show by measurements taken from your diagram in what proportion the stereoscopic range of the observer has been increased.

Describe briefly some optical instrument in which this principle is incorporated.

47. A person with inter-ocular distance 60 mm. uses a prismatic binocular the objectives of which have focal length 20 cm., their optical axes being separated by 100 mm. The eyepiece focal length is 3 cm.

If the person's stereoscopic acuity is 15 seconds of angle, find the smallest difference between the distances of two clear objects, at a mean distance of 400 metres, that can be appreciated when they are observed through the instrument.

48. With what percentage accuracy can the range of objects at 1500 metres be estimated by a person of stereoscopic acuity 20 seconds of angle when using a stereoscopic rangefinder the base length of which is 1 metre and magnification 14 ? Assume the person's inter-ocular distance to be 60 mm.

49. Write an essay on: Stereoscopic vision through binocular instruments. (S.M.C.)

50. What is " Listing's Law " ? Discuss its importance in the mechanism of binocular vision. (S.M.C. Hons.)

51. Explain what is meant by horopter. Indicate the normal shape of its trace in a horizontal plane when the eyes fix a median point in the horizontal plane.

Discuss some of the factors which would alter the shape of the trace. (S.M.C.)

52. What is stereoscopic vision ? What conditions must be fulfilled to obtain the appearance of stereoscopic relief from a pair of photographs ? (B.O.A.)

53. With many observers the pupillary apertures are displaced temporally or nasally off the axis of the eye and for nearly all observers the visual axis is not coincident with the optical axis. Explain how these conditions affect the apparent distances of differently coloured objects. (B.O.A.)

OCULO-MOTOR IMBALANCE

CHAPTER XIII

HETEROPHORIA

We have seen that binocular vision depends upon the fulfilment of certain requirements concerned with the presentation of two suitable uniocular impressions and the projection and fusion of these into a single binocular percept. Conditions may exist or may arise in the visual apparatus which interfere with the fulfilment of these requirements and so prevent the full exercise of binocular vision. The interference may be of such a nature as to render it impossible for the oculo-motor system to achieve binocular fixation, or to achieve it only with difficulty and to the accompaniment of symptoms of strain or discomfort. On the other hand, binocular fixation may be attained in the normal manner but the subject experiences difficulty in appreciating the stereoscopic relief of the external field or obtains a distorted percept of the field.

Thus we may divide anomalies of binocular vision into two classes:

A. Oculo-Motor Imbalance: difficulties associated with achieving or maintaining binocular fixation.

B. Anomalies of Space Perception: distortions in binocular projection and stereoscopic relief.

The second class will be dealt with in Chapter XV. In the present chapter and the next, however, we are concerned *only* with the first class, oculo-motor imbalance.

13.1. Grades of Simultaneous Vision.

It is necessary to bear in mind the differences between simultaneous macular vision, fusion, binocular fixation and binocular vision. A person, such as a squinter, who cannot direct both visual axes to a common point in the field, may nevertheless be able to see with both eyes simultaneously.

If two separate objects, such as points on the two slides in a stereoscope, placed one on each visual axis, are seen at the same time by such a person, there is SIMULTANEOUS MACULAR VISION. If the objects are those of Fig. 14.1 and the vertical line of each is placed on this subject's visual axis, then the vertical lines will be superimposed one on the other.

If now one or both of the objects is displaced laterally and the subject makes a corresponding movement of convergence or divergence in order to maintain the single impression of the vertical line, this is evidence that the separate images are being *fused* in the cortex and that the oculo-motor system is forced by the fusion impulse to make the requisite movement. That is, FUSION is present.

Such an individual may not be able to direct both visual axes on to one common object, however. If this can be accomplished, BINOCULAR FIXATION is present. Another individual may have binocular fixation, but no power to fuse the two images into a single mental percept, the images being merely superimposed and not interpreted as a single view of the object. If a prism be placed before one eye of such an individual, creating diplopia, no vergence effort will be made to regain single vision. Binocular fixation is present; but fusion, and hence binocular vision, are absent.

The individual who, possessing binocular fixation, also moves the eyes in the appropriate direction to overcome such an obstacle as the prism, has an active fusion sense and BINOCULAR VISION. Even this individual may not possess the capability of blending the two retinal images of the object and its surroundings in proper stereoscopic relief, or may do so inefficiently. In which case full STEREOSCOPIC VISION is absent, or defective.

There are many shades of difference even among people who do possess this highest grade of binocular vision, namely stereoscopic vision. Some fuse stereoscopic pairs very quickly and attain considerable accuracy in seeing the objects in their correct relative positions or in using instruments such as a stereoscopic rangefinder; while others have to "grope" for some time before fusing a stereoscopic pair and are not accurate observers with stereoscopic instruments.

People who have macular vision in the two eyes simultaneously may thus be sub-divided into the following grades :

A. Simultaneous macular vision (1) without binocular fixation.
(2) with binocular fixation.

B. Simultaneous macular vision with fusion
(1) without binocular fixation.
(2) with binocular fixation; i.e. binocular vision.

C. Stereoscopic vision.

The above classification includes only those people who can see with both foveæ *at the same time.* When dealing with heterotropia in the next chapter we shall see that there is a certain class of squinters who can see with either eye *alternately*, but not with both simultaneously, the vision in the temporarily non-seeing eye being mentally suppressed. At any given moment such vision is monocular. Also, there are squinters who can see with both eyes simultaneously, but who do not use the *fovea* of the squinting eye; such people have simultaneous vision, but not simultaneous *macular* vision.

13.2. Definitions. Orthophoria and Motor Imbalance.

The student should recapitulate the definitions of fixation position and passive position given in §5.2.

Active Position : when the attention is actively directed to an object and no obstacle is presented to the eyes, the fusion impulse is free to assume control; the full resources of the oculo-motor system are in operation and it assumes a condition of active equilibrium. The position taken up by the eyes in this condition we will call the active position.

In most individuals the active position is the fixation position; under the direction of fusion the eyes achieve the desired binocular fixation. Usually binocular single vision and an adequate degree of stereoscopic depth of perception are also attained, but this *may* not be the case.

Orthophoria. In the great majority of people the functional rest position is one in which the eyes are gazing straight ahead in the general direction of the median line. There is, however, a rare group of individuals whose eyes both deviate equally *in the same direction* from the median line when they are in the condition of functional rest. In this rest condition their eyes are turned to the right or left, or up or down; to observe an object lying straight ahead, such people must turn the head, and with it the median line, in one direction or another to achieve fixation.

From the standpoint of the attainment of binocular fixation, the ideal state is orthophoria. When the condition of the oculo-motor system is such that:

(a) *in the condition of functional rest the eyes are directed along the median line of the head*;

and

(b) for any given object position *both the active position and the passive position of the eyes coincide with the fixation position*, the condition is *orthophoria* for that object position.

In such a case of perfect motor balance the eyes remain in the fixation position when one eye is occluded or when fusion is suspended in some other way.

The individual may not be orthophoric for other positions of the object. To be completely orthophoric the eyes must satisfy the condition (b), not only for objects, both distant and near, in the median plane, but for all objects in the common binocular field. Such a theoretically ideal state of affairs is probably never attained.

The orthophoric position for distance is the primary position. In a person orthophoric for distance the passive position, or functional rest position, is the primary position.

It is to be noted that orthophoria is the ideal condition only so far as binocular fixation is concerned. It is possible for a person to attain this and yet be deficient or defective in the attainment of the highest grade of binocular vision, i.e. stereoscopic vision. There may be obstacles (such as unequal ocular images) of a nature not interfering with the perfection of motor balance but yet capable of causing error in binocular projection and the perception of space.

Motor Imbalance: any departure from the perfectly balanced condition of orthophoria is called motor imbalance. In classifying this condition we have firstly to distinguish between those people whose functional rest position is disposed symmetrically about the median line and those, already mentioned, in whom both eyes turn away in the same direction from the median line in functional rest. This second class is of very rare occurrence and we will not discuss it.

The first class is of far greater importance since the vast majority of imbalance cases belong to it. Since in this class the eyes deviate *with respect to one another* as they do in the vergence movements (§12.13), we may describe all such cases as *vergence* imbalances. It is to this class *only* that we refer in dealing with the subject of motor imbalance.

Within this class there are two main divisions of imbalance called respectively:

Heterophoria
and *Heterotropia*, or *Strabismus*, or *Squint*.

HETEROPHORIA: in this condition of motor imbalance the active position of the eyes coincides with the fixation position, but the passive position deviates from it. The eyes deviate when fusion is prevented, and diplopia occurs; but as soon as the fusion mechanism regains control they move into the fixation position. Thus heterophoric subjects obtain binocular fixation, and usually binocular vision; to do so, however, they have to exert a fusional *effort*, in moving the eyes from the passive to the fixation position, which is not required in the case of orthophoria. This effort may give rise to discomfort and strain, as we shall see.

HETEROTROPIA, OR STRABISMUS, OR SQUINT: in this condition of motor imbalance neither the passive position nor the active position coincides with the fixation position. Even when fusion is free to operate, the eyes do not take up the fixation position and the subject, consequently, cannot achieve, or maintain, binocular vision. Thus one eye or the other deviates, even in ordinary vision. The subject *may* have simultaneous vision, however.

In some individuals the degree of imbalance remains constant for different directions of fixation, the object distance, and hence accommodation, remaining constant; the heterophoria or squint, as the case may be, is then termed CONCOMITANT. On the other hand the degree of imbalance may change as the gaze is shifted from one part of the field to another; or there may be orthophoria in one direction and imbalance in another; in these cases the heterophoria or squint is described as NONCOMITANT or PARALYTIC (or paretic).

In cases of squint the deviation of one eye or the other is generally manifest to the examiner, unless it be small in amount or confused by the existence of the angle alpha. In heterophoria there is no deviation in ordinary vision; to reveal the deviation, the eyes must be dissociated by suspending fusion. Heterophoric deviations are therefore sometimes referred to as *latent* deviations in contra-distinction to the *manifest* deviations of squint. Indeed heterophoria is largely considered as a latent condition of, or a tendency towards, heterotropia; the word is derived from the Greek root φορα meaning *a tending.*

In this chapter we will deal with heterophoria of the concomitant variety. When heterophoria is referred to without further qualification, the concomitant variety is intended. It is only this variety that can be treated by optical and educative measures, the paralytic type of heterophoria requiring medical attention.

HETEROPHORIA—CONCOMITANT

13.3. Classification according to Direction.

We are indebted mainly to STEVENS for the nomenclature of motor imbalance now generally adopted. In this text we follow the broad lines of his scheme, though departing from it in certain particulars.

In heterophoria the deviations of the two eyes, when passive, are in opposite senses. The fixation lines or primary vertical meridians may deviate from the orthophoric position in any of the six directions corresponding to the disjunctive or vergence movements numbered 7 to 12 in the table of binocular movements given in §12.13. When fusion is suspended there is a deviation of one fixation line, or of one primary vertical meridian, *with respect to* the other; and consequently there is diplopia. In esophoria, for example (see accompanying table) the fixation lines when passive deviate inwards to a convergent position relative to the desired object of fixation, and the subject experiences homonymous diplopia; in exophoria they deviate outwards to a divergent position producing crossed diplopia.

TABLE. CLASSIFICATION OF HETEROPHORIA

NATURE OF CONDITION	NATURE OF DEVIATION when eyes are passive
ESOphoria.	Inwards.
EXOphoria.	Outwards.
R. HYPERphoria.	Right eye upwards.
L. HYPERphoria.	Left eye upwards.
INCYCLOphoria.	Primary vertical meridians converge upwards : Λ
EXCYCLOphoria.	Primary vertical meridians diverge upwards : V

In hyperphoria one fixation line assumes a position higher than the other, giving rise to diplopia in the vertical direction. In each of these cases the primary vertical meridians are in their correct fixation positions ; but in cyclophoria the eyes rotate in opposite directions, in or out, around their fixation lines when, fusion being suspended, they fall into the passive position. The term cyclophoria we owe to George PRICE and G. C. SAVAGE.

A horizontal phoria and a vertical one may exist simultaneously ; thus if the passive position is one compounded of inward deviation and an elevation of the right eye over the left, the condition is esophoria with right hyperphoria ; and so on.

MADDOX considered that the phorias are due to disturbances of the innervations 7 to 12 of the Table, §12.13.

Exophoria occurs more frequently than the other kinds of heterophoria.

13.4. Diplopia.

In heterophoria the fixation lines are moved into the correct fixation position, and maintained there, by the exertions of the fusion impulse. The greater the deviation the greater must be the fusion effort and the more likelihood there is of symptoms of strain. It is necessary, therefore, to determine the nature of the deviation and to measure its amount. We can do this conveniently in the various conditions of heterophoria by determining the kind and extent of the diplopia that arises when the eyes are rendered passive, since the diplopia is governed by the deviation. The diplopia is, as it were, a measuring stick for the imbalance and its importance justifies a brief recapitulation of certain portions of the previous chapter.

From the discussions in §§ 12.3, 12.5 and 12.19 we have learnt that *the projections of the two foveæ are conceived as one point in space.* In Fig. 12.2, with the fixation lines intersecting at the point O as shown, a single object at O is seen singly. Two equal objects at A and B (Figs. 12.5 and 12.6) will be fused into a single object at the point A′B″, Fig. 12.5, or B′A″ Fig. 12.6. Thus, returning to Fig. 12.2, a *single* object at any other situation than O must appear double so long as the fixation lines remain in the position shown. A spot of light placed at M_L will be seen centrally by the left eye, but to the right eye it will appear in the left visual field ; the extent of the diplopia, reckoned in the frontal plane M_LM_R containing the object *is the separation* M_LM_R *of the two foveal projections.* A " muscle light " at m_L will also be seen in diplopia, homonymous diplopia in this case. In both cases the extent of the diplopia is a measure of the deviation of the right eye, the deviating eye, from the fixation position.

The diplopia that arises in normal binocular vision, as explained in §12.3, is physiological diplopia. Diplopia caused by a motor imbalance or other disorder will be called generally pathologic diplopia, which is accompanied by mal-projection of objects in the visual field. We may summarise the characteristics of the two types thus :

PHYSIOLOGICAL DIPLOPIA

(*a*) The object of fixation is seen singly.

(*b*) The doubling of objects nearer or more remote than the object fixed does not ordinarily obtrude itself as such and does not cause confusion.

(*c*) The objects seen double appear shadowy and insubstantial or " transparent ".

(*d*) The diplopia disappears immediately the doubled object is fixed.

PATHOLOGIC DIPLOPIA

(*a*) The object of fixation is seen double, one projection being distinct and one indistinct.

(*b*) The noticeable diplopia of practically all objects in the field of view causes confusion.

(*c*) The diplopia remains in spite of changes of convergence.

Both these types of binocular diplopia are easily distinguished from monocular diplopia since the diplopia disappears on closing one eye ; the single object remaining is, or becomes, clear provided the vision of the uncovered eye is good. If the double objects are close together they may not be recognised by the subject as two, but may be interpreted as a single object seen indistinctly.

Dealing now with pathologic diplopia, the disposition of the two foveal projections will vary with the direction of the motor imbalance ; they may be side by side, one above the other, tilted, or a combination of these ; giving us three kinds of diplopia namely lateral, vertical and cyclo diplopia. Purely for convenience of expression we will specify these in terms of the position subjectively occupied by the projection of the right eye relative to that of the left eye, which we will suppose to be the fixing eye. In adopting such a convention it must be stressed that disorders of motor balance are essentially binocular in character and the method of specification is merely for simplicity. Thus, according to the positions of the two projections, *as seen by the subject*, we may classify as follows :

Pathologic Diplopia

1. *Lateral.*

   Right eye projection to the right—homonymous or uncrossed diplopia.

   Right eye projection to the left—heteronymous or crossed diplopia.

2. *Vertical.*

   Right eye projection lower—right inferior diplopia.

   " " " higher—right superior diplopia.

3. *Cyclo.*

   Right eye projection tilted clockwise—right clockwise diplopia.

   Right eye projection tilted anticlockwise—right anticlockwise diplopia.

The kind of diplopia obtained by individuals with the various subdivisions of heterophoria is given in the following table. That the individual with exophoria obtains crossed diplopia when fusion is suspended will be understood by referring back to §12.3 and Fig. 12.2. Suppose the object to be at the point B and the visual axes to lie for a moment along the directions N_LO and N_RO, divergent with respect to B. To the left eye, the positions of objects will be judged with reference to the projection M_L of its fovea, so that B (or the projection of the retinal image b′) will lie apparently to the right. To the right eye B will lie apparently to the left of its foveal projection M_R. Hence the diplopia will be crossed.

In practice the eyes would remain in this situation only for a moment since the object is not seen distinctly by either eye. They would immediately execute a version movement until one eye fixes the object B to see it clearly. Whether this movement would be to the right or to the left depends upon such factors as which is the dominant eye and which eye has the dissociating element* placed in front of it. Supposing the movement is to the right so that the left eye fixes; the visual axes are then in the positions shown in Fig. 13.1, in which the angles ON_LB and ON_RM_R, through which the eyes have respectively rotated from their previous position, are equal. To the left eye the object appears centrally placed; to the right eye it appears to the left by twice the previous amount. The total diplopia is the same as it was before. In the frontal plane containing the object B it is given by the distance M_LM_R which is proportional to the angle of deviation of the right eye, BN_RM_R.

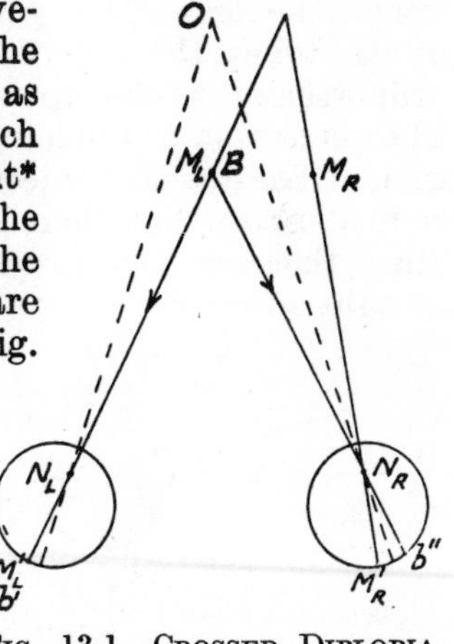

Fig. 13.1—Crossed Diplopia in Exophoria. B is the Object.

Type of Heterophoria.	Diplopia exhibited when fusion is suspended.
Esophoria.	Homonymous or uncrossed.
Exophoria.	Heteronymous or crossed.
R. Hyperphoria.	Right inferior.
L. Hyperphoria.	Right superior.
In-cyclophoria.	Right clockwise.
Ex-cyclophoria.	Right anticlockwise.

* §13.7.

Although in clinical practice the testing distance of 6 metres is considered " distant ", it is to be observed that there is convergence of each eye of one sixth metre angle when the eyes fix an object at 6 metres, just as there is accommodation of one sixth dioptre ; total convergence is one prism dioptre.

Consider a case of right hyperphoria with fusion suspended, the left eye fixing the object (Fig. 13.2). The right visual axis is directed upwards in the field and so the right fovea is below the plane of fixation and the image b″ of the object, although in the fixation plane, is formed above the fovea M'_R. With respect to the projection M_R of the fovea the object appears low by an amount M_RB, proportional to the upward deviation, M_RN_RB, of the eye. The projection of the left eye will appear in its true position at B. The foveal projections M_R and M_L are conceived as coincident so that there is diplopia of the single object B. Since the right eye projection of B is below, the diplopia is right inferior.

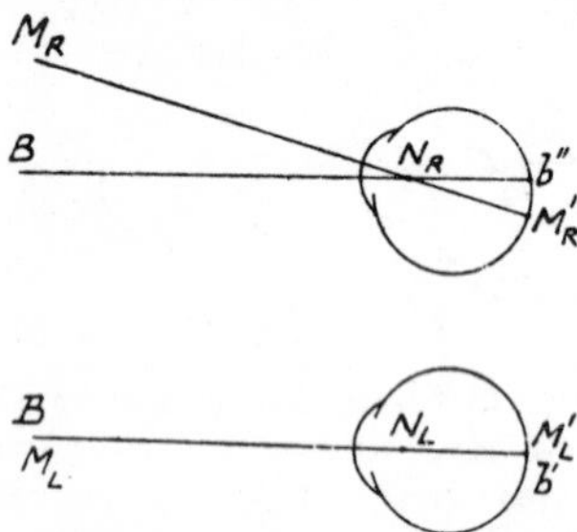

Fig. 13.2—Right Inferior Diplopia in Right Hyperphoria.

If fusion is rendered inoperative in a case of cyclophoria the eyes will rotate, each around its visual axis, and a vertical line, or a horizontal line, object will appear as two, inclined to one another. There will probably be no conjugate movement of both eyes to restore one of them to its proper fixation position. If the condition is incyclophoria, the upper extremity of the primary vertical meridian of, say, the right eye will lean nasal-wards. The image of the lower portion of a vertical line object will be formed in the upper half of the retina, to the temporal side of this tilted meridian. Projected outwards, the lower end of the line will appear displaced to the left, and the upper end to the right; i.e. to the right eye the vertical line will appear rotated clockwise.

Diplopia of any kind is a disagreeable and confusing condition and to most people is intolerable. It is instinctively avoided in low degrees of imbalance by means of fusion movements. If the imbalance is of high degree or the fusion powers weak, efforts are still made to avoid the resulting diplopia.

13.5. Prisms and Diplopia.

We have already seen* that prisms of certain strengths can be overcome by individuals possessing normal fusion powers; also that when the prism is too strong the motor system abandons the attempt to overcome it, the eyes settle down to their position of passive equilibrium, and diplopia is established. The image formed in one eye is removed from the fovea and the condition is analogous to pathologic diplopia. The direction of the diplopia depends upon the direction of the prism, as follows:

Strong Prism before right eye	*Diplopia produced*
Base in – – – – –	homonymous—uncrossed
Base out – – – –	heteronymous—crossed
Base up (or down before left eye)	right inferior
Base down (or up before left eye)	right superior

Two prisms of 6△ base in, one before each eye, are equivalent to one prism of 12△ base in before either eye separately; and 4△ base up before the right eye can be applied as 4△ base *down* before the left eye, or as 2△ base *up* before the right combined with 2△ base *down* before the left.

If the subject be orthophoric, the displacement of the retinal image from the fovea in the one eye will be proportional to the prism deviation; hence the observed diplopia will be equal to the prism deviation when the object is distant. (The diplopia will be equal to the *effective* prism power when the object is near.)†

When the subject is heterophoric the eyes will move from the fixation position they occupied before the application of the prism into their passive or phoria position. The resultant diplopia will then be compounded of the effect of the prism and the movement of the deviating eye. For example, suppose a 15△ prism be placed base in before the right eye of a subject who is exophoric by 5△ at distance, the subject observing a distant object such as the muscle light at 6 metres. The prism is too strong to be overcome; the left eye will fix the light and the right eye will diverge through an angle of 5△ to the passive phoria position.

* §5.4. † §5.1.

The light enters this eye at an angle of 15△ to the fixation direction and so will be incident on the retina at a point distant 10△ from the fovea, expressing the distance in angular measure. To the right eye the object will appear to the right (uncrossed) by 10 cm. for each metre distance of the object; that is, 10 × 6 = 60 cm.

In Fig. 13.3, the right eye diverges from its first fixation position M'_0 shown by the dotted line to the position PM′, the angle M'_0NM' being 5△. The light is deviated by the prism along DNb″, the angle M'_0Nb'' being 15△.

Where the same prism applied to a person *eso*phoric by 5△, the diplopia would be 20△, uncrossed; and the object would appear to the right eye 120 cm. to the right of its position as seen by the left eye.

Suppose now the subject had right hyperphoria to the extent of 3△ for distance. On interposing the same prism before the right eye the eyes would be dissociated, the right eye moving upwards by 3△. The retinal image would thus be 15△ nasal-wards from the fovea because of the prism and 3△ above the fovea due to the eye's own elevation. The diplopia would be homonymous right inferior; to the right eye the object would appear 90 cm. to the right of, and 18 cm. below, its true position as seen by the left eye.

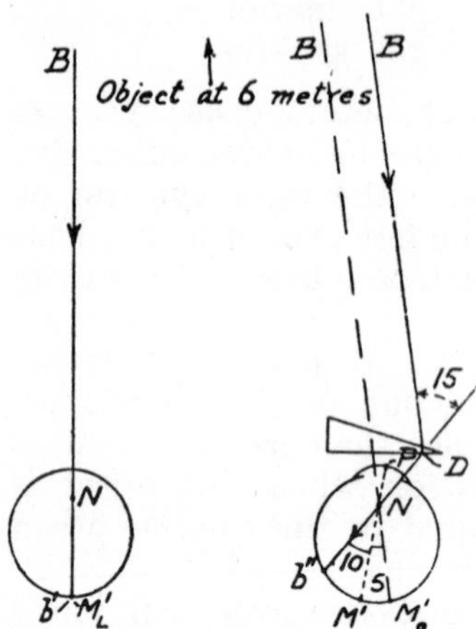

FIG. 13.3—EXOPHORIA OF 5 △ WITH 15 △ BASE-IN PRISM UNCROSSED DIPLOPIA OF 10 △.

Since prisms (of sufficient strength) produce diplopia they may be used to correct or measure it. Thus in the last example above, the 15△ prism has been instrumental in dissociating the eyes so that they fall into their passive position, which turned out to be one of right hyperphoria. Apart from the lateral separation of the projections caused by the prism, the vertical separation reveals the presence of the phoria. Since the right eye projection is low, we know the right eye has rotated upwards. To annul the vertical diplopia we must bring the retinal image in the right eye (e.g. b″, Fig. 13.2) down to the level of the fovea by means of a 3△ prism base *down* before the right eye; or we may raise the image b′ in the left eye to a position correspondingly higher than the fovea with a 3△ prism base *up* before this eye. In either case the projections will then appear to lie on the same level and the 3△ prism has annulled and measured the hyperphoria.

The 15△ prism which is responsible for preventing fusion, or in other words dissociates the eyes from one another, we will call the *dissociating prism*. If we wish to measure the resulting deviation by annulling it, the second prism required to do this (the 3△ prism above) we call the *measuring prism*. Whether this measuring prism is placed before the deviating eye (the one with the dissociating prism) or the fixing eye, *its apex points in the direction of the relative deviation*. It is to be noted that when, the eyes having been dissociated, a measuring prism is applied, the eye behind the prism does not rotate, but the light is deviated by the prism to fall into the position on the retina necessary to annul the diplopia in the given direction.

Prisms cannot be used as above for neutralising and measuring cyclo diplopia.

DETECTION AND MEASUREMENT OF HETEROPHORIA: DISTANCE

13.6. General Principle and Subdivision of Methods.

The same general principle underlies all methods of detecting and measuring heterophoria. In some way or other the fusion of the uniocular impressions has to be prevented; no active attempt will then be made to obtain binocular fixation and the eyes will deviate from the fixation position in a direction depending upon the type of heterophoria present. The eyes are then said to be "dissociated". The extent of this deviation from the fixation position has to be measured in some way.

It is assumed that, when thus freed from the effort of maintaining binocular fixation, the eyes fall back into their passive position, which is the functional rest position when testing the motor balance at distance. Although this assumption may be open to question,* experience indicates that we do not go far wrong in making it; and in any case there appears to be no other alternative.

---

* See also §12.14.

It will be gathered from §12.6 and from our study of the effects of strong prisms that fusion may be prevented in various ways. In general, we have to create a diplopia too large to be overcome, or render the two retinal images so dissimilar that fusion will not be attempted. Tests for heterophoria consequently arrange themselves into four main groups :

1. *Exclusion or Cover Tests.*
2. *Diplopia or Displacement Tests.*
3. *Distortion Tests.*
4. *Tests with Independent Objects.*

The cover tests are objective and the remainder subjective.

Innumerable tests and appliances have been suggested, but they all fall into one or other of these groups.

In changing from distance vision to near vision complicated readjustments of the accommodative and motor mechanism of the eyes have to be made and so it is desirable to test the state of the motor balance at distance, 6 metres, and at the near working distance, usually 33·3 cm.* We will deal with distance tests first.

A complete test includes two parts : firstly, the detection of the presence and the kind of heterophoria ; and secondly, the measurement of its amount. The latter is the angle of deviation of the eyes, when dissociated from the correct fixation or orthophoric position and is usually expressed in prism dioptres, or frequently in degrees in the case of cyclophoria.

Except perhaps when using the cover test, the motor balance is investigated with the subject wearing his refractive correction ; it is *most important* that the lenses be very carefully centred and that this centring be maintained during the test. Unless care be taken it is easy for the trial frame or other holding device to become displaced as the test proceeds. It does not require much decentration of a correcting lens of moderate power to introduce prismatic effect comparable with a heterophoria that may be producing symptoms in a susceptible individual, especially in the vertical direction.

The refractive correction is worn in order to eliminate the disparity between accommodation and convergence which, as we have already seen,† itself tends to set up an imbalance of the motor system. In some cases, useful information

---

* §6.4. † §5.2.

concerning the accommodation-convergence relationship can be gleaned by testing the motor imbalance without and then with the refractive correction.

When the eyes have been dissociated, in one of the ways about to be described, a diplopia of the test object, of a kind and amount depending on the heterophoria present, becomes manifest to the subject, the right and left eye projections appearing separated or, in the case of cyclophoria, inclined to one another. This separation, or relative inclination, has to be measured. It is frequently found, however, that the diplopia fluctuates in amount, indicating that the eyes are not remaining stationary in their passive position, but are oscillating round about it. It is to be remembered that when accommodating at 6 metres, the eyes are not really in a static state. The fluctuations may be due to a small amount of anisometropia outstanding, even after refractive correction, the eyes focusing the object alternately and affecting horizontal vergence in so doing. The measurement of the phoria should consequently be made in such cases immediately upon uncovering the eye provided with the dissociating device, it having been covered for a number of seconds. These fluctuations are more troublesome in near testing, however.

As with prisms, the dissociating device may be placed before either eye. It is sometimes found, however, that the amount of the imbalance measured differs somewhat according to which eye is left to fix and which to deviate. This again, when present, is due to a small amount of anisometropia still existing, so that the accommodation called into play when looking at the test object varies according to which eye is the fixing eye. Small amounts of anisometropia may sometimes be revealed in this way.

It is presumed that, before commencing to investigate the subject's heterophoric condition it has already been ascertained that he has, in fact, vision in both eyes and the power of binocular fixation. If this is not the case, the subject is suffering from heterotropia, not heterophoria, and the case will be investigated as explained in the next chapter. The presence or absence of binocular fixation may be determined by tests described in §§ 14.6 and 14.7.

13.7. Group 1. Exclusion or Cover or Screen Tests.

If, when both eyes are fixing an object and obtaining single vision of it in the normal way, one eye is occluded, binocular vision is rendered impossible and the covered eye immediately deviates if heterophoria be present. The uncovered eye continues to fix the object.

The subject observes a small light, the muscle light, at 6 metres. The examiner covers one eye with a card and this eye deviates to the passive position. On suddenly withdrawing the card, binocular vision is again possible and the eye returns to its correct fixation position. The return movement is visible to the examiner and thereby provides an objective means of discovering the presence and type of the heterophoria. This is a useful test (except

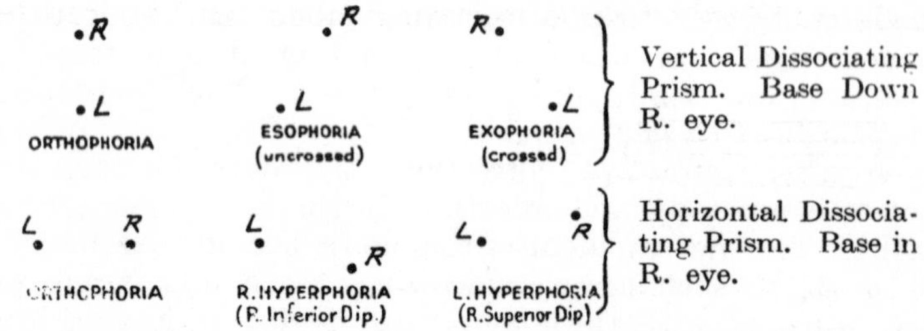

FIG. 13.4—SINGLE DISSOCIATING PRISM. APPEARANCES TO SUBJECT

with nervous subjects) on account of its extreme simplicity. It cannot be used to determine the degree of phoria present and is not reliable in the case of low degrees since the small movements are difficult to detect; but it serves to guide the examiner to investigate the condition more fully by other means.

13.8. Group 2. Diplopia or Displacement Tests.

In these methods fusion is suspended by creating an insuperable diplopia.

(*a*) SINGLE PRISM.

This method was suggested by von GRAEFE (*ca.* 1860) who was responsible for considerable pioneer work in the investigation of motor imbalances. If a fairly strong prism, 6△ or so, be placed base down before the right eye, the subject will see two projections of the distant muscle light, the right projection being higher than the left. Fusion is impossible as this prism is too strong to be overcome by the supravergence powers of the eyes, which will consequently assume their passive position. If the eyes are orthophoric horizontally, the two projections will be seen vertically one above the other. If a horizontal imbalance be present, the projections will not lie on a vertical line but will appear to the subject as indicated in Fig. 13.4.

To reveal the presence of any vertical phoria that may be present we can create an insuperable diplopia in the horizontal direction by means of a prism, base in, of about 10△, which is too strong to be overcome by the divergence capabilities of the eyes. The appearances of the light will then be as indicated in Fig. 13.4, the extent of the vertical separation being a measure of the vertical phoria.

As explained in §13.5, the degree of heterophoria thus made manifest by the dissociating prism can be measured

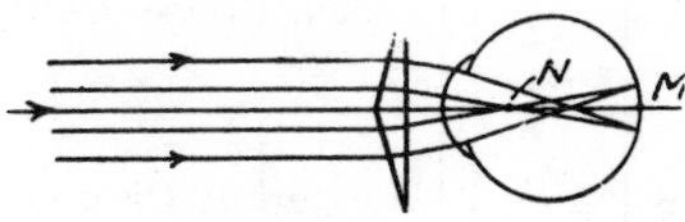

FIG. 13.5—DOUBLE PRISM (MADDOX) CREATING MONOCULAR DIPLOPIA.

by a second prism, placed before either eye. Suppose that, with the vertical dissociating prism before the right eye, esophoria is revealed; if the base-out prism required to restore verticality of the spots is one of 5△, this is the amount of the esophoria.

The carrying out of the test is simplified by placing a coloured glass, say red, before one eye. The examiner then asks the subject whether the red spot appears to the right or left, or above or below, the white spot.

When using single prisms as above, any inaccuracy in setting the prism will upset the findings. If the base-apex direction of a vertical dissociating prism is not set truly vertical before the eye, a horizontal displacement of the two projections will be introduced by it, and this would affect the measurement of any horizontal phoria there may be. To remedy this defect MADDOX proposed his double prism.

(*b*) DOUBLE PRISM.

This consists of two prisms each of 4△ to 6△ deviation, arranged in one cell (and usually of one piece of glass) with their bases adjacent and their B.A. lines lying along a common direction, Fig. 13.5. When this device is placed before one eye so that the junction of the two prisms bisects the pupil, artificial monocular diplopia is produced in that eye. Suppose it to be placed before the right eye with the common B.A. line vertical, the subject observing the spot of light at 6 metres through his distance correction. With the left eye a single spot is seen and with the right eye two spots respectively above and below the true position. If the double prism is correctly placed, the two right eye projections will lie vertically one above the other. Fusion is suspended and the eyes take up their passive position. The appearance to the subject in the various horizontal and vertical conditions of imbalance will be as indicated in Fig. 13.6.

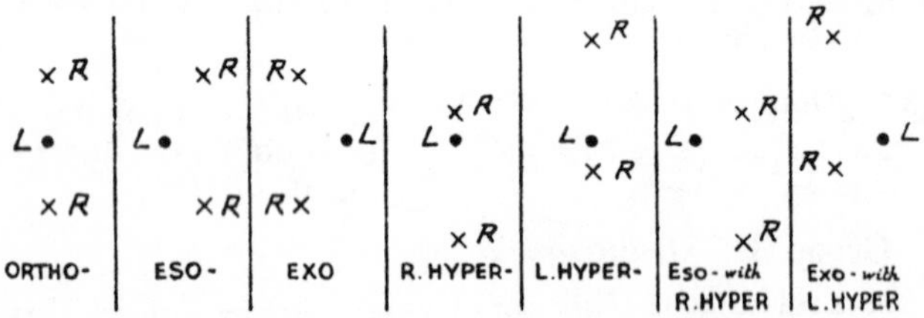

Fig. 13.6—Double Dissociating Prism. Subjective Appearances

To prevent a tendency to fusion between the single projection of the left eye and either of the two projections of the right eye, and also to facilitate the questioning and answering by examiner and subject, it is usual to place, say, a good red glass before the right eye and a complementary green glass before the left.

The kind of phoria present, if any, is ascertained from the subject's description of the relative positions of the green spot and the two red spots. The appearance characteristic of orthophoria may then be obtained by interposing prisms with their B.A. lines in appropriate directions to neutralise the diplopia due to the heterophoria. These measuring prisms may be single prisms placed in the trial frame ; or a special device called a *prism battery* containing a series of prisms of gradually increasing strength which can be introduced conveniently one after another ; or a rotary prism device such as Risley's ;* or the phorometer.

If the small spot of light be replaced by a single well defined horizontal line on a large white background, we

* §5.7.

can investigate cyclophoria. The right eye will see two lines parallel to one another, the single line seen by the left eye lying between them. In the absence of cyclophoria the three lines will appear all parallel; otherwise the appearances indicated in Fig. 13.7 will be obtained. This procedure reveals the presence of cyclophoria (without measuring its amount), if it be sufficiently marked.

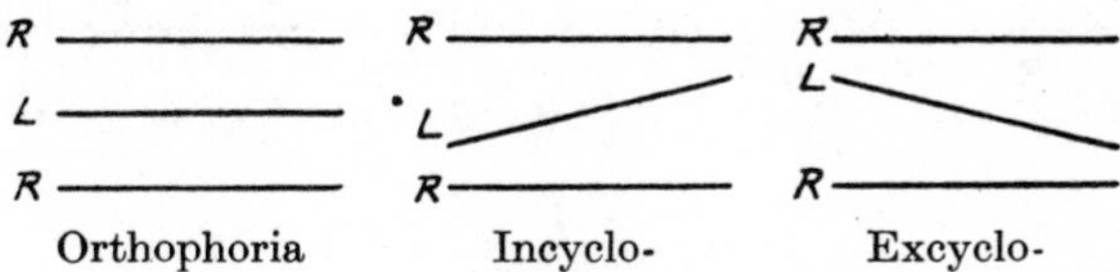

FIG. 13.7—DOUBLE DISSOCIATING PRISM. SUBJECTIVE APPEARANCES IN CYCLOPHORIA.

13.9. Group 3. Distortion Tests.

In the methods of this group the similarity between the two images is destroyed by some device so that fusion is not attempted.

MADDOX ROD OR GROOVE

The simplest and most effective device for distorting one image is the cylindrical glass rod introduced by MADDOX in 1890. It is probably the most generally useful of all methods of dissociation and possesses the advantage that it may be used for detecting and measuring cyclophoria,

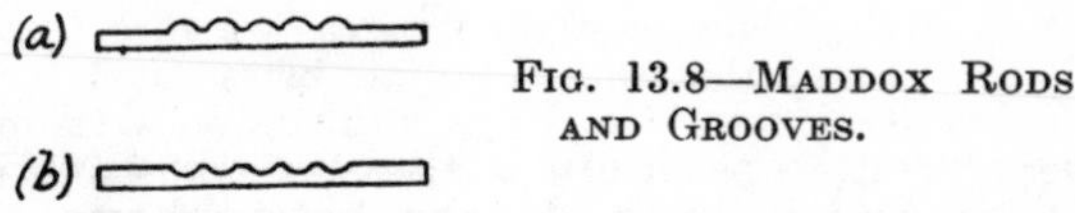

FIG. 13.8—MADDOX RODS AND GROOVES.

which cannot be done with some of the devices used. In its original and simplest form the device consists of a cylindrical glass rod about 20 mm. long and 3 mm. diameter mounted in a disc that can be inserted in the trial frame. Seen through such a powerful cylinder held close to the eye, a spot of light appears as a long streak *perpendicular* to the axis of the cylinder. A brighter and better defined streak is obtained by using a series of such rods parallel to one another as indicated in Fig. 13.8 (a) or a similar series of grooves as in (b); one of these forms is usual nowadays. They are generally made of red glass, to enhance still further the difference between the white spot as seen by the one eye and the red streak seen by the other.

MADDOX discarded the double prism in favour of the glass rod on the suggestion of BERRY, who pointed out that the rounded edge of the double prism produced a streak. The student will understand why, although a positive cylinder produces a real focal line *parallel* to its axis, the observed streak is perpendicular thereto, in the following way; hold a disc of Maddox rods (or grooves of good quality glass,

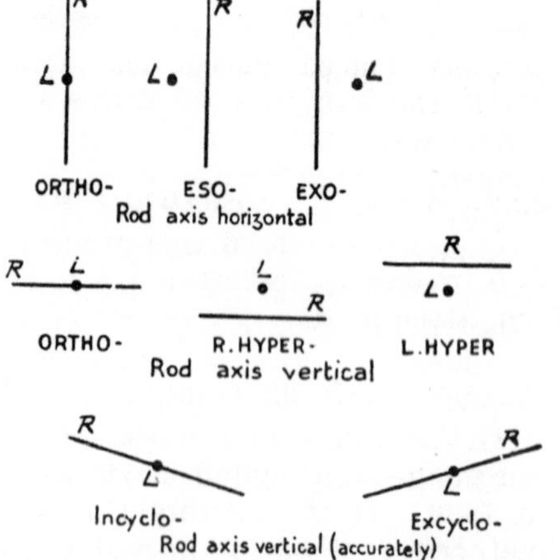

FIG. 13.9—MADDOX ROD SUBJECTIVE APPEARANCES. ROD BEFORE RIGHT EYE.

preferably) at arm's length a metre or so away from the muscle light. Each rod or groove of the disc will be seen to produce a short focal line parallel to itself. Now slowly approach the disc towards the eye; it will be observed that each focal line blurs out in a direction perpendicular to its length, the blurs ultimately overlapping and forming a long streak perpendicular to the axes of the rods and of a width determined by the diameter of your pupil. On retreating from the light, with the rods close to the eye, the streak lengthens and sharpens somewhat.

The rods, or grooves, must not exhibit any prismatic effect along their length. Although the disc with multiple rods or grooves is usually employed, we will refer to it simply as the Maddox rod, for convenience.

To test for horizontal imbalances the rod is placed with axis horizontal before one eye, say the right. Wearing his distance correction the subject, observing the muscle light at 6 metres, sees a white spot with the left eye and a vertical red streak with the right eye. These cannot be fused and the eyes will retire to their passive position, the left eye fixing the light and the right eye deviating. The relative positions of spot and streak in horizontal phorias are indicated in Fig. 13.9. With the rod vertical and streak horizontal, the relative positions in vertical imbalances are also shown in the figure. The student should make himself familiar with these subjective appearances so that he may decide at once as to the condition when the subject describes them.

13.10. Measurement of Motor Imbalance by Tangent Scale.

When the eyes have been dissociated we may measure the amount of any heterophoria revealed by an appropriately placed measuring prism as already explained; or, if the subject's acuity permits, we may use a large tangent scale. This consists simply of a uniform scale graduated in both directions from the zero, at which is situated the muscle light. The divisions are, most conveniently, at such a distance apart as to read the diplopia, and thus the heterophoria, in prism dioptres. Thus for use at 6 metres, they will be 6 cm. apart for each prism dioptre. It may be arranged that the scale can be rotated around the muscle light so as to occupy either a horizontal or a vertical position; or two scales may be provided as indicated diagrammatically in Fig. 13.10.

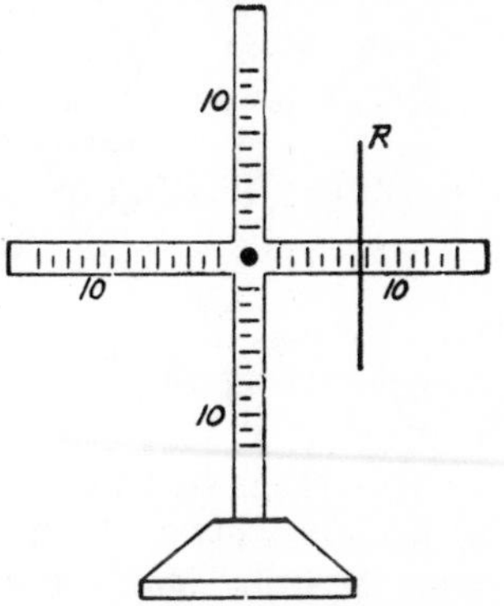

Fig. 13.10—Tangent Scale; for measuring Heterophoria and Heterotropia (7·5△ of Esophoria indicated).

If the subject, with a Maddox rod horizontal before the right eye, sees the vertical streak as indicated, the condition is exophoria of 7·5△.

13.11. Group 4. Independent Objects. Phoriagraphs.

Suppose we can arrange that of two adjacent objects, such as an arrow head and a scale as depicted in Fig. 13.11 (a), only the scale can be seen by the left eye and only the arrow head by the right eye, no other object being in either field of view. We could arrange this by using a stereoscope, for example. The dissimilarity prevents fusion, the eyes are dissociated and will take up their passive phoria position. Suppose the left eye is fixing the zero mark of the scale; then to a subject with exophoria of such an amount that his right fovea is projected to the point M_R, this point and the zero of the scale (which is the projection M_L of the left fovea) will be conceived as coincident.* With reference to the scale seen by the left eye, anything seen by the right eye will appear displaced to the left, as shown in (b). The arrow head will apparently point to the division 5 on the left, indicating 5 units of exophoria; the unit will

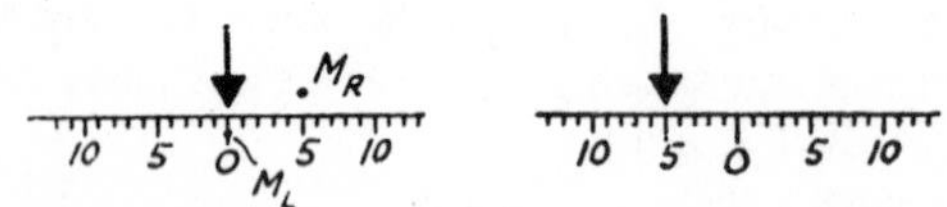

(a) Actual scale and pointer; (b) as seen by subject with 5△ of exophoria. M_R is foveal projection of right eye.

FIG. 13.11—DISSOCIATION BY INDEPENDENT OBJECTS. ARROW SEEN BY RIGHT EYE.

be the prism dioptre if the size of the divisions is one hundredth of the testing distance; e.g. 6 cm. divisions for testing at 6 metres.

Apparatus of this kind, in which one of the independent objects is a scale which serves to read off the phoria directly, may be called *phoriagraphs.* The instruments vary according to the method employed to secure dissociation. Diaphragms may be used for this purpose, as in the *Maddox wing test* to be described later; the stereoscope may be adapted as in the *synoptophore*; or it may be arranged that the objects are differently coloured and are observed through plano glasses of complementary colours so that only one object is seen by each eye.

(*a*) PHORIAGRAPH WITH DISSOCIATION BY COMPLEMENTARY COLOURS.

Two small lights are mounted in sliders on two long parallel rods (Fig. 13.12). One is covered with red glass and the other with complementary green. The lights can be moved independently along the rods, which are graduated to read in prism dioptres, usually at 6 metres.

* §13.4.

The subject wears plano glasses (in addition to his correction) of the same colours, one before each eye. If the red glass is before the right eye and the green before the left, then the right eye can see the red light only and the left eye the green light only, and the eyes are dissociated. The rods can be rotated into the vertical position or the horizontal position.

To test for vertical imbalance the rods are disposed vertically, the subject provided with the red and green planos, and the lights both placed together at the zero of their respective scales. To the subject with left hyperphoria the red light will appear above the green. The

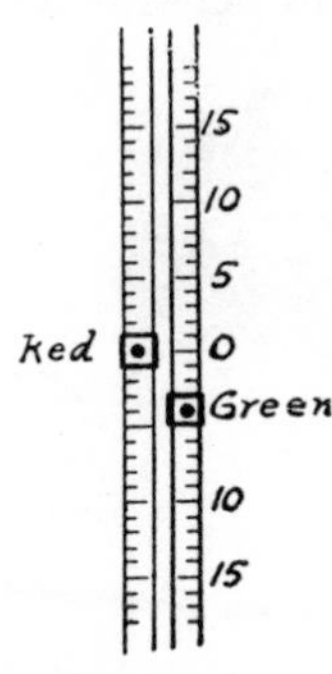

FIG. 13.12—INDEPENDENT OBJECTS. DISSOCIATION BY COMPLEMENTARY COLOURS; WITH RED GLASS BEFORE RIGHT EYE AND GREEN GLASS BEFORE LEFT EYE. DIAGRAM INDICATES MEASUREMENT OF 4△ OF RIGHT HYPERPHORIA.

red light is moved down its rod, or the green light moved upwards until they appear at the same level to the subject. The number on the scale occupied by the displaced light indicates the vertical imbalance. Horizontal imbalance may be measured in the same way with the rods disposed horizontally. With the two lights placed at zero, the red will appear to the right of the green in esophoria, and to the left in exophoria.

Care must be taken that the general illumination of the apparatus is low and that the subject sees nothing but the two coloured lights. Any object visible to both eyes may cause the subject to fuse it, or attempt to do so.

(*b*) THE SYNOPTOPHORE.*

The independent and dissimilar objects may be provided by means of the two slides in a stereoscope. The mirror stereoscope of WHEATSTONE (Fig. 12.19) is conveniently adaptable for our present purpose, as also for measuring

* The *Synoptiscope* is a similar instrument with very similar functions.

the lateral, vertical and cyclo vergences of the eyes* and further, as we shall see later, for exercising them in certain conditions. When it is to be used for such purposes as these the two arms of the stereoscope are arranged to be independently rotatable around the centres of projection, CC, of the eyes (Fig. 12.19). In this way the objects A′B′ and A″B″ can be presented in such positions that the eyes have to vary their convergence in order to observe them directly; and accommodation can be varied, when required, by moving the objects in or out along the axes of the arms, or by inserting lenses of appropriate focal length between the eyes and the mirrors. The instrument then becomes one to which HERING, and JAVAL, applied the general term

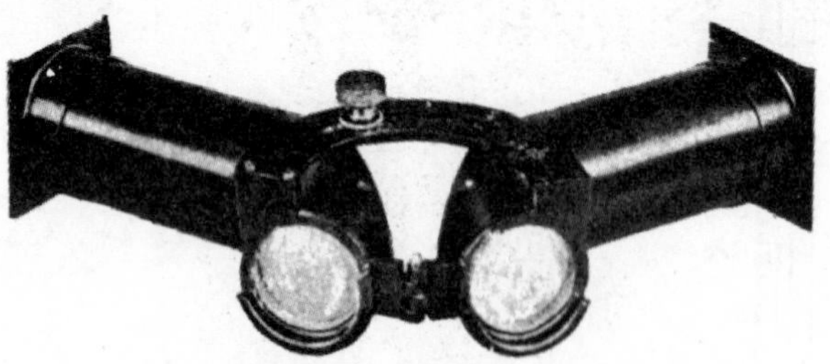

FIG. 13.13—WORTH'S AMBLYOSCOPE.

HAPLOSCOPE. Usually lenses are fitted permanently, in front of the mirrors, of such power that the object slides lie in their focal planes; the objects are then virtually at infinity and are viewed with relaxed accommodation. When it is required to use the instrument for a test at the near working distance, lenses of power – 3 D can be inserted in front of the permanent lenses.

Many instruments of this type, varying in detail, have been proposed from time to time. The AMBLYOSCOPE, introduced by WORTH in 1895, is a well known example. Its design and general mode of action will be gathered from Fig. 13.13. It is intended primarily for fusion training.

A successful modern example, possessing many ingenious adjustments which make it suitable for most purposes, is the SYNOPTOPHORE.† A rear view of the instrument is

* §5.4.

† Due originally (1914) to the late Dr. W. ETTLES. The account given here applies also to the synoptiscope.

A still more recent instrument of this type is the Lyle Major Amblyoscope, illustrated in Fig. 13.14 (A).

illustrated in Fig. 13.14. The slides L, when inserted in their rectangular carriers, are illuminated uniformly by lamps at M if they are transparent, or by lamps at K if they are opaque. The slides may be moved vertically, or rotated, in their carriers by slow-motion

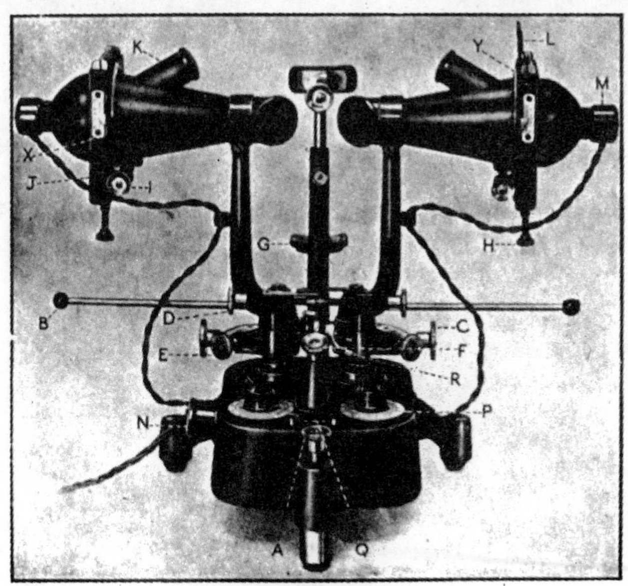

Fig. 13.14—The Synoptophore.

screws H and I. Each arm can be rotated independently around the rigid vertical columns; or by means of clamping screws they may be rotated together (version) at equal speeds. The rotations are carried out by the subject through the agency of the handles B and the amount of rotation is registered on scales divided into degrees and prism dioptres. Thus the instrument provides a means of presenting pairs of independent objects in various states of horizontal, vertical and cyclo vergence and of moving one or both objects smoothly in any of these directions.

Fig. 13.15 shows the essential parts of the two arms diagrammatically. The lenses L_1 and L_2 of focal length about six inches, are designed to provide a flat field so that the object slides A′B′ and A″B″ in their focal planes are seen clearly and undistorted from one side to the other.

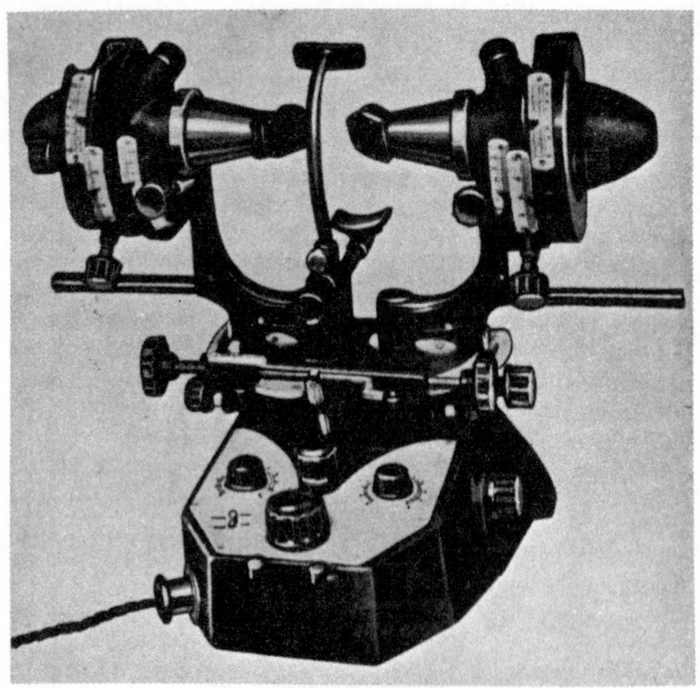

Fig. 13.14(a)—Lyle Major Amblyoscope.

In the figure the left arm is shown in its zero position and the right arm rotated through an angle of 30° around the point C, which will be occupied by the centre of rotation of the eye when the subject's head is in position, supported by the chin rest G (Fig. 13.14) and the forehead rest.

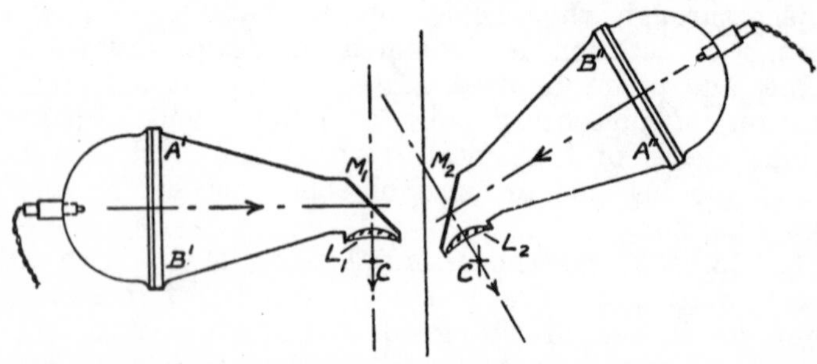

Fig. 13.15—The Synoptophore. Diagram to show rotation of right arm around the eye's centre of rotation.

By inserting a pair of slides presenting dissimilar objects we may measure horizontal phoria by rotating the arms and vertical phoria by raising or lowering one slide. Cyclophoria may be revealed, and measured, by using two horizontal lines as objects, one on each slide, and separated vertically by an amount sufficient to prevent fusion. If they do not appear parallel to the subject, one line may be tilted by means of the tangent screw I (Fig. 13.14) until parallelism is attained ; the rotation necessary to produce this result measures the cyclophoria.

Glasses of different colours may be inserted in the optical paths to act as a still further deterrent to fusion, if required.

DETECTION AND MEASUREMENT OF HETEROPHORIA : NEAR

13.12. Uncertainty of Findings.

When investigating the motor balance at near, the subject's attention is directed to some kind of test object at $33\frac{1}{3}$ cm. distance. The eyes are dissociated by means that are essentially the same as those adopted for distance. The eyes then fall into what we have called their (near) passive position and, as for distance testing, it is assumed that the diplopia then appearing to the subject is a measure of the imbalance of the oculo-motor system at near. This assumption is more doubtful than the similar one made concerning distance testing.* The passive position is not one of functional rest as it is for distance ; accommodation is most probably in force, and perhaps fluctuating ; and generally it is a somewhat dynamic, and not a rest, position. The general trend of modern thought is that there is a separate and complex innervation for near work ; an innervation that distributes nervous energy in due proportion for all the processes—accommodation, convergence, fusion, etc.—necessary for near vision. If, by suspending fusion, we eliminate the incentive for the operation of this governing innervation, it appears likely that it may not operate normally in respect to any of its components, such as convergence and accommodation. There is thus an element of uncertainty as to what we really are measuring when we undertake to investigate the motor balance at near.

---

* §13.6.

Although, on account of this uncertainty, we must not draw hasty conclusions from the discovery of small departures from orthophoria at near, the results of our tests, combined with other information such as the subject's vergence or fusion capabilities, are of some value.

The fluctuations of the diplopia when the eyes are dissociated, already mentioned in connection with distance testing, are more troublesome in near testing. They are due to the same causes, small outstanding differences of refraction between the two eyes, their greater influence probably being due to the more dynamic state of the motor system. They may be overcome by covering and uncovering one eye, as already explained.* The same precautions are to be observed, too, concerning low general illumination and preventing any object other than the test object or objects being seen by the subject.

We will briefly describe a few methods of testing, in the same order as for distance. The subject wears his near correction, carefully centred† for the distance of the test. This distance will usually be $33\frac{1}{3}$ cm., but may be smaller or larger than this in certain cases depending upon the nature of the near work the subject is to be engaged upon.‡ The subject's head and eyes should be depressed below the horizontal, in the position naturally taken up when reading or executing close work. Most of the devices used ensure that this attitude will be adopted.

13.13. Tests for Heterophoria at Near.

Group 2. The Double Prism.

This is sometimes suggested for investigating cyclophoria at near, using as object a horizontal line on a white card. The method is the same as the one already described for distance testing and is open to the same criticism.

Group 3. The Maddox Rod.

This may be used exactly as for distance testing. The test object may conveniently be a small hole in the middle of a card with a light behind it. The card may have a horizontal and a vertical scale of divisions (3·33 mm. apart to read in △ at 33·33 cm.), the illuminated hole being the zero for each scale.

---

* §13.6.

† Especial care in this respect is needed when measuring hyperphoria—see also §13.19.

‡ §6.4.

GROUP 4. PHORIAGRAPHS.

Probably the most useful devices for measuring the near motor balance belong to this group.

(*a*) THE MADDOX WING TEST.

The independent objects are provided by means of the ingenious piece of apparatus illustrated in Fig. 13.16, which was introduced by MADDOX in 1912 as the wing test. The plate marked out with the scales and pointers is situated 33⅓ cm. from the two slits through which the subject looks. The two diaphragms are arranged in such a way that nothing but the two scales is visible to the left eye and nothing but the two pointers to the right eye. The pointers actually point to the zero marks of their respective scales, as shown in the figure. As already

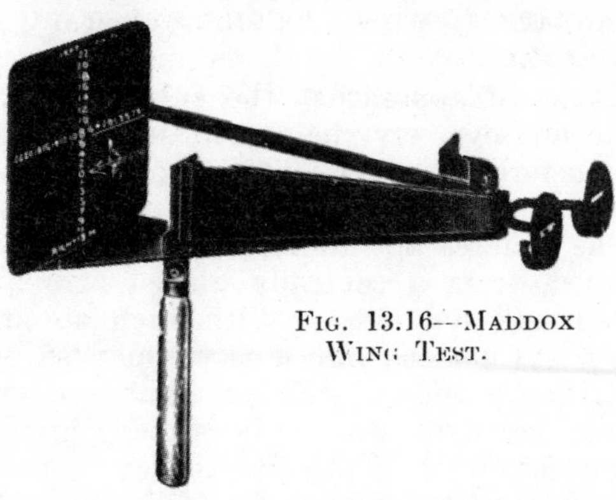

FIG. 13.16—MADDOX WING TEST.

explained,* the eyes are dissociated when looking through such an arrangement. The pointers will appear to point to the zero marks to a subject with no lateral or vertical heterophoria ; and the long horizontal limb of the arrow pointer will appear parallel to the horizontal line running along the horizontal scale if he has no cyclophoria. If any lateral or vertical phoria exist, the pointers will appear to point to some division on the respective scales the number opposite which indicates the amount of the phoria in prism dioptres—the divisions are 3·33 mm. apart.

If any cyclophoria exists, the arrow will appear inclined to the horizontal line. The right hand extremity of this arrow can be displaced up or down over a short scale marked in degrees, thus tilting the arrow, the head of

* §13.11.

which is fixed. When the extremity is so placed that the arrow and horizontal line appear to the subject parallel, the cyclophoria may be read off from the degree scale. The measurement is, however, not accurate.

The vertical scale and horizontal arrow are usually coloured red; the horizontal scale and vertical pointer, white; all on a black background.

In order to ensure that the subject accommodates as precisely as possible for the 33·3 cm. distance, the scale numbers should be very small so that they will not be distinguished otherwise. If the accommodation wanders, so may the fixation lines, in which case a false reading of horizontal phoria will be obtained. The scale numbers on the usual commercial instruments are too large. Also the black plate carrying the scales and index marks should be large so that its edges will not be easily seen by both eyes and so will not constitute an incentive for fusion.

(*b*) Phoriagraph with Complementary Colour Dissociation.

In this type of apparatus* the subject, wearing a red glass before one eye, say the right, and a complementary green glass before the other, observes a white card marked out in squares by means of vertical and horizontal lines in red. The squares are numbered to right and left, and up and down, from a centrally placed zero at which is mounted a small red light. With such an arrangement the left eye sees nothing but squares, marked out in *black* on a green background; and the right eye sees nothing but the small red light, the red lines being invisible on the wholly red background. Thus dissociation is secured and the horizontal and vertical phorias are indicated to the subject according to the square that appears to be occupied by the red light. Cyclophoria is not revealed by this apparatus.

The card may be held at various distances from the eyes, 25, 33·33, 40 cm., etc., as desired. The imbalance in prism dioptres may then be calculated. Thus if the size of the squares is 1/3 cm., each represents one prism dioptre when the testing distance is 33·33 cm.; 1·33△ when 25 cm., and 0·833△ when 40 cm.

(*c*) The Synoptophore.

This may be used for investigating cyclophoria at the near working distance by inserting −3 D spheres before the front faces of the reflecting prisms and proceeding as already explained for distance.

* A neat practical form has been introduced (1934) by H. Rosen, of London

CONCOMITANT HETEROPHORIA. SYMPTOMS AND CAUSES

13.14. Symptoms.

Whereas the symptoms vary according to the variety of heterophoria present, each of which will be briefly considered separately below, certain general symptoms accompany all varieties.

Visual symptoms: blurred vision, particularly in near work when there is insufficiency of converging power; momentary diplopia may occur and there may be difficulty in maintaining steady gaze at objects, especially moving objects, as at cricket and football matches, etc. A certain amount of distortion of objects may occur in high degrees of cyclophoria, with difficulty in judging distances, causing trouble in descending steps, etc. The subject may adopt unusual postures of the head and wrinklings of the forehead.

The eyes may feel uncomfortable and strained and may be difficult to control. Pain may be experienced, referred to the muscles; or frontal headaches may appear, especially towards the end of the day, or when otherwise fatigued. There may be dizziness, especially with hyperphoria. Many of these symptoms are relieved when one eye is closed. Neurasthenia may be accentuated and the subject may become morose and depressed. There may be conjunctival hyperæmia or blepharitis.

Hyperphoria is the form most liable to give trouble, even in relatively small amounts, since the verging powers of the eyes are small in the vertical direction.

13.15. Analysis of Causes.

If any of the four basic requirements for binocular vision stated in §12.1 are violated, then the attainment of binocular vision will be interfered with, the nature and extent of the interference depending upon the nature and severity of the violating cause. The latter may be such that binocular vision is quite impossible, as in heterotropia; or it may allow of binocular fixation and fusion, and hence some measure of binocular vision if not good stereoscopic vision, but only as the result of unusual effort and discomfort, or unnatural position of the head, on the part of the subject.

(1) Assuming there are no gross malformations interfering with the orbits or the forward direction of the eyes and

no obvious disease putting one eye out of action; that is, assuming no anatomical or pathological condition sufficient to violate the first basic requirement of binocular vision, the latter may yet be absent or defective or difficult from three main causes, namely;

(2) Violation of the second requirement for binocular vision: that is, interference with the characteristic binocular reception of visual stimuli by the brain.

(3) Violation of the third requirement: interference of some kind with the oculo-motor system so that the eyes are badly positioned, or do not execute correctly their conjugate and disjunctive movements, or do so with difficulty, or do so only in restricted regions of the total field.

(4) Violation of the fourth requirement: defect, inherited or acquired, interfering with fusion and co-ordination in the brain.

It will be understood that these main causes may react on one another. Thus, although the musculature of the eyes and their connections with the nuclei may be sound, inefficient ocular movements may result from a weakened power of fusion in consequence of which the *incentive* to carry out the complicated movements necessary for single vision is absent or defective. On the other hand, the arrangements for fusion and higher processes in the cortex may be perfect, but defects in the motor system may prevent their proper functioning or may arrest their development during the early formative years.

These interdependencies complicate the diagnosis of any given condition of imbalance; nevertheless, we may attempt a broad classification which should be of service, somewhat as follows:

(2) Reception: interference with the formation of the retinal images or with the transmission along the afferent paths to the brain.

(3) Motor System:

A. Interference with the transmission from the cortical centres along the efferent paths through the subcortical co-ordinating stations to the oculomotor nuclei.

B. Interference of a refractive nature: ametropia or accommodational disturbances upsetting the relationship between accommodation and convergence or affecting other movements.

C. Defect in the motor nuclei or their efferent connections with the muscles.

D. Anatomical defects or weakness in the muscles.

(4) FUSION: interference with the process of fusion and co-ordination.

A. *Ocular Inequality*: (a) anisometropia; (b) unequal ocular acuities (amblyopia, fundus disease, opacities); (c) unequal ocular images (aniseikonia, luminosity differences).

B. Defective fusion and co-ordination ability, congenital or acquired.

C. Suspended fusion: to relieve discomfort from some other cause.

To obtain binocular vision with comfort, the visual apparatus must be able to execute all conjugate movements and adjustments of accommodation and convergence on any object up to and within the near working distance and must fulfil the requirements concerning reception and fusion. The movements must be effected without undue effort and with the head held in a natural position. There should be adequate amplitude of vergence—horizontal, vertical and cyclo—at every point in the field, not only when looking straight ahead at objects on the median line, but also when looking in other directions, particularly downwards as in reading and close work. The passive position should not lie so far removed from the desired fixation position that the fusion powers of the individual shall be unduly taxed in securing binocular fixation and fusion. It must necessarily lie within the extreme positions CA and CZ (Fig. 5.3) to which the eyes can respectively diverge and converge; and similarly between the limits of vertical and cyclo vergence.

If the receptive and fusional processes are defective, whether the motor system be normal or not, the stimulus to the motor nuclei will be absent or inadequate and binocular fixation will not be achieved, or at least will not be maintained, through lack of incentive. One eye or the other, or perhaps one eye and the other alternately, will deviate from the fixation position producing a condition of heterotropia or squint. The image of the object then falls on the fovea of the fixing eye and on a point removed from the fovea of the deviating eye and diplopia results, unless and until such time as the extra-foveal image in the deviating eye is mentally suppressed.* When this is so, only monocular vision, by the fixing eye, is present. Thus concomitant squint is to a large extent an anomaly of or a check in the development of the receptive and fusion processes. We will deal with squint later, however.

There may be an imbalance, but if it is not too large and if the above conditions for comfortable binocular vision hold, there will be binocular vision and no symptoms. Heterophoria of this order is quite common, the rule rather than the exception in near vision, and requires no treatment. On the other hand the imbalance may be considerable, but if the reception and fusion of the visual stimuli are normal and the stimulus despatched to the motor nuclei adequate, binocular vision may still be achieved. The effort to move the eyes and effect fusion may now produce troublesome vision and symptoms, however. Whether this is the case depends upon the cause of the heterophoria, upon its direction and magnitude and the relation to these of the vergence powers, and upon the general condition of the subject. In any event since, in spite of the imbalance, binocular vision *is* achieved, the fusion impulse must be generally adequate; and the imbalance is due to some cause amongst those producing interference with the motor system. That is, *heterophoria is a motor anomaly*.

In the above classification we have subdivided the motor anomalies into four groups which we will consider briefly in order.

3A Interference in the region between the cortical centres and mid-brain co-ordinating centres is likely to cause a general insufficiency of innervation and hence a general deviation from orthophoria, i.e. a concomitant imbalance. Lack of tone due to general debility and illness would probably have this effect. A defect in one or other of the subcortical regions, on the other hand, is more likely to give rise to noncomitant heterophoria, since in this region the innervation may have been subjected to directional control.

3B. The tendency towards excessive convergence in hyperopia, and towards deficient convergence in myopia,

* §14.4.

has already been noted.* The sequence of events in the former, which usually develops in early childhood, is the onset of esophoria followed by intermittent convergent squint for near objects and, later, for distant objects.† The limited calls on accommodation in myopia may lead correspondingly, as the child approaches about twelve years of age, to exophoria and divergent squint. The dissociation between accommodation and convergence may also affect, or be affected by, vertical imbalances. We have seen that all the muscles are concerned in all eye movements and unusual efforts in one direction may upset the general balance and so lead to faulty execution in another direction. Assuming that the imbalance has not progressed to the condition of manifest squint, the imbalance and its accompanying symptoms, if any, may lessen or entirely disappear when the refraction is suitably corrected. On this account these refractive or accommodative heterophorias are regarded by some as not *essentially* heterophoria at all.

3C and 3D. Defects under these subheadings are situated at or below the motor nuclei, in which area the innervations have already passed through the process of distribution by the co-ordinating stations, and so the effect will be confined to one muscle or a small group of muscles and generally the heterophoria will be noncomitant.

Broadly, noncomitant or paralytic heterophoria (and squints) are due to causes situated at or below the level of the nuclei; concomitant heterophoria to disturbances above the nuclei, or to refractive conditions.

CONCOMITANT HETEROPHORIA. TREATMENT.

13.16. The Motor System in Heterophoria.

From the previous paragraph it appears that heterophoria is brought about by a disturbance of the normal functioning of the oculo-motor system. Our analysis of such disturbances appears to indicate that the cause of concomitant heterophoria is to be sought above the motor nuclei or in an upsetting of the equipoise between the refractive system and the motor system of the eyes (3A and 3B). The treatment to be adopted, when the condition is accompanied by symptoms, is not yet firmly established. Our

* §5.2. † See also §14.3.

knowledge of the subject, even of the restricted aspect of it concerning the accommodation-convergence relationship,* is incomplete.

It may be that the lack of equipoise between the refractive and motor systems could be restored either by correcting the refractive error or by treating the heterophoria. Usually the refractive error of itself requires some measure of correction, however; in myopia to provide clear distance vision; in hyperopia to lessen the incidence of accommodative strain, which may be contributory to the symptoms complained of; in astigmatism for both reasons probably. But the refractive or presbyopic correction may require modification in the presence of imbalances of the motor system, as was indicated when describing methods of determining these corrections in Chapters III, IV and VI.

In those cases where the symptoms are not relieved by the refractive correction, it appears to be necessary to investigate the motor system by measuring the vergence powers and the relative vergence powers of the eyes: and to take such steps as we can to augment the vergence powers if they are found to be subnormal or to modify the distribution of the relative vergence powers if these are still unsymmetrical after refractive correction. Any hyperphoria present should be corrected before the horizontal vergence is measured; and if any cyclophoria exists, the object slides in the synoptophore should be tilted accordingly.

The procedure at present available for improving the performance of the motor system is to subject it to certain binocular exercises, which will be described below.

We will first consider the vergence and relative vergence amplitudes in relation to heterophoria.

13.17. Heterophoria, Convergence and Relative Convergence.

Just as ciliary strain is likely to arise if more than one half to two thirds of an individual's amplitude of accommodation has to be exercised continuously in near work,† so with convergence; a certain proportion of the total amplitude of convergence should always be in reserve. LANDOLT suggested that the total amplitude should bear

---

* §5.2. † §6.4.

to the convergence in use the ratio 3 : 1; and this seems to have stood the test of clinical experience. Thus: to read at 33·33 cm. an orthophoric person has to exert 3 metre-angles of convergence, measured from his functional rest position, which is also in his case the primary position; to carry out continuous work at this distance the individual should possess a total amplitude of 9 metre-angles, leaving 6 metre-angles in reserve. As we have seen, most people can converge more than this and consequently experience no trouble in near work if their accommodation also has adequate reserve—the corresponding ratio in accommodation is 3 : 2.

Exophoria and Convergence.

The functional rest position of an exophoric person lies on the divergent side of the primary position. Since the eyes settle down to this position when not activated by the desire for fusion, the amount of convergence to be brought into action in order to fix a given object should be reckoned from this passive position. Thus in the case of an individual with 16△ of exophoria at distance, the one eye has to converge by $8 + 9 = 17\triangle$ or $5\frac{2}{3}$ metre-angles, in order to do close work at 33·33 cm. Assuming his measured total amplitude of convergence, reckoned from the passive or phoria position, has about the normal value of 12·5 metre-angles,* the ratio between the total and the amount in use is 12·5 : 5·67 or about 2·2 : 1. According to LANDOLT'S ratio, there is a possibility here of trouble in continuous near work; and the exophoria is likely to be greater at near than at distance. The near point of convergence is 12·5—2·67 metre-angles, or rather more than 10 cm. from the inter-ocular base line, which exceeds the normal 8 to 9 cm.

The accommodation-convergence diagram for an exophoric person, corresponding to Fig. 5.3 which applies in orthophoria, might be somewhat as represented in Fig. 13.17. CP_D is the functional rest or distance phoria position; CB the fixation position for reading; CZ the limit of convergence. The lettering of the diagram corresponds to Fig. 5.3. The convergence in use when fixing B is the angle $P_DCB = 17\triangle = 5\cdot67$ M.A. The total convergence from functional rest shown on the diagram is

* §5.1.

angle P_DCZ = about $9\frac{1}{3}$ M.A., which is less than normal. The amount BCZ in reserve is insufficient. Even if the total amplitude were normal at 12·5 M.A., the amount in reserve would be less than LANDOLT'S value. The near point of accommodation M_P is supposed to be 4·5 D in the case illustrated.

This is a case where exercises, aimed at stimulating the powers of convergence, are prescribed in current practice.

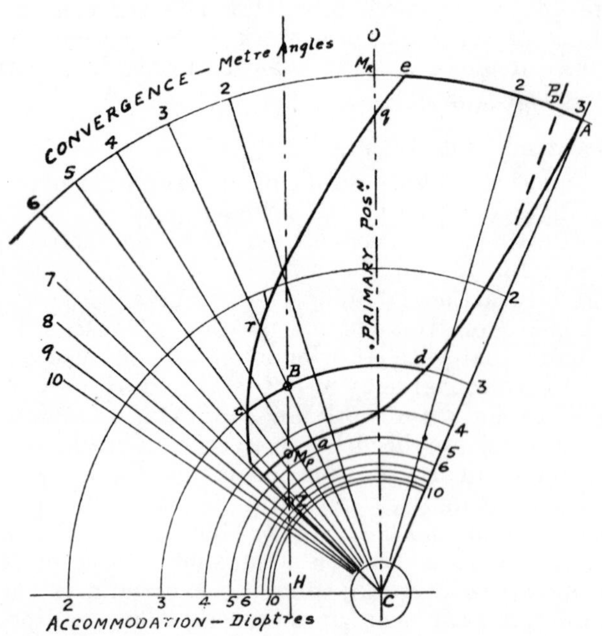

FIG. 13.17—ACCOMMODATION—CONVERGENCE DIAGRAM. DISTANCE EXOPHORIA OF 16△ (8△ EACH EYE). NEAR POINT OF ACC. 4·5 D. COMPARE FIG. 5.3.

If the convergence near point Z can be brought nearer to the eyes, the total amplitude and the amount in reserve are increased. And if, in addition, any presbyopic addition that is required for near work is kept as low as possible, convergence is stimulated still further.

It is likely that had the convergence amplitude P_DCZ been 17 M.A. or so, bringing the near point Z to within 8 or 9 cm., there would have been no symptoms in the above case. Such cases of exophoria occur. Had symptoms been complained of in spite of such ample convergence resources, it is unlikely that convergence exercises would improve matters; in which case attention should be directed to an examination of the range of *relative* vergence or fusion breadth, at distance and near.

Exophoria and Relative Convergence.

It is conceivable that discomfort may arise because of the manner in which the exophoria effects the positioning of the amplitude of *relative* convergence. Thus, suppose that although the total convergence extending from CP_D to CZ (Fig. 13.17) be adequate, the convergence cannot be increased beyond the position Ce without a corresponding increase of accommodation (to Cq) coming into action, or at least without the distant object becoming subjectively indistinct. The efforts to relax accommodation to see clearly would induce divergence which would produce diplopia; this could not be tolerated and the refractive and motor systems might fluctuate around the desired fixation position CO and cause fatigue and distress.

It was maintained by PERCIVAL* that the situation of the fixation position CO relative to the region eA of *relative* convergence is important; and similarly for near, of the fixation position CB in the region cd. He states that, for comfort, the fixation position should lie within the middle third of the amplitude of relative convergence. It clearly does not so lie, either at distance or near, in Fig. 13.17. In Fig. 5.3 the near fixation position CB satisfies this condition, but not the distance fixation position CO.

Experience with heterophoric cases with symptoms supports this view. In some cases the near point of convergence Z may lie in the normal position, but the relative amplitudes are unsymmetrically disposed about the fixation positions CO and CB, as in Fig. 13.17; the symptoms are relieved by taking steps to shift these amplitudes until the fixation lines lie within the middle thirds of their extents. This shift can sometimes be accomplished, at least partially, by modifying the spherical portion of the refractive correction; by undercorrecting 0·50 D or so in hyperopia and fully correcting in myopia, in exophoria cases. Some measure of shift can also be brought about by submitting the subject to a form of ocular exercise on such an instrument as the synoptophore, as explained later.

---

* A. S. PERCIVAL: *The Prescribing of Spectacles*; John Wright, 1928.

Esophoria

Fig. 13.18 illustrates an accommodation-convergence diagram for an esophore of 8△ (4△ each eye). The whole area is depicted as rotated towards the convergent side along with the functional rest position CP_D. The distance fixation position CO almost reaches the extreme divergence

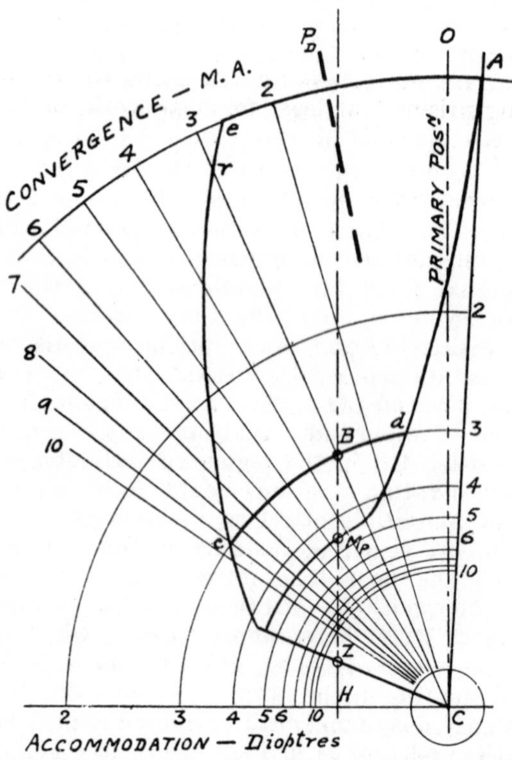

FIG. 13.18—ACCOMMODATION—CONVERGENCE DIAGRAM. DISTANCE ESOPHORIA OF 8△ (4△ EACH EYE). NEAR POINT OF ACC. 4·5 D. COMPARE FIG. 5.3.

position CA and it would appear that difficulties might arise in maintaining single vision of distant objects.

In near vision there is ample reserve convergence within the fixation position CB and the relative convergence range cd is not too badly distributed around CB. On the basis of the considerations advanced above, therefore, near vision should be comfortable.

If symptoms are complained of, exercise with the synoptophore, in the divergent direction, may be tried; but since divergence is not ordinarily called upon in everyday vision, it is a movement not readily susceptible of development and exercises are generally of little or no avail.

In those cases, of exophoria or esophoria, where the convergence and relative convergence are normal or have been made so by exercise, but in which symptoms still persist, current practice is limited either to the prescribing of relieving prisms,* at least for near work, or to referring the subject for medical attention.

13.18. Cyclovergence.

Disjunctive torsional movements of the eyes in the interests of binocular vision have been referred to in §5.6 and in Chapter XII, but some further description may be given here.

The eyes take up a position of excyclovergence when they accommodate and converge to bring near objects under observation.† The full extent of the possible in- and excyclovergence movements as the eyes observe a given object may be measured by means of the synoptophore, the objects being a pair of straight lines—one presented to each eye—which, while being fused, may be rotated in opposite directions around their mid-points. The greatest extent to which the lines can be rotated relatively to one another and still be fused into a single line, measures the cyclovergence of the eyes. As we shall see immediately, the lines must be horizontal and not vertical.

Suppose the objects in the synoptophore consist of two vertical lines, one visible to each eye. They are fused into a mental percept of a single vertical line. If the line objects are oppositely tilted through a small angle in the vertical plane, they are still fused into a single line which appears to be sloping away from the observer. It has been found‡ that the fusing of such "skew vertical" lines is not accomplished by cyclo rotations of the eyes, but that successive points of the lines are fused as the eyes sweep over them from one end to the other, varying convergence in doing so.

* §13.19. † §§ 12.4 and 12.13.

‡ From experiments at the Northampton Polytechnic, London; see footnote to §12.10.

The vertical version movements of the eyes were measured objectively with a microscope while they fused the skew verticals (presented in a haploscope arrangement) and it was found that their vertical excursions were directly proportional to the lengths of the test lines. Measurements to determine the limiting value of the angle of tilt between the test lines for which fusion was still just possible showed that this angle is dependent upon both the length of the test lines and their distance from the eyes. It decreases with increase of object length and increases with object distance; its value is such that the separated extremities of the test lines subtend a constant angle at the mid-point between the centres of rotation of the eyes.

Thus it appears that the eyes fuse two skew vertical lines in somewhat the same way as they view a single line object leaning away from them in space. In the latter case, however, accommodation changes, as well as convergence, as the gaze is shifted from one end of the line to the other; and there is no limit to the extent of the leaning away of this line; it may be a horizontal line running directly away from the observer, in which case the projection of it seen by each eye is a horizontal line and the angle between the projections is 180°. In the case of the two skew lines, they cannot be inclined to one another by anything like this amount, probably due to the fact that all parts of the lines are at the same distance from the eyes and there is consequently a restriction on the play of accommodation.

When the test lines were disposed horizontally, however, it was found (*a*) that the extent of the possible relative inclination of the lines, the eyes still fusing them, was very much less than with the vertical lines; (*b*) stereoscopic relief in the blended projection was not observed; and (*c*) the fusing of the lines was achieved by cyclovergence movements of the eyes, as demonstrated by the fact that the limiting angle of tilt of the test lines was independent of their distance from the eyes.

The experiments indicate that the cyclovergence powers of the eyes cannot be measured by means of vertical test lines, but that the lines must be disposed horizontally. By gradually rotating such horizontal lines, in a stereoscopic instrument, so that their outer* extremities are lowered, we measure the excyclovergence of the eyes. By reversing the direction of tilt we measure the incyclovergence. The average values found in the case of the few subjects tested in the above experiments were: incyclovergence about 7°; excyclovergence about $3\frac{1}{2}$°—total for both eyes in each direction—these values being constant for all distances of the test lines.

13.19. Ocular Exercises. Relieving Prisms.

Mention was made above of the possibility of improving the performance of the oculo-motor system by some form of binocular exercises in those cases where symptoms

* The left extremity of the line seen by the left eye and the right extremity of the right.

persist after refractive correction. The somewhat empirical methods at present available will probably be modified as our knowledge of oculo-motor imbalance is extended.

Since vergence movements in the vertical direction and cyclo movements are not voluntarily executed in normal vision, exercises are generally useless in the vertical and cyclo directions and are scarcely ever attempted. And in the horizontal direction little can be done to amplify the divergence powers, for the same general reason. Such exercises as are attempted are consequently limited to convergence and to relative convergence. They are frequently called *orthoptic* exercises.

Amplitude of Vergence.

The exercises may be carried out with *adverse prisms.* While the subject observes binocularly an object such as the muscle light at 6 metres or so, a prism may be interposed before one eye with its *base* in the direction of the heterophoric deviation ; e.g. base out in exophoria. The subject is made aware of the diplopia and asked to fuse the two projections. To do so he must exert verging power in the opposite direction to his deviation, just as he does in viewing a distant object in ordinary vision, but to a greater extent. This is repeated at intervals of a few seconds. If he succeeds, the prism strength is gradually increased, step by step, being divided equally between the two eyes in all but the weak starting prisms. The task thereby increases in difficulty and presently a stage will be reached at which the diplopia is insuperable.

Provided with two or three prisms of different powers the subject is instructed how to continue these exercises at home. The procedure is then repeated, but for near objects, after which the subject's own home exercises alternate between distant and near objects, situated at the sides as well as in the median plane.

The gradually increasing strength of prism may be applied by means of a variable rotary prism device such as the prism verger or the variable prism stereoscope. Or the exercises may be carried out equally well, both for distance and near, with a haploscope device such as the amblyoscope or the synoptophore.

In the case of exophoria, convergence exercises may be executed in the absence of any apparatus, the subject gazing intently at a small object, such as the tip of a pencil.

while it is brought towards the nose and then carried away, repeatedly. Or the subject may practise daily reading aloud (aloud to maintain concentration) bringing the book nearer and nearer until the print is too blurred to see clearly ; the process to be repeated for some few minutes. Relaxation is obtained by occasionally looking away into the distance.

Amplitude of Relative Convergence.

Exercises intended to extend the range of relative convergence could be conveniently carried out with the synoptophore. Similar object slides containing suitable detail are inserted in the instrument and the subject discriminates and fuses them with the arms of the instrument set in a comfortable position. The arms are then rotated in the direction requiring convergence on the part of the subject until the object either "breaks"* or becomes indistinct. The procedure is repeated a number of times at each sitting, the subject endeavouring to hold on to clear and single vision as long as possible at each rotation, the extent of which is, if possible, gradually increased. By such means it is hoped to extend the range of relative vergence, eA at distance, and cd at near, Fig. 13.17, until it is more symmetrically distributed around the fixation position CO or CB respectively.

Relieving Prisms.

Assuming that exercises have proved of no avail or that the case is one in which exercises would have been of no service, we can yet fall back on the device of attempting to give the subject relief from his symptoms by means of relieving prisms. This step should not be taken, except in hyperphoria, until the previous remedies have been given a fair trial and should even then be considered as only a temporary measure. The prisms prescribed should be reduced in strength by stages, if at all possible, on subsequent occasions.

A relieving prism is placed with its apex in the direction of the deviation. The eyes may then take up an easier position approaching the passive position and the symptoms induced by the previous efforts to maintain fixation against the tendency to deviate will tend to be relieved. In esophoria, for example, base-out prisms would be prescribed,

* §5.5.

divided equally between the two eyes. The eyes will then take up a definite position on the convergent side, which is the passive side, of the object of fixation; they are thereby relieved of some of the fusional divergent effort they have previously been forced to make. With regard to the strength of the prism, this should be kept as low as will produce the desired relief. Frequently quite a weak prism will suffice even in cases of large degrees of heterophoria. Base-in prisms may similarly be prescribed, usually for near work only, in exophoria giving rise to symptoms which persist after other measures have failed.

Relieving prisms may be prescribed for constant wear in hyperphoria with much less hesitation. Hyperphoria, with symptoms persisting after refractive correction, may be treated at once with relieving prisms of a strength equal to two thirds or the full value of the deviation, to be worn continuously. In right hyperphoria the prisms will be base down before the right eye and base up before the left.

Prisms are of no avail in cyclophoria.

In those cases where a refractive correction is worn, the relieving prisms may be incorporated in the correction by appropriately decentring the lenses.*

Strong prisms cannot be used because of their weight and the distortion they produce. These effects will probably be prohibitive in prisms exceeding 5△ deviation, total for both eyes. In such cases the only means available for relieving the condition is by means of the fifth step, namely surgical operation.

13.20. Summary of Treatment.

We may now briefly summarise the general steps to be taken in clinical practice.

The refractive error is determined and, the subject wearing his correction, the motor balance is determined for distance and near. The correction must be carefully centred for the distance of the test; the presbyopic correction, if any, is worn for near. The near point of convergence is also determined.

If appreciable exophoria or esophoria are found, the spherical portion of the refractive correction is modified, as explained. If the convergence near point does not

---

* *Ophthalmic Lenses;* Ch. VII.

reach the normal position of 8 to 9 cm., simple convergence exercises are prescribed.

In many cases any symptoms previously existing will now disappear and no further treatment is required. If, after wearing of the correction for two or three weeks, the symptoms persist, the heterophoria for distance and near and the convergence near point are re-determined. The amplitude of relative convergence at distance and near are also determined with the synoptophore. As explained in the previous paragraphs, sufficient information is then available to decide whether orthoptic exercises are likely to prove beneficial. If not, relieving prisms may be prescribed.

In a case where exercises may be expected to be of service, these are prescribed if the subject's general health is satisfactory. If not, this should receive medical attention and for a period reasonable rest should be given to the eyes, near work especially being curtailed, particularly with children.

13.21. Cyclophoria. Oblique Astigmatism.

A few separate remarks may be made concerning this particular form of heterophoria. It appears to be infrequently encountered and symptoms on account of it are rarely complained of. When cyclophoria is found, it is usually in association with appreciable degrees of horizontal or vertical imbalance or with a squint condition; and then it often disappears if, and when, the accompanying condition is disposed of. It has already been noted* that a certain amount of excyclophoria at near is normal and unimportant, when the plane of fixation is in certain positions.

When symptoms are present they take the form of persistent headache and giddiness, perhaps accompanied by such visual symptoms as disturbances of perspective and difficulty in estimating distances in the upper and lower fields of vision, so that the subject experiences awkwardness in moving about, in descending stairs, etc. If the phoria is paretic there is a marked tendency to cyclodiplopia in the upper or lower portions of the visual field.

In concomitant cyclophoria very little can be done by optical means. It is possible to rectify the leaning of vertical lines to some extent by taking advantage of the

---

* §12.13.

distortion produced by prisms when these are angled around their base-apex lines.* Thus a pair of base-out prisms with their upper edges tilted away from the eyes will rectify vertical lines that appear to lean outwards, although they will also be curved. Such measures, or the wearing of concave cylinders set at symmetrically oblique axes before the two eyes, are but clumsy expedients at the best, however. Relief can be obtained by covering one eye.

In the presence of these difficulties it may be worth while attempting to develop the cyclovergence powers by exercises with horizontal lines, as already mentioned.

Tests for cyclophoria should be made with the subject wearing his full ametropic correction and the horizontal and vertical phorias relieved by prisms.

It is frequently stated that a condition of cyclophoria, or pseudo-cyclophoria, is set up by oblique astigmatism, but this seems scarcely possible. An astigmatic system produces an undistorted though blurred image in a plane containing one of the focal lines, or in that region. Thus, although a cylinder or sphero-cyl. lens produces the well-known scissors effect on a crossline when rotated around the visual line into an oblique position relative to the cross line, the lines being apparently shifted towards the meridian of greater power, this effect is zero when the lens is held at the object or at the eye. Each individual point of the object is, of course, blurred out in the direction of one or both of the principal meridians of the lens, but with the lens held close to the eye the object as a whole is not distorted; the crosslines continue to appear vertical and horizontal as the lens is rotated. In the presence of extremely high oblique astigmatism of the eye, there may be a very slight distortion since the astigmatism must reside either in the cornea or the crystalline lens, neither of which is at the principal point of the combined system; but this can scarcely be noticeable.

Further than this, any slight tilt of the image on the retina will vary according to the orientation of the corresponding object line. Hence, if there were any tendency for the eyes to execute a cyclovergence movement in order to rectify such image tilt, every retinal meridian would need to be rotated a different amount.

---

* *Ophthalmic Lenses*; Chap. VI.

It is possible, however, for a sphero-cyl. correction of high cylinder power to introduce some distortion since the correcting lens is placed some distance in front of the eye. The spectacle magnification* is different in the two principal meridians and an object in the form of a square with sides parallel to these meridians will be imaged on the retina as a rectangle. The retinal image of a diagonal of the square, or of any line oblique to the principal meridians, will be tilted from its true orientation.† Subjectively, however, these effects will be very small and will probably disappear after a period.

The discomfort sometimes experienced for a while after correction of oblique astigmatism may be due to the change from retinal images possessing directional blurring to unfamiliar clear images.

EXERCISES. CHAPTER XIII.

1. Describe carefully the conditions designated by the following terms, making clear the differences between them: simultaneous macular vision, fusion, binocular fixation, binocular vision, stereoscopic vision.

2. In relation to the use of two eyes in binocular vision, explain clearly the meanings of the following terms: fixation position, passive position, active position, orthophoria, heterophoria. Illustrate your answer with an explanatory diagram.

3. Explain carefully the terms heterophoria and heterotropia. Presented with an object such as a "muscle light" at 6 metres, what would subjects with these conditions be expected to see when in the passive position and in the active position?

Explain briefly the terms concomitant and noncomitant as applied to the two conditions.

4. Explain clearly, in relation to one type of heterophoria, just how the diplopia arises. Give a diagram showing the eyes with the foveæ, the projections of these in relation to the object of regard, and indicate the extent of the diplopia.

5. Compare physiological diplopia and pathological diplopia. With the aid of diagrams explain the kind of diplopia experienced, in the passive position, by a person with (*a*) esophoria, (*b*) left hyperphoria, (*c*) excyclophoria.

6. In connection with the investigation of the condition of motor balance of the eyes, explain what is meant by a dissociating prism and by a measuring prism.

A spot of light at 6 metres is observed binocularly with an 8△ prism base up before the right eye. (*a*) If the person is exophoric 5△ for distance (6 metres) what is the relative position of the two projections seen by the person? (*b*) If a 4△ prism be placed base out before the left

---

* §3.13. † §10.16.

eye what will then be the positions of the projections ? (c) If the 4△ is removed, what prism before the left eye will " measure " the phoria ?

7. A person with left hyperphoria of 4△ observes a spot of light at 6 metres through a base-in prism of 12△ placed before the R.E. Give a diagram, with dimensions, showing the appearance to the subject.

What appearance is to be expected when the base-in prism is replaced by a base-out prism of equal strength ? Give reasons.

Explain, with a diagram, *why* a person with esophoria obtains homonymous diplopia when the eyes are dissociated.

8. A person with normal motor balance observes binocularly a muscle light at 6 metres. Explain the appearance of the light and give careful diagrams showing the course of light into the eyes and the positions of the foveæ, when prisms as below are placed in turn before the right eye :—

(*a*) 12△ base in ; (*c*) 12△ base out ;
(*b*) 3△ base in ; (*d*) 12△ base up.

In case (*d*) what would be the appearance observed by a person with 5△ of exophoria ?

9. A person with 4△ of esophoria observes binocularly a spot of light at 6 metres, an 8△ prism being placed base down before the right eye. Show on a diagram the appearance to the subject, giving dimensions. The prism remaining before the right eye, what will be the effect of placing before the left eye (*a*) an 8△ prism base out ; (*b*) an 8△ prism base down ?

If the spot of light be replaced by a long bright vertical line, show the appearance by diagrams in this case.

10. What is meant by dissociating the eyes ? Explain briefly the condition of the oculo-motor system when dissociation is in operation.

Describe the four types of methods of dissociating the eyes when testing for heterophoria.

What preliminary measure must be taken before setting out to investigate the heterophoric condition of the subject ?

11. What is meant by heterophoria ? Discuss various methods of measuring it, along with the precautions to be taken. How is the condition differentiated from heterotropia ? (S.M.C.)

12. Survey the advantages and disadvantages of using metre-angles as units of measurement. Describe other units which may be used in their place and indicate how they are all related.

What inferences can be drawn from the following measurements ?

At 6 m. testing distance:
emmetropia and orthophoria.
At 33 cm. testing distance:
1 metre-angle exophoria ;
3 metre-angles prism divergence ;
3 metre-angles prism convergence.

(S.M.C.)

13. Describe, with a diagram of its construction, the Stevens' phorometer and explain carefully how it may be used to measure horizontal heterophoria and vertical heterophoria.

Mention any precaution to be observed in using the instrument.

14. Compare the single prism and the double prism for the purpose of dissociating the eyes when seeking to measure heterophoria. Describe

briefly instrumental devices for measuring the degree of heterophoria made manifest by the dissociating device.

15. Describe the condition called cyclophoria and explain the type of diplopia experienced by a subject with ex-cyclophoria when his eyes are rendered passive.

Explain how the condition may be detected and measured, for distance and for near, using a double prism. Is the method accurate ?

16. Describe in detail how the Maddox groove causes a point of light to appear as a streak. Draw two carefully constructed diagrams to show the cross-sections of the beam entering the eye (*a*) in a plane through the light and axis of a groove ; (*b*) in a plane at right angles to the groove axes and containing the light. (S.M.C.)

17. Explain how the Maddox rod or groove may be employed in detecting and measuring (*a*) vertical imbalances, (*b*) cyclophoria.

With a Maddox rod before the right eye a person observing a light binocularly at 5 metres, sees the streak :

(*a*) 10 cm. to the right of the spot ;
(*b*) 6 ,, ,, ,, left ,, ,, ,,
(*c*) 1·5 ,, above the spot.

Write down the heterophoric condition in each case.

18. When a Maddox groove, axes vertical, is placed in front of the right eye, and the left eye fixes a point source of light at a distance of 10 metres, describe the appearances in the following cases :—

(*a*) both eyes in horizontal plane, visual axes parallel ;
(*b*) both eyes in horizontal plane, visual axis of right eye directed upwards ;
(*c*) right eye 3 mm. higher than left, visual axes parallel.

If the position of the point be altered to one metre distance, what alterations would you expect in each of the conditions specified ? (S.M.C.)

19. Explain, with the aid of a diagram, why the streak observed through a Maddox rod is perpendicular to the axis of the rod.

With the rod axis horizontal before the R.E., the streak is observed to lie 42 cm. to the left of the spot, testing at 6 metres. What is the heterophoric condition and what will be the direction and strength of prism before the L.E. to measure the defect ?

If the measuring prism were a rotary prism consisting of two equal prisms, of 12Δ deviation each, mounted in one cell, how far must they be rotated from the starting position to measure the above phoria ?

20. In the distance passive position the visual axes of a subject lie in the horizontal plane but are inclined to one another at a divergent angle of 4 degrees. What heterophoric condition will be registered on a tangent scale at 6 metres if a Maddox rod, axis horizontal, is before the right eye and a 2Δ base out prism before the left eye ? The subject's P.D. is 60 mm.

Compare briefly the Maddox rod and the double prism as dissociating elements in testing heterophoria.

21. A myope of 10 D, wearing his full distance correction in a frame 3 mm. too wide, is tested for lateral heterophoria at 5 metres. With the Maddox rod before his left eye, the streak appears 15 cm. to the right of the light. Is there any true lateral heterophoria in this case ? If there is,

state the type and amount that would exist if the glasses were centred correctly.

22. When tested with a Maddox rod for motor balance at near ($\frac{1}{3}$ metre) the visual axes of the subject take up a position inclined to one another at 5 degrees (convergent). The subject's P.D. is 60 mm. What is the near heterophoric condition ?

Describe a phoriagraphic method of testing motor balance at near.

23. Explain *why*, when one eye of a subject is allowed to see only a scale and the other eye only a pointer which is actually pointing to the zero of the scale, the pointer appears to be directed towards some other part of the scale when the subject is heterophoric.

Describe a form of phoriagraph using complementary colours for dissociating the eyes. Explain clearly how the dissociation is brought about and precautions to be observed in using the device.

24. Explain the general method of dissociating the eyes by means of independent objects, making clear why the reading given by the instrument is a measure of the subject's heterophoria.

Describe briefly an instrument of the stereoscope type that has been adapted for investigating conditions of motor balance.

25. What is a haploscope ? Explain briefly how such an instrument may be applied to investigate the accommodative-convergence relationship of an individual. For what other purpose, connected with binocular vision, may instruments of this type be used ? Sketch a form of the instrument.

26. Explain why the findings of motor balance tests in near vision are to be used with caution.

Explain the fluctuations in the extent of the diplopia observed by a subject whose eyes have been dissociated, particularly when the motor balance is being investigated at near.

Describe briefly one method of testing heterophoria at near.

27. Sketch and describe the Maddox Wing Test for investigating the condition of motor balance at the reading distance. How is cyclophoria indicated by the instrument ?

28. Describe briefly the following types of diplopia. In each case show on a diagram the appearance of the test object to a subject who is suffering from the diplopia and explain what heterophoric condition would be responsible for the diplopia :—heteronymous diplopia ; right superior diplopia ; right clockwise diplopia.

29. Write down the type and amount of the heterophoria in each of the conditions enumerated below. (N.B. The student should perform this and similar exercise tests mentally) :—

(*a*) Test at 6 metres ; Maddox rod horizontal before R.E. ; subject sees vertical streak 24 cm. to right of spot.

(*b*) Test at 5 metres ; Maddox rod vertical before L.E. ; horizontal streak seen 8 cm. above spot.

(*c*) Horizontal line test object at $\frac{1}{3}$ metre ; double prism before R.E. ; double line tilted anticlockwise to subject.

(*d*) Test at 6 metres ; red glass before R.E. and green before L.E. ; subject sees red light of phoriagraph 18 cm. below green light ; and also sees red light 15 cm. to left of green light when tested horizontally.

(*e*) Test on synoptophore with single horizontal line in left carrier and double horizontal line in right; subject sees single line tilted clockwise relative to double lines; rotation of each carrier through 5 degrees (in opposite directions) restores parallelism.

In this last case, in which direction must the carriers be tilted to restore parallelism ?

30. Explain how you would use an instrument of the haploscope type, such as the synoptophore, (*a*) to measure cyclophoria in a given subject; (*b*) to measure the cyclovergence powers of the eyes. What would you use as test object slides in each case ? Give reasons.

31. Describe with the aid of well drawn diagrams how the amblyoscope (or any other instrument of similar principle) can be calibrated to measure muscular anomalies. (S.M.C.)

32. Name four different types of instruments used for measuring degrees of muscular anomalies. Indicate briefly how each is used and give a detailed optical theory of one. (S.M.C.)

33. Describe apparatus for measuring vertical imbalance at reading distance—not Maddox rod. Why does this imbalance sometimes differ from that for distance vision ? Why is its determination of importance ? (B.O.A. Hons.)

34. Explain the meaning of the following and the conditions under which they are used: (*a*) dissociating prism; (*b*) measuring prism; (*c*) relieving prism; (*d*) adverse prism.

35. State the basic requirements for binocular vision; hence give a classification of the cause of heterophoria based upon the violation of these requirements. Differentiate between concomitant and paralytic heterophoria from the standpoint of their causation.

36. A subject with refractive error and a heterophoric condition is usually supplied with optical correction for the former, but not always for the latter. Write a short account of the reasons for this. In what circumstances will the heterophoria need treatment and what, briefly, is the trend of the treatment that may reasonably be followed ?

37. What effect has esophoria and exophoria in cases of hypermetropia and presbyopia; and how would such correction (condition ?) affect the correction you would order ? Give reasons for the procedure you would adopt. (B.O.A.)

38. How do you interpret the findings of muscular imbalance tests at distance and near ? When do you apply these tests and to what extent do the measurements influence your final prescription ? (S.M.C.)

39. How would you carry out an investigation into the binocular functions at the reading distance ? Describe the instruments you would use and discuss their limitations. State what anomalies you would look for, how you would detect and measure them, and the treatment you think necessary. For what conditions would you suggest base-in prism and how would you determine the amount to be incorporated in the prescription ? (B.O.A. Hons.)

40. What trouble would you expect a patient to experience who was suffering from one prism dioptre of (*a*) exophoria, (*b*) esophoria, (*c*) hyperphoria ? To what extent would you correct each ? Give reasons for your answer. (B.O.A. Hons.)

41. Why is a slight hyperphoria so much more troublesome than a horizontal imbalance ? When should it be corrected ; are exercises likely to be of any use ? Give reasons for your replies. (B.O.A. Hons.)

42. Explain carefully how to deal with cases in which there is both ametropia and heterophoria. Is it advisable to prescribe lenses combined with prisms in cases of this kind ? Give full reasons.

43. Describe carefully how esophoria for distance and near vision may be detected and measured. Explain fully what influence, if any, this condition may have upon the actual lenses to be prescribed for distance or for near work, and upon the fittings of the frames. (S.M.C. Hons.)

44. Give an account of the information you would need to have available in order to decide upon the advisability of prescribing ocular exercises in a given case of heterophoria. Explain how such information is obtained and give particulars of a chosen case, with such diagrams as may be necessary, in which you consider exercises might reasonably be expected to be of some benefit.

45. Draw an accommodation-convergence diagram for an emmetropic person aged 45 years who has 12△ of exophoria at distance ; total amplitude of convergence of 11 metre-angles, measured from the passive or phoria position ; amplitude of relative convergence at distance 2 M.A. ; far point of convergence $33\frac{1}{3}$ cm. behind the eyes ; P.D. 60 mm.

Discuss the condition of this person in relation to his reserve of (*a*) accommodation and (*b*) convergence. How much, if any, lens power would you prescribe for near work at $33\frac{1}{3}$ cm.? Would you prescribe any treatment for the exophoria ? Give particulars.

46. Explain the circumstances that might lead to the prescribing of relieving prisms and discuss the base direction and degree of prism for such conditions as exophoria and left hyperphoria. Describe briefly the steps of the examination and treatment up to the stage of the decision to try relieving prisms.

47. A subject is found to have right hyperphoria with esophoria, for distance. Describe a method by which this condition and its amount could have been ascertained and discuss the question of proceeding to treat it.

48. Draw a clear diagram showing the relation between accommodation and convergence for a person aged 20 years, who has 3 D of hypermetropia and 8△ of esophoria—total in both eyes. From your diagram give the following particulars :

(*a*) amplitude of convergence ;
(*b*) amplitude of relative convergence ;
(*c*) amplitude of accommodation ;
(*d*) far point and near point of convergence.

49. Describe in detail any instrument which provides optical training in cases of muscular imbalance. Discuss to what extent such exercises can be satisfactorily applied in such cases. (B.O.A. Hons.)

50. Describe the condition cyclophoria and explain how it may be detected and measured. Discuss the possibility of optical treatment.

It is sometimes stated that a condition of cyclophoria or pseudo-cyclophoria may be set up by oblique astigmatism. Discuss this.

51. Give a general definition of exophoria and use it to distinguish between " distance " and " near " exophoria.

If exophoria is found both at distance and near tests, what inferences can you deduce and how do you apply the information ? (S.M.C.)

52. A person shows six prism dioptres apparent exophoria at six metres using a tangent scale, when corrected with + 5·0 D spheres, right and left eyes, placed 25 mm. in front of the centres of rotation in a frame which is 4 mm. too wide (P.D. of eyes 60 mm.). What is the angle between the visual axes ? (S.M.C.).

NOTE : the test object may be assumed to lie either on the median line or on the primary line of one eye. The student can verify for himself that the result is the same in both cases.

OCULO-MOTOR IMBALANCE

CHAPTER XIV

HETEROTROPIA

(OR STRABISMUS OR SQUINT)

14.1. Introductory. Definitions.

IN this second main division of motor imbalance the subject cannot attain binocular fixation even when the oculo-motor system is in its active condition with the fusion sense free to assert control. The subject cannot therefore obtain binocular single vision. One eye or the other deviates from the fixation position, the fusion impulse being unable to overcome the deviation, which is consequently apparent, except in certain cases, to an outside observer. One eye, the FIXING EYE, is used for fixation while the other, the DEVIATING OR SQUINTING eye, is directed to some other point in the field. The angle between the fixation lines is the ANGLE OF DEVIATION or angle of squint.

Although only one eye deviates, heterotropia is a binocular disorder ; one eye is kept " straight " by the desire to see objects distinctly, the other eye bearing the deviation of the two.

If the angle of squint varies as fixation is shifted to different parts of the field, the heterotropia is *noncomitant* or paralytic.* The angle varies because the paralysed muscle or muscles interfere with the movements of the affected eye in certain directions. Many such subjects suffer from persistent diplopia, which increases in the direction of action of the paralysed muscle ; the false image may, however, be ignored when the paralysis has lasted some years, or even after a much shorter period in some cases. Paralytic squints, being due to local disturbances in the co-ordinating system,† and the accompanying muscle paralysis, usually require medical treatment.

We will confine our attention to *concomitant* heterotropia, in which the deviation remains constant in all directions of the gaze—for a given state of accommodation. When

---

* See §13.2. † §13.15.

heterotropia is referred to without further qualification the concomitant type is intended. Concomitant squint is due generally to a handicap or disorientation of the motor equilibrium situated above the motor nerve nuclei and so may be amenable to optical and educational treatment.

Although the deviating eye remains directed to a point in space removed from the object of attention fixed by the fixing eye, it does not follow that this object is seen in diplopia since the image formed in the squinting eye is almost invariably mentally suppressed. Vision is consequently monocular. If the deviation of the squinting eye and the suppression of its vision are allowed to persist, its vision gradually deteriorates, at a rate dependent upon the age of the subject, and the eye acquires amblyopia—*amblyopia ex anopsia.*

Not only is the subject deprived of binocular vision, but he is afflicted with the disfiguring appearance of a squint. Although we shall be continually referring to the whole condition in terms of the manifest squint accompanying it, yet it must be noted that the squint is but one of the symptoms of the condition.

As we shall see, squints usually arise in children, during the early period in which the fusion sense and binocular equilibrium are in process of development. Success in their treatment also largely depends upon commencing remedial measures while the subject is young. Hence many of the devices and tests to be described will be found to be simple in character, since they must be capable of attracting the interest and co-operation of children.

The deviations of the eyes met with in heterotropia are generally much greater than those found, when the eyes are passive, in heterophoria. Squints of 45° (100$\triangle$) are frequently encountered. Angles of these dimensions are better measured and expressed in degrees.

The terms heterotropia, strabismus and squint are all used to describe the condition we are discussing. By some authors the terms are used quite synonymously; others adopt the term heterotropia when referring to the concomitant condition and strabismus to the paralytic condition. To obviate a multiplicity of terms we will refer to the condition generally as heterotropia or squint, so that we may have either concomitant heterotropia or squint, or paralytic (noncomitant) heterotropia or squint. We will, nevertheless, incline to the use of the word heterotropia when referring to the condition and of the word squint when referring to the deviation of the eyes accompanying the condition.

HETEROTROPIA—CONCOMITANT

14.2. Classification according to Direction.

The classification and table of §13.3 may be applied to heterotropia as to heterophoria.

It is found that cyclotropia is so rare in practice that authors such as WORTH, who have devoted many years to the clinical study of motor imbalances, scarcely refer to the term, if at all. We are left, therefore, with :

ESOTROPIA or CONVERGENT SQUINT, in which the fixation lines deviate inwards :

EXOTROPIA or DIVERGENT SQUINT, in which the fixation lines deviate outwards :

R. Hypertropia or *R. Supravergent Squint*, in which the fixation line of the right eye deviates upwards :

L. Hypertropia or *L. Supravergent Squint*, in which the fixation line of the left eye deviates upwards.

The hypertropias by themselves are also comparatively rare. When they occur they are, in most instances, either not strictly concomitant but paralytic in character, or they are found as accompaniments of a horizontal tropia and usually react to the treatment accorded to the latter.

Although we must maintain an open mind as to the possibilities of hypertropia and cyclotropia occurring, and requiring further investigation as our knowledge of this difficult subject of squint progresses, we are practically limited at present to the consideration of the horizontal imbalances: esotropia (convergent squint) and exotropia (divergent squint), of which the former is by far the more common.

14.3. Classification according to Continuity.

Whatever the direction of the squint may be, whether convergent or divergent or otherwise, it may be further subdivided according as the one eye deviates constantly or as the deviation is transferred from one eye to the other alternately. Or it may be that the squint occurs only at intervals, separated by periods in which the eyes are orthophoric. From this point of view we may subdivide heterotropia into:

A. INTERMITTENT
  (1) *Occasional*; (2) *Premonitory* or *Incipient*

B. CONTINUOUS OR ESTABLISHED
  (1) Unilateral
  (2) Alternating: (*a*) *Essentially* or *True* Alternating
  (*b*) *Accidentally* Alternating.

A.1. *Occasional Heterotropia.*

This condition, in which the eyes occasionally deviate for a few seconds only, may be observed in normal infants during the first few months of life, frequently when the infant is disturbed by gastric or other troubles. The deviations are not usually constant either in direction or degree. They are fleeting in character and in many cases are merely examples of heterophoria. They gradually disappear as the fusion faculty develops, or with the correction of refractive errors.

A.2. *Premonitory or Incipient Heterotropia.*

This condition is more common than the occasional variety and the deviation usually persists for longer than a few seconds, recurring frequently in the same eye. It is the forerunner of continuous heterotropia, becoming established after a few months.

In this category might be included what is sometimes called *accommodative squint*, which appears only when the subject's attention is fixed and increases when the object of fixation approaches the eyes. Such occasional lapses are not noticed by the parents for some time as the child's head is usually inclined when looking at near objects such as toys, etc. The squint probably appears because the child is hyperopic; accommodation has to be excessive, and convergence acts in association. Gradually a new association is built up between accommodation and convergence; there is heterophoria for distance and squint at near. The subject may sometimes remain in this condition as he attains adult life; alternatively the condition progresses to continuous convergent squint in distance, as well as near, vision.*

* See also §13.15—Class 3B.

B.1. *Continuous Unilateral Heterotropia.*

Here the squint is constantly present and it is, as the name implies, always the same eye that deviates. The angle of deviation may vary from time to time, however. Thus in right unilateral convergent squint the left eye fixes and the right eye continuously turns inwards. When the fixing eye is screened the deviating eye turns to fix the object of attention, if it still possesses the power of central (macular) fixation; the previously fixing eye deviates by the same amount as that originally manifested by the (previously) deviating eye. When the cover is removed the squinting eye may continue to hold fixation for a little while, but most often it will turn at once to its original squinting position and the fixing eye will fix.

The deviation of the squinting eye when both eyes are uncovered is called the *primary deviation*; and that of the fixing eye when it is covered, the previously deviating eye now fixing with its true macula, is the *secondary deviation*. In concomitant heterotropias with which we are dealing the primary and secondary deviations are equal.*

B.2. *Alternating Heterotropia.*

As the name implies the deviation alternates from one eye to the other in this condition, the eyes being more or less equal in refraction and acuity. The subject fixes with either eye indifferently and does not give preference to either. At one moment the left eye fixes and the right eye deviates in (or out) by a certain amount; at another moment the right eye fixes and the left eye deviates in (or out) by the same amount. Alternating squinters are much less common than unilateral squinters, in the proportion of about 1 to 5 or 6 (WORTH). Two distinct classes of alternating cases are found:

B.2.(*a*) *Essentially Alternating.*

In some cases of alternating squint the two eyes are approximately the same (no anisometropia), there is little or no refractive error and the visual acuity is normal, or even better than normal, in both eyes. Nevertheless these people can never be made to see both pictures in a stereoscope simultaneously; for some reason it appears to be

* Except perhaps in a case of uncorrected anisometropia, in which the accommodation may vary according to which eye is called upon to fix.

impossible, or at least it is extremely difficult, to break down suppression in these subjects; at any rate with the means at present at our disposal. The term essentially alternating heterotropia has been applied to these cases and the view is generally held that they have a congenital inability to acquire fusion; and that consequently no treatment other than operation, aimed merely at removing the deformity and so improving the appearance of the subject, is possible. These so-called essentially alternating squints appear in early infancy and are rarely met with.

It may be, however, that this apparent absence of fusion ability is nothing more than a manifestation of a firmly established habit of suppression; and that these cases differ from accidentally alternating heterotropia (below) not in character but only in degree.

B.2.(*b*) *Accidentally Alternating.*

Here too the vision is good, usually about 6/6, and approximately equal in the two eyes. Otherwise these cases do not differ essentially from unilateral squints; if untreated they may develop into unilateral squints, the subject consciously or subconsciously forming the habit of fixing continuously with the one eye.

14.4. Characteristics of Concomitant Heterotropia.

Suppression of Vision.

In individuals with normal vision a deviation of one eye from the correct fixation position results in diplopia; and it is probable that diplopia exists in the earliest stages of heterotropia when the child is in its infancy. Diplopia is so disagreeable and confusing, however, that great efforts will be made to avoid it. The normal way to do this is to position the eyes by muscular action until they are both directed to the object of attention. If the oculomotor system and fusion powers are in proper condition, the child gradually learns to fix binocularly and to fuse the uniocular images into a single mental perception. If some condition is present, or arises, to interfere with this normal process of development, the attempts to direct the fixation lines correctly may be unsuccessful, in which case diplopia, or alternations between diplopia and single vision, are encountered by the subject. The subject seeks for a way to minimise the confusion and learns to *suppress* one of the two neural images. It is easier to do this when the retinal image in one eye is removed considerably from the macula, for in this position the image is much less distinct; and so one eye is allowed to deviate from the orthophoric position and a squint has developed. Henceforth vision is practically monocular.

In the presence of conditions unfavourable to the proper development of binocular vision, such mental suppression is often easily and quickly learned. Suppression is indeed practised regularly by normal individuals; in ordinary vision the images of innumerable objects formed on peripheral portions of the retina are mentally put on one side, as it were, during our examination of one particular object in the field; the microscopist, looking into his instrument with both eyes open, learns by experience to suppress the image in the eye not applied to the microscope. Some people appear to have more difficulty than others in suppressing, a fact that may have a bearing on the subsequent development of the individual's binocular vision.

In the case of a child whose developing heterotropia is unilateral, the suppression becomes a continuous process and the vision in the deviating eye rapidly deteriorates to amblyopia. If the tropia is alternating, the subject acquires the ability to suppress the image of either eye indiscriminately to a remarkable degree. In both the unilateral and the alternating cases binocular, and consequently stereoscopic, vision has been sacrificed for the comfort of monocular vision.

The suppression does not always extend over the whole field of vision of the deviating eye. Objects within the extreme temporal field (L or R, Fig. 12.1) can be seen, although they may not be accurately located; this is useful to the squinter in avoiding accidents and catching moving objects.

In individuals of the kind just described the powers of fusion have never properly developed. In others it is possible that the squint arises after binocular vision and fusion have developed in the normal manner, due to the incidence of some other condition which makes binocular vision impossible or uncomfortable. Such an individual possesses a developed power of fusion which in the meantime, has been inhibited.

Simultaneous vision and diplopia may be aroused, at least in cases of unilateral and accidentally alternating squint, and unless the amblyopia is too deep-seated, by presenting differently coloured objects to the eyes. This will be referred to later when discussing treatment.

Eye Movements.

In convergent squint the movements of the eyes considered separately are normal except that in a few cases of long standing there is a restriction of external rotation due probably to anatomical changes that take place in the muscles and check ligaments of the squinting eye following the development of the squint.

The conjugate movements of the eyes are also normal. A movement of the fixing eye is accompanied by an equal movement of the deviating eye, so that the angle between them remains constant over the entire binocular field—hence the term concomitant. (An exception to this may be found in cases of moderate and high degrees of myopia, when owing to the restriction of movement caused by the larger globes, movements in the periphery of the field may depart from concomitancy.)

The normal association between accommodation and convergence also holds. Thus there is no motor defect in concomitant convergent squint, but there is a constant " zero error ", the eyes commencing their excursions from an initial crossed position instead of from the orthophoric position of parallelism of the fixation lines.

In divergent squint the power of convergence is deficient and varies capriciously from time to time. There is only a feeble association between accommodation and convergence; a subject who can usually voluntarily correct the divergence of the squinting eye often allows this eye to diverge when he brings accommodation into operation for near vision. The movements of the eyes considered separately are usually normal except that inward rotation may be restricted in cases of long standing.

Variation of the Angle of Squint.

Nervous excitement, emotion and hysteria may increase a squint temporarily, the disorientation of the innervations in the oculo-motor system resulting in some motor centres being stimulated more than others. This is to be kept in mind during the measurement of a squint.*

---

* §14.8.

Amblyopia.

It is to be noted that the amblyopia referred to is a partial blindness that is not accompanied by anything abnormal in the media or fundus; the ophthalmoscope reveals nothing.

As already explained the deviating eye in unilateral squint becomes amblyopic; this is so in nearly all cases of unilateral *convergent* squint but not so frequently in divergent squint. It does not occur in alternating squint. In the amblyopic eye central vision deteriorates so far that some subjects can scarcely count fingers held close to the face. It is only the macular and near-macular region that is thus affected; there is no restriction of the peripheral field. The central scotoma extends further towards the blind spot than in the opposite direction; in extreme cases it may include a total extent of 25° to 30°, within which area there may be bare perception of light.

The younger the child is when the unilateral tropia develops the more rapidly is the amblyopia acquired. According to Worth amblyopia is seldom acquired to any extent after six years of age.

In a few cases of squint the amblyopia may be congenital. In these rare cases the acuity is usually higher than 6/18 and never lower than 6/60, which differentiates them from the amblyopia-ex-anopsia cases.

Abnormal Retinal Correspondence, or False Association.

Although the subject with concomitant heterotropia does not experience diplopia in everyday vision since the image in the deviating eye is suppressed, simultaneous vision and diplopia may be elicited by special means. Indeed simultaneous vision must be aroused during the course of treatment before further measures can be taken to assist the subject to attain binocular vision. The diplopia then experienced subjectively will often correspond, in magnitude and direction, to the deviation. A subject with, say, a convergent squint of 20°, will normally have homonymous diplopia in which the projection of the squinting eye, say the right eye, lies 20° to the right of the (true) projection of the left eye.

There are cases, however, in whom this normal correspondence between the two eyes has been upset. The point of the retina of the squinting eye which has habitually received the images of objects, or a region between this point and the fovea (albeit the images have been suppressed), seems to acquire* enhanced sensitivity during the time that the acuity of the fovea itself has deteriorated to amblyopia; and a false correspondence exists between the true fovea of the good eye and this extra-foveal region (false association area) of the deviating eye. This abnormal correspondence reveals itself in clinical practice in two main ways which we may call abnormal retinal correspondence:

(*a*) *with eccentric fixation*,
(*b*) *without eccentric fixation.*

It is only recently that the frequent occurrence of these conditions has come to be realised. When DUANE drew attention to them some years ago, referring to them as cases of *incongruous diplopia*, he considered them to be rare. It is found, however, that they occur, in different degrees of severity, in at least 50 per cent. of squinters of a few years' standing. It is too early yet to make definite statements as to their ætiology or to relate the condition to the magnitude of the deviation; as to the latter, conflicting views are held by practical workers in the field of squint. The condition probably depends upon the absoluteness of the concomitancy; on the ground that the more constant is the angle of deviation the more likely will be the acquisition of the habit of using a fixed area of the peripheral retina of the deviating eye for fixation. It may be noted that this condition of abnormal retinal correspondence does not arise in occasional or periodic squints.

(*a*) ECCENTRIC FIXATION.

Because it reveals itself easily in diagnosis, this condition has been familiar for some time. It can occur only in unilateral squinters. When the fixing eye is covered, the deviating eye takes up monocular fixation of the test object without moving. The image is received on that part of the retina which habitually receives the images of objects in everyday vision. This area of the retina has, in a way, usurped the functions of the true anatomical fovea; it was at one time customary to refer to it as a false macula. In monocular vision with this eye the subject projects always with reference to this eccentric area and not with reference to the true fovea.

---

* There are two views, (*a*) that it is innate; (*b*) that it is acquired. Whereas the second view is most favoured, the first warrants attention. The condition may perhaps be due to some anatomic defect and may even be considered as the cause of the squint in large angle cases. Most squints under 15° have normal correspondence.

Further, in circumstances when both eyes are in use, the subject has acquired the habit of associating the true fovea of the non-deviating eye with this eccentric area of the deviating eye. On being requested to superpose two slides in the synoptophore* he does so, and attains simultaneous vision, with the tubes set at zero, as would a non-squinter. This abnormal correspondence sometimes appears to be as strongly established as the normal correspondence between the two true foveæ in a normal person.

The larger the angle of squint, the less acute will be this eccentric area. It would be expected therefore that this condition of abnormal correspondence with eccentric fixation would be less likely to develop in cases with a large angle of squint; especially when this angle exceeds 25 degrees or so, for then the image on the retina will be diminished in intensity, if not completely prohibited, by the iris.

(b) Abnormal Correspondence without Eccentric Fixation.

These cases may be either unilateral or alternating. Monocular fixation, with the deviating eye as well as the fixing eye, is always taken up by the true fovea. If a test object be presented and the fixing eye then covered, the deviating eye will turn through the angle of squint to receive the image on the anatomical fovea. If a subject of this class, capable of simultaneous vision, is placed before a synoptophore with tubes set at the true angle of squint, so that the images are formed on both foveæ, he will see the slides *in diplopia.* (A squinter with no abnormality of correspondence would see them superimposed.) If now the subject is requested to set the tubes of the instrument until the pictures appear superimposed, he will reduce the angle between them to a value that varies in different cases, but is usually somewhat less than half the angle of squint. Moreover, there will be some hesitation in executing the setting; and the settings will vary in several attempts, as though in binocular vision the true fovea of the fixing eye may be used in association with any part of an appreciable area of the retina of the deviating eye extending from the place that habitually receives images to a position about midway between this and the true fovea.

---

* §13.11.

DUANE attempted an explanation of abnormal retinal correspondence. He supposed that some squinting individuals, although seeing with eyes open, do not project binocularly; that is, do not conceive the projections of the two foveæ as coincident or, alternatively, do not project from the binoculus. They make, or attempt to make, an allowance for the mis-direction of the visual axis of the squinting eye as they would in monocular vision, perhaps because they are overcoming part of the deviation by unconscious effort. In such cases the brain becomes imperfectly aware of the true direction of the deviating eye and the diplopia subjectively experienced is smaller than that corresponding to the deviation.

DUANE pointed out that monocular projection is of earlier phylogenetic development than binocular projection, which is founded upon the association between the two forward-looking eyes in convergence, for which movement the innervation is discharged equally to the two eyes; and that consequently incongruous diplopia represents a reversion to the primitive type of vision.

On an instrument of the synoptophore type a normal individual superimposes the two pictures (and fuses them if they are sufficiently alike) when the tubes are set at zero. As we have seen, a person with what we have called eccentric fixation does likewise, since he has acquired the habit of associating the true fovea of the fixing eye with the localised eccentric area of the other eye; and he fixes monocularly with this false area. It appears as if the quality of local sign has been transferred in these individuals from the true fovea as origin to the false eccentric area as origin. In cases of abnormal correspondence without eccentric fixation, such complete transference has not taken place. It appears as if there exists in the brain a state of rivalry between the true fovea and the false area as origin of local sign, the perceptual processes striking a mean between the two—a common phenomenon in psychological acts. The fact that the tubes of the synoptophore are set at various angles between zero and half the angle of squint would appear to illustrate varying degrees of preponderance of the false area over the true fovea.

It may be that in squinters who exhibit normal correspondence the fovea has become firmly established as origin before the squint developed.

14.5. The Power of Fusion.

It will be explained later (§14.12) that there is a stage in the investigation of a squint case, after certain initial obstacles have been overcome, when it is necessary to determine whether the subject possesses any power of fusion. This can usefully be done by means of the amblyoscope or synoptophore. At the stage of the squint investigation referred to, cases of abnormal correspondence have either been eliminated or corrected; the subject possesses simultaneous macular vision, grade A.1, and can see both slides of the pair illustrated in Fig. 14.1 at the same time with the tubes of the synoptophore set in a position corresponding to his angle of squint.

The image of the vertical line passes through the fovea in each eye.

It is necessary to take precautions to ensure that the subject really sees with both eyes. It will quite likely be necessary to illuminate the slide presented to the poorer

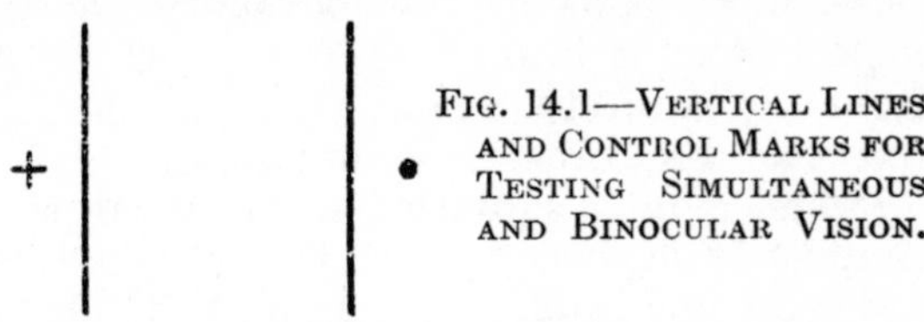

FIG. 14.1—VERTICAL LINES AND CONTROL MARKS FOR TESTING SIMULTANEOUS AND BINOCULAR VISION.

eye to a greater intensity than the other slide; means of varying the illumination intensities on the slides are provided in the instruments. The small cross and dot alongside the respective vertical lines are intended as control marks to verify simultaneous vision. The subject may see a single vertical line, not as the result of superposition of two retinal images, but because he is seeing with one eye only; but if he also sees the cross *and* the dot, this is evidence of simultaneous vision with both eyes.

There is still the possibility, however, that although the cross and dot are both seen, there is absence of simultaneous

FIG. 14.2—STEREOSCOPIC PAIR FOR TESTING STEREOSCOPIC VISION.

foveal vision, for the images of the cross and dot are formed on extra-foveal regions of the retinæ. It would be better to have, as control marks, short horizontal lines projecting out from the vertical lines themselves, to the left in the case of one vertical line and to the right in the other.

Assuming that simultaneous macular vision is established with the arms of the instrument in some position, if the singleness of the vertical line can be " held " by the subject while the arms are converged and diverged to some extent from this squint position, then the subject also possesses grade B (1) vision; for the singleness of the line could not be held unless the eyes, under the direction of an alert fusion sense, were following the movements of the tubes. If the single picture is broken up as soon as the tubes are moved from the subject's squint position, then fusion is, at least in the meantime, not functioning and grade B vision is absent. Many squinting subjects will show little, if any, amplitude of fusion in this test. And most will have no stereoscopic ability, i.e. grade C vision, and will be unable to see and describe correctly the stereoscopic relief in such stereoscopic pairs as those illustrated in Fig. 12.18 or Fig. 14.2.*

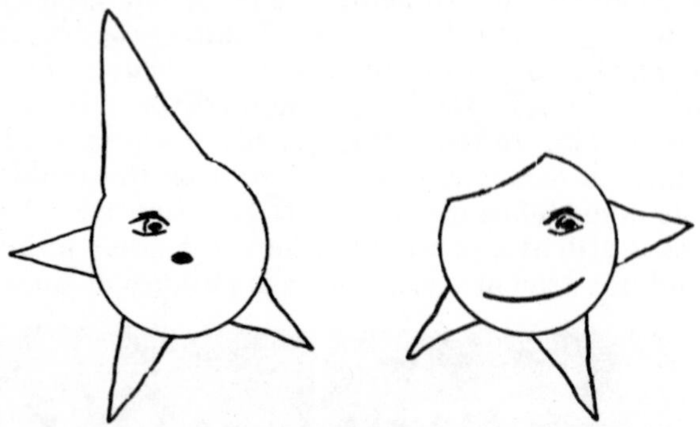

Fig. 14.3—Grade B slides for children.

More interesting slides will be required when testing young children. For the grade A test the slides may consist of a bird on one slide and a cage on the other; a rat and a trap; and so on. For grade B, slides such as Fig. 14.3 may be used; the picture seen by the subject is incomplete and confused unless fusion is in operation. The stereoscopic pairs may be such as fuse into a picture of a common object such as a ball, a bucket, etc. in which the stereoscopic effect will be extremely vivid when the slides are properly fused.

If, using the slides of Fig. 14.1, the vertical line is seen single, together with both control marks, when the tubes

* These slides are so made that the different objects, when fused, appear at varying distances. The subject is asked to name the objects in order according to their distances, as they appear to him.

of the instrument are parallel, then the subject possesses grade A (2) vision, the eyes being directed in the orthophoric position; and thus there is no squint. Hence the instrument might sometimes be used, instead of the cover and corneal images tests, for determining the existence of a squint and its magnitude.

BERRY's slides, Fig. 14.4, are useful when investigating, and attempting to stimulate,* the stereoscopic sense. On each slide the smaller inner circle can be given a lateral displacement within the outer circle. When the two inner circles are in the positions indicated in full lines the two slides are in a condition to be fused into a truncated cone with the narrower end appearing nearer than the base.

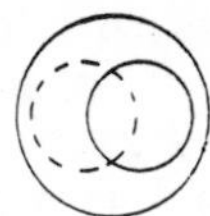

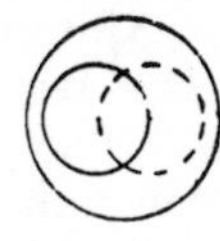

FIG. 14.4 — BERRY'S STEREOSCOPIC PAIR.

When they are moved to occupy the dotted positions the fused picture is changed to one giving the appearance of a hollow cone (or bucket) with the narrow end further away than the wide end. When the centres of the inner circles coincide with those of the larger circles the two slides are exactly similar and fuse simply into a flat picture of two concentric circles. The alteration in the appearance of depth thus obtainable is very useful when testing a subject's stereoscopic capabilities.

14.6. Other Tests for Simultaneous Vision.

The state of the subject as to simultaneous or binocular vision, whether absent or, if present, its grade, is most satisfactorily determined by the methods just described, or by means of the diploscope or separator.† Such methods would ordinarily be adopted when dealing with a subject known to be heterotropic. We will digress for a moment to notice one or two other methods of checking the presence or absence of simultaneous vision and binocular fixation in subjects generally. It is necessary to do this, for example, in all subjects when the distance and near refractive corrections have been determined, in order to decide whether to proceed to test for heterophoria or whether it

* §14.13. † §14.12–2 (ii).

is, or appears to be, a squint case. In anisometropic cases* it is specially important to check and, if necessary, further investigate the state of binocular vision. Although a subject may have exhibited good visual acuity in each eye separately, this does not establish that vision is binocular, nor even simultaneous. To prove conclusively that a person has simultaneous vision in the two eyes is not such a simple matter as might be imagined.

Innumerable tests for simultaneous vision have been proposed from time to time. Some of these, such as SNELLEN'S "FRIEND" test and WORTH'S "four dot" test, depend upon presenting red and green objects or letters to a subject provided with a red glass before one eye (say the right) and a green glass before the other.† According to the statement of the subject as to what he sees when both eyes look at the test object, it is decided whether both eyes are seeing. Thus in the FRIEND test, the letters F, I and N are green and R, E and D are red.

If the subject reads only RED, it is concluded that the left eye is not seeing; and that if the left eye only is seeing, the words FIN will be read; also that if both eyes see, the whole word FRIEND will be read. Such tests cannot always be accepted as conclusive, however. A person who does not see ordinary objects with both eyes may possibly use both eyes together when presented with the unusual combination of different colours to the two eyes. Such a test then may prove that both eyes *can be made* to see simultaneously, but not that they do so in ordinary circumstances. Also it is conceivable that this test might be passed by a person who is using the eyes alternately.

Another type of test consists in interposing between the subject's eyes and some printed matter held at, or about, the reading distance, an opaque obstacle such as a vertical ruler or pencil (*bar reading*). If the printed matter is read right across from left to right without hesitation, and without moving the head or the obstacle from side to side, it is concluded that vision is binocular, or at least that it is simultaneous. Great care must be exercised by the examiner to rule out the possibility of the subject using the eyes alternately, however. Carefully watching the subject's eyes during the reading, it would be difficult to detect a case of alternating squint with a not too appreciable angle

* Ch. XVI. † See §§ 13.11 and 13.13.

of deviation. The Bishop Harman *diaphragm test* is of this type.

The sudden interposition of a prism before one eye when the subject is reading the test chart with both eyes free, is another method sometimes employed. The principle is: a subject who is really using both eyes simultaneously in binocular vision (e.g. a heterophore), will be immediately confused by the diplopia that arises when a prism (say 4△) is suddenly introduced before one eye. If only one eye is seeing, nothing will happen if the prism is placed before the non-seeing eye; a displacement of the test object, but not diplopia, will take place if the prism is interposed before the seeing eye. This test can be taken as tolerably conclusive as to the existence of simultaneous and of binocular single vision when diplopia is elicited by the prism; although, here again, there is just a possibility of error. For the eye suddenly presented with the prism may be a non-seeing eye in ordinary circumstances but, when the image of an object is formed on an area of its retina not usually stimulated similarly to and simultaneously with the macula of the fellow eye, it may see; especially when the prism is placed with its base-apex line vertical.

Great care must be exercised by the examiner in the case of a subject who is *malingering*, i.e. pretending that one eye is blind, perhaps in order to claim compensation for accident, etc. It is necessary to employ tests such as the above in a manner calculated to confuse the subject. For example: if, when the prism is inserted before the supposedly blind eye, the other eye makes an associated movement, the former is a seeing eye.

DETECTION AND MEASUREMENT OF CONCOMITANT HETEROTROPIA

14.7. General Procedure.

The remarks under this and subsequent headings of this chapter will be brief. For details of procedure the student is referred to books on clinical practice.

In heterotropia one eye deviates. If the deviation be large, its presence and its convergent or divergent character will be apparent by simple inspection.

Although we do not have to employ means to dissociate the eyes, we have to determine the character of the squint;

whether concomitant or paralytic; and assuming a concomitant case, whether convergent or divergent, unilateral or alternating.

Certain tests can be employed to distinguish between paralytic and concomitant cases. At this stage we will assume that such tests have revealed the tropia to be concomitant.

To come to a decision as to the type of the concomitant squint and as to the best course of treatment to be followed; whether, for example, "squint training" is likely to prove successful, it is desirable to collect systematic information under the following headings concerning it:

1. History.
2. Central vision and refractive condition of each eye.
3. The character of the heterotropia and the power of fixation, including detection of abnormal correspondence, if any.
4. The movements of each eye.
5. Measurement of the angle of squint.

(2) Central Vision.

If the subject is old enough, the vision of each eye is tested on the ordinary letter chart and recorded. If the child is under school age a special chart containing pictures of animals and common objects, in various sizes, may be used. Still younger children, including those with amblyopia may be tested by means of Worth's *ivory balls*, or some similar test that is sufficiently interesting to engage the attention of children.

(3) Character of Squint and Power of Fixation.

If the magnitude of the squint is too small for its character to be determined by simple inspection, the following tests may be applied:

(*a*) *Exclusion or Cover Test.*

This provides only a rough indication and may be difficult to apply to young children. The subject's attention is directed towards a small object or light. When his gaze is fixed on it one eye, say the left, is *suddenly* covered with a card. If the other eye, the right eye, makes no movement it is probably fixing correctly. The test is repeated with the right eye covered, the left eye being closely observed for any signs of movement. If no movement is observed, the left eye is probably fixing correctly. If, on covering the right eye, the left makes a movement outwards to fix the object, it was previously squinting inwards; if its movement is inwards, it was previously deviated outwards.

There are three conditions in which there will be no movement of either eye: (*a*) binocular fixation that is quite normal—no squint; (*b*) a squint with eccentric fixation; (*c*) a squint with loss of the power of central fixation in the deviating eye.

In (*a*) the corneal reflexes (see below) will be symmetrically situated; in (*b*) and (*c*) they will be unsymmetrical. To distinguish between (*b*) and (*c*), we examine the movements of the deviating eye. In (*b*) the unsymmetrical position of the reflex in that eye remains unchanged, since the eye steadily follows the light; in (*c*) the following movements of the deviating eye are erratic and consequently the reflex position varies.

The difference between the interpretation in this cover test and the one described for detecting heterophoria* must be noted. In heterophoria, binocular fixation exists before covering, and it is the *covered* eye we observe for signs of movement.

In squints of high degree it can be determined whether they are unilateral or alternating. If, after covering the fixing eye for a few moments and then uncovering, the other eye continues to hold the fixation it has taken up, the squint is alternating. But if fixation is immediately transferred back to the originally fixing eye, it is unilateral.

The above observations can also be made using a near fixation object.

(*b*) *Corneal Reflex Test.*

In this method, due to PRIESTLEY SMITH, an ophthalmoscope is used to direct light into the subject's eyes from a distance of about one third of a metre. The subject is asked to fix the sighthole of the mirror. By rotating the mirror the light is reflected first into one eye and then the other in rapid succession. Through the sighthole the examiner views the corneal reflexes. If the subject is a normal orthophore, the corneal reflexes will be seen symmetrically disposed within the cornea as indicated in

* §13.7.

Fig. 14.5. They will be slightly to the nasal side of the pupil centre in the usual case possessing a positive angle α, but may be more central than indicated in the diagram if this angle is small. Lack of symmetry between the two reflexes indicates squint and it may be seen which is the deviating eye.

This test is more certain, especially for slight squints and in children, than the cover test. As the subject fixes the mirror sighthole, the visual axis of his seeing eye coincides with that of the examiner, and the small reflex spot marks out the point of the cornea traversed by the subject's visual axis.

By watching the corneal reflex in the deviating eye it can be observed whether this eye, after taking up fixation when the fixing eye is covered, maintains its fixation for

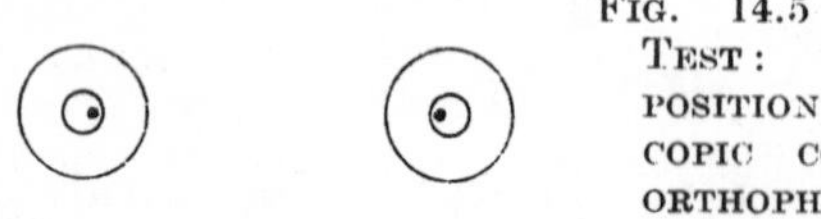

FIG. 14.5—CORNEAL REFLEX TEST: SYMMETRICAL DISPOSITION OF OPHTHALMOSCOPIC CORNEAL IMAGES IN ORTHOPHORIA.

some time when the fixing eye is uncovered. If this happens the squint is alternating; otherwise unilateral.

It is important in deciding upon the subsequent course of treatment to have some knowledge of the power of central fixation in the deviating eye. For this purpose, after noting the position occupied by the reflex in relation to the cornea of the fixing eye, this eye is covered and it is observed whether the deviating eye takes up fixation with precision and with the corneal reflex in corresponding position, in which case we have central fixation. There may be unsteadiness in the reflex indicating a wandering eye, or it may occupy an unsymmetrical position, indicating that fixation has been taken up by an extra-foveal part of the retina, i.e. abnormal correspondence.

If, after the above tests, it is found that there is no squint, but the subject possesses binocular fixation, the case will be examined for heterophoria as explained in the last chapter.

The Placido disc may be used in a similar manner to the ophthalmoscope above. If the subject be asked to fix binocularly the centre of the disc, the position of the reflected images of the rings relative to the pupil centres can be observed.

(4) SEPARATE EYE MOVEMENTS (Monocular Field of Fixation).

Knowledge of any limitations of the normal excursions of the eye in various directions, or of any irregularities in such movements, are of interest principally in determining whether the squint is concomitant or paralytic.

14.8. (5) **Measurement of the Angle of Squint** (Strabismometry).

HAPLOSCOPE METHOD.

If simultaneous vision can be elicited and the squinting eye possesses the power of central fixation, the most satisfactory way of measuring the deviation is by means of the amblyoscope or synoptophore as already described. With a pair of dissimilar objects in the instrument, the tubes are rotated until the subject sees the objects superimposed. The angle between the tubes then gives the deviation required. The examiner should see that the corneal reflex of the light from the tube in the squinting eye is symmetrical with that in the fixing eye, so as to ensure as well as can be, that the vision in the squinting eye is macular vision.

This method cannot be applied, however, to subjects in whom simultaneous vision cannot be elicited or to young children without sufficient intelligence to carry out the test. In these cases it is necessary to adopt some objective method depending upon the use of the cornea as a spherical reflector.

PERIMETER METHODS.

1. *JAVAL'S Procedure.* The subject is arranged so that his deviating eye D is accurately situated at the centre of the perimeter arc—Fig. 14.6 (a). Directly in front of D and 5 metres distant is a small light S, which is fixed by the fixing eye, F. A second small light E, such as the lamp of a luminous ophthalmoscope, is moved round the arc of the perimeter, the examiner keeping his eye just behind this light. When the reflected image of E appears to lie in the centre of the cornea of the deviating eye, the angle ODE is read off. The line DE is practically the *optical* axis* of the deviating eye; were it fixing the same

* §10.3.

object S as the fixing eye, its *visual* axis would lie along DOS. Thus the indicated angle ODE includes the angle of squint and the angle alpha* ; a positive angle alpha is to be added to ODE.

The angle alpha need not be considered at all if the position E is found, not by arranging that the reflex in the deviating eye is central, but in a similar position to that occupied by the reflex of S in the fixing eye. This position of the reflex in the fixing eye could be determined by observing that eye along the direction SF before making the measurement.

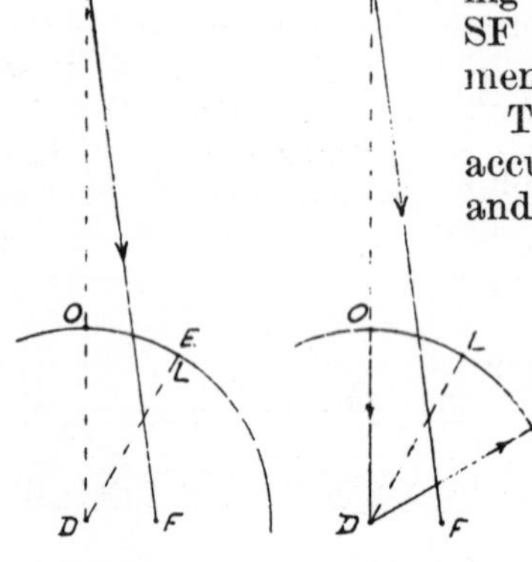

(a) JAVAL. (b) CHARPENTIER.

FIG. 14.6—MEASUREMENT OF ANGLE OF SQUINT WITH PERIMETER.

This method is reasonably accurate, but it takes some time and also has the disadvantage that when the angle of squint is small, the examiner's head and the second light E obstruct the subject's view of the distant source S, particularly in convergent squints. This difficulty is to some extent overcome in the following manner.

2. *CHARPENTIER'S Procedure.* The second light is kept stationary over the zero fixation spot, O, of the perimeter, the subject regarding the distant source S with his fixing eye as before. The examiner moves round the arc until he arrives at a position E in which the reflex of O occupies the centre of the cornea of the squinting eye —Fig. 14.6 (b). It is then assumed, from the fact that the angles of incidence and reflection are equal, that the deviation is half of the indicated angle ODE, allowance being made, as before, for the angle alpha. The angle of squint ODL has been drawn equal in the two diagrams.

There is a source of error in this method.† The corneal reflex will be situated rather less than 4 mm. behind the anterior corneal surface and on the line joining the source O and the centre of curvature of the cornea. It will therefore lie a little behind the apparent plane of the iris. If the examiner moves to a position in which the image

* For measurement of angle alpha, see §10.3. † See also §10.3.

occupies the centre of the iris, as is probable, the angle read off will be more than twice the angle of squint. Moreover, if the squint is appreciable, the reflection at the corneal surface is oblique and the image will not lie at the paraxial image point but at a point of the caustic surface removed eccentrically therefrom—producing another source of error.

Sometimes a perimeter is not available in which case a "tangent scale" method may be employed; one of these will be briefly described.

THE TANGENT STRABISMOMETER (MADDOX).

The subject is placed facing a tangent scale at a distance of one metre. The examiner places his head in the space between the subject and the tangent scale and a little below a small light at the zero of the scale. He views the reflection of the light in the subject's deviating eye. The subject is requested to fix successively the numbers on the tangent scale until the corneal reflex in the squinting eye is seen in the centre of the cornea.* The scale number fixed by the fixing eye then gives the angle of squint—in prism dioptres if the divisions are one centimetre apart. If the tangent scale already available for testing heterophoria is used,† with divisions 6 cm. apart for use at 6 metres, the number must be multiplied by six to give the deviation in prism dioptres.

CONCOMITANT HETEROTROPIA—CAUSES AND TREATMENT

14.9. Analysis of Causes.

Mainly because of the disfiguring squint that accompanies it, the condition of heterotropia has attracted attention from the earliest times. Many curious suggestions have been made as to its cause and various methods, such as the wearing of an opaque "gnomon" or septum between the eyes, horn spectacles with central perforations, etc., proposed for its treatment. Occluding of the good eye in order to force the squinting eye to function was proposed as early as 1743 by BUFFON, thus providing a first step in rational treatment.

---

* When the angle a is already known, the experienced practitioner can make allowance for it, and so obtain a reading of the deviation uninfluenced by the angle a, by obtaining the reflex, not in the centre, but to one side of the centre by an amount representing the angle alpha. This applies also to the other methods described.

† §13.10.

A period in which squint was attributed entirely to defects in the muscles themselves, particularly to a shortening of the medial recti, the treatment consisting correspondingly in cutting the muscles, terminated when A von Graefe (*ca.* 1857) turned his attention to the investigation of motor imbalance.

Following Boehm, who discovered (1845) a frequent association between convergent squint and hyperopia, Donders developed his theory (1864) that heterotropia depends upon refractive and accommodative anomalies. Convergent squint is so frequently found in hyperopes and divergent squint in myopes that Donders considered these tendencies to be the main *cause* of heterotropia. The view is strengthened by the fact that convergent squint usually makes its appearance between the ages of two and six when the child is beginning to use accommodation more than before, for picture books, etc.; and that the condition tends to diminish with age, as does the amplitude of accommodation ;* and by the fact that one class of divergent squint appears first at about ten or twelve years of age, and tends to increase with age—myopia also being, not a congenital condition, but one that develops during the growing period.

There is little doubt that ametropia plays a large part in the ætiology of unilateral squints and the ametropia should always be carefully tested and considered.

On the other hand some cases of heterotropia are not associated with ametropia; there are subjects with convergent squint and myopia, and others with divergent squint and hyperopia. Further, most ametropes do not develop squint at all. Hence, although refractive errors are undoubtedly predisposing causes, and Donders performed a great service in demonstrating their effects, at a time of much confusion of thought on this subject, they are not the sole factors in the causation of heterotropia. Valuable work on the problem was later carried out by Javal.

Heredity also plays its part; in over 1,300 cases of convergent squint, Worth found a history of squint, in parent, grandparent, brother or sister of the subject, in 50 per cent. of the cases.

Unilateral esotropia or convergent squint and accidentally alternating squint are the most common varieties. Divergent

---

* Consider, however, §6.2, in which the view is expressed that the physiological accommodative *effort* does not diminish.

squint is much less common than convergent and, from the point of view of its ætiology, may be divided into two main classes: *myopic* and *essential*. The former type is associated definitely with myopia, but refractive errors do not constitute a predisposing factor in the latter type.

Thus the older muscular theory as to the origin of squint has been entirely superseded by the view that the defect is generally in the central nervous system. Further proof of this is supplied by the fact that in practically all cases of concomitant convergent squint, for example, the deviation disappears under general anæsthetic.

WORTH maintained that the essential cause of squint is a defect of the fusion impulse; and that in the presence of this fundamental cause the eyes, being in a state of unstable equilibrium, will develop a squint if some other predisposing anomaly, such as refractive error, anisometropia heredity, etc., exists at the same time.

The analysis of §13.15 led to a somewhat similar view, that squint arises from defective functioning of the fusion powers. This, in turn, may originate in various ways. Some ocular inequality or defect of reception or other condition may have existed or have arisen during childhood, which interfered with the normal development of binocular vision and fusion; (4B) of §13.15. The train of events leading to such mal-development of fusion may be started suddenly by some illness such as whooping cough, or by fright or convulsions; or by the resultant lowering of the general health during the period of development of binocular vision. In most cases the subject completely recovers from the illness and regains normal health so that his powers of fusion, although perhaps in a backward state, are nevertheless capable of full development by appropriate educational treatment. With some individuals, however, the recovery is incomplete in that there remains a permanent obscure derangement of fusion, which is apparently not capable of improvement by educational measures.

The defective fusion may, on the other hand, be the result of an adaptative process (4C) aimed purposely at suppressing fusion because of discomfort arising in binocular vision from some other cause, the suppression having been carried out below the conscious level. Or again, it may be due to arrested development of the binocular character of the visual apparatus before birth (4B), leaving the eyes to a greater or less extent independent of one another;

in which case, when the individual character of each eye is marked, an essentially alternating squint is likely, the eyes doing the work alternately.

Thus, on the one hand we may have a fusion sense which has never developed, either because of congenital defects, maybe inherited, or defects appearing in infancy; and on the other hand a developed fusion sense purposely put out of action or suspended.

TREATMENT

14.10. Introductory.

The ideal to be aimed at in the treatment of heterotropia is to correct the deformity of the squint and also to restore binocular and stereoscopic vision. This ideal is by no means always achieved. Following on the suggestion by BUFFON to occlude the good eye, ocular exercises of a kind were practised in squint cases during the latter half of the eighteenth century; but in the absence of reliable knowledge as to the nature of the complaint they appear to have been unsuccessful, and neglected. Interest was revived by GRAEFE and the investigations continued by many ophthalmologists anxious to relieve this troublesome malady. Amongst these may be noted DONDERS and especially JAVAL, who laid the foundations of the course of treatment that is being attempted to-day. MADDOX and WORTH were also especially active in this sphere of work.

The methods about to be described are to be looked upon as the best of which we are capable in the existing state of our knowledge. The present is a period of much activity in the treatment of squint and practical clinical information is continuously accumulating. The data have not yet been systematically analysed and related to the classification of possible causes however. There is little doubt that when this has been done by competent investigators and when the significance of the subconscious and conscious acts of perception are more clearly understood, a more rational system of treatment will be evolved. Meanwhile our present methods are largely empirical and sometimes rather crude.

Unless the squint is congenital, it appears during childhood when the binocular functions are in process of development and remedial measures are far more likely to be successful if *commenced* during this early period than if postponed to a later date, when the sense of fusion has lain dormant and, in the case of unilateral squints, amblyopia ex anopsia has progressed considerably in the squinting eye. It is therefore of the utmost importance to take active preliminary steps as soon as the squint has been noticed. In those cases where it is found to be necessary to carry out the full treatment in the attempt to secure complete restoration of binocular vision, the later steps are usually best undertaken when the subject is somewhat older, say between the ages of ten to twenty years. If he is too young, it will be difficult to secure his co-operation in performing the tests and exercises that have to be imposed. But we must at least arrest the further progress of the amblyopia or the habit of suppression while he is still young. If possible we should go further and improve the vision of the squinting eye and, maybe, attain simultaneous macular vision. Then later, when the time is opportune, the treatment is to be continued in the endeavour to make both eyes work together and so awaken and train the fusion sense, without which binocular vision is impossible. Continuing the treatment we must attempt to strengthen the fusion powers and the oculo-motor system until the eyes can achieve binocular fixation without discomfort in any part of the common binocular field.

The treatment is to be undertaken only if the subject's general health is satisfactory. It consists of two main stages. The first might be described as an exploratory or selective stage, largely concerned in getting rid of obstacles that stand in the way of fusion so that we can decide whether to proceed, and if so, in what manner. This is the stage to be undertaken as soon as possible in infancy. It can be divided into three steps. Sometimes it is found that the obstacles are too serious to be overcome or at least not likely to be surmountable except after a prolonged and tedious treatment, which may be impracticable.

In the second stage, which could reasonably be called the fusion training stage, we attempt to " straighten " the eyes and assist the subject to develop or re-awaken his powers of fusion and stereoscopic sense and to hold these in all parts of the field.

The general sequence of the steps of the treatment may be set down as follows. The scheme applies generally to unilateral and alternating squinters, both convergent and divergent. Each will receive separate mention as occasion requires.

FIRST STAGE.

1. Correction of refractive errors and treatment of abnormal retinal correspondence, if any.
2. Establishment of simultaneous vision.
   (i) Removal of amblyopia—unilateral cases.
   (ii) Breaking down of suppression—alternating cases.

   These steps to be followed, if the amblyopia or suppression respond to treatment, by
3. Establishment of simultaneous macular vision, grade A.1, and examination of the power of fusion.

   If grade A.1 vision is attained within a reasonably short period and if the fusion power is satisfactory (see later) we proceed to the

SECOND STAGE.

4. Development of fusion—grade B.1.
5. Elimination of the deviation—grade B.2.
6. Training of the stereoscopic sense—grade C.
7. Version and vergence exercises ; to assist in maintaining the resultant binocular vision throughout the whole field.

In heterophoria, exercises are designed to stimulate the verging powers of the oculo-motor system and so assist an already active fusion sense to retain binocular vision without undue strain. In heterotropia, on the other hand, we have first to re-awaken, as it were, a fusion sense which has been out of action for a period and which was perhaps never properly developed.

There is some conflict of opinion concerning the order of the fourth and fifth steps in the above sequence. By some it is maintained that, after simultaneous vision has been elicited (step 3), the eyes should be straightened (step 5) before setting out to encourage the development of fusion (step 4).

14.11. First Stage of Treatment.

PRELIMINARY SELECTION OF CASES.

As already remarked, many squint cases are found to be unresponsive to educative orthoptic treatment, at least in the present state of our knowledge. It is not, however, until certain steps have been taken that the inability to respond becomes evident; and some cases can be decided upon earlier than others. Consequently the process of selection of cases suitable for orthoptic treatment is a continuous one; "acceptances" and "rejections" occur at each step of the treatment. And in those cases which survive the first few steps, we cannot usually decide whether they are likely to be responsive until the subject has acquired simultaneous macular vision.

Experience shows that congenital and hereditary squint cases are rarely responsive to treatment and are usually eliminated at this stage.

It is assumed that we know the character of the squint (whether unilateral or alternating, etc.), the angle of deviation, the central vision of the deviating eye and whether there has developed an abnormal retinal correspondence or eccentric fixation.

Some degree of false association occurs in quite an appreciable proportion of squint cases and it is an extremely troublesome condition to deal with. It is found that existing technique is in practically all cases inadequate to break down a well-established eccentric fixation (which occurs only in unilateral squints) and such cases are usually eliminated from the list of those who are to be submitted to orthoptic treatment. Surgical operation is sometimes tried, but this has to be carefully considered since it brings difficulties in its train. A suspicion is growing that cases of marked eccentric fixation gradually revert to eccentric fixation again after the operation.

Other cases of false association, however, in which a marked eccentric fixation is not present, are frequently found amenable to certain orthoptic measures, which will be described later, as a result of which the abnormal retinal correspondence can be replaced by normal correspondence between the two anatomical fovea.

We have now eliminated cases of hereditary squint and established eccentric fixation and are left with

squinters, both unilateral and alternating, with normal retinal correspondence,

squinters with abnormal retinal correspondence (*b*),

squinters with eccentric fixation not too pronounced,

and we are now in a position to discuss the first stage of

the treatment to which these accepted categories will be submitted.

14.12. First Stage of Treatment.

(1). CORRECTION OF ABNORMAL CORRESPONDENCE AND REFRACTIVE ERRORS.

Whether the heterotropia is unilateral or alternating, the refractive correction is carefully determined. In convergent cases the determination may be made under atropine in order to estimate the optimum amount of positive addition that we should attempt to apply during the treatment.

First we will consider the cases in which abnormal correspondence has been discovered. If the squint is unilateral, the refractive correction is prescribed for use before the fixing eye only ; it seems logical in such cases to refrain from improving the quality of the retinal image on the falsely associating area of the deviating eye, and so no correction is provided for that eye at this stage. Moreover, during the first few weeks of the attack on false association, the deviating eye should be occluded.

If the squint is alternating, the full refractive correction is to be worn constantly. There is here no question of eccentric fixation, either eye being capable of fixing correctly. During the first few weeks an occluder should be worn for one week at a time before each eye alternately.

Whether unilateral or alternating, the subject should attend the clinic as frequently as possible during the first two weeks or so of the occlusion period in order to undergo certain forms of training now to be described. It is to be understood that the suggested exercises are but in the experimental stage and may quite likely be modified as further experience accumulates. They have nevertheless proved successful in breaking down the abnormal correspondence in the majority of cases.

Three variations of the procedure may be tried, in each of which an instrument of the synoptophore type is employed. Firstly : conspicuous slides are inserted in the instrument ; e.g. one slide may consist of a circle in red and the other of a prominent blue square the internal width of which just exceeds the diameter of the circle. The synoptophore tubes are set at the true angle of squint, the setting being checked by observing the subject's corneal reflexes.* The subject with abnormal correspondence will now see the slides in diplopia. With the tubes clamped in this position the illumination of the slides is switched off and on, first from one slide and then the other in rapid alternation. After a few periods of such treatment, each occupying a few minutes, it is sometimes found that the diplopia begins to decrease.

Secondly: a unilateral squinter is requested to fix one slide with his fixing eye; the tube containing this slide is clamped. While the subject steadily fixes this stationary picture, the other tube is rapidly rotated back and forth over a range of two or three degrees so that the retinal image of this picture moves onto and off the anatomical macula of the deviating eye. This exercise is continued until the subject has arrived in the condition in which he sees the pictures superimposed when the tubes are set at his angle of squint. In the case of an alternator the left tube of the instrument is clamped at one sitting and the right tube at the next sitting; and so on alternately.

Thirdly: the synoptophore tubes are set at the angle of squint and clamped in this position so that they can be made to execute version movements. The subject observes the slides, which he sees in diplopia. The tubes are then slowly moved together (version) back and forth over a range of 10 degrees or so. It is frequently found that, although with the tubes stationary the subject experiences diplopia, this disappears and the slides are seen superimposed during version movements of the tubes.

Any or all of the above three variants are tried until the subject sees the two pictures superimposed with the instrument set at his angle of squint. It may be found advantageous to use slides of the " moving picture " type, as these are more effective than stationary objects in overcoming suppression. These are slides which, by means of an extra mechanism that can be fitted to the synoptophore, present pictures in which some object or objects are given in a continuous movement across the field of view. For example: the picture may present a number of fish swimming in a glass bowl. It is suppression of the image formed on the true anatomical fovea of the deviating eye that the above exercises are intended to overcome. If, as suggested above, the subject is seen frequently,

*§14.8.

signs that the abnormal correspondence is giving way to treatment should be in evidence during the first fortnight or so.

A unilateral squinter will not be provided with the refractive correction for his deviating eye until the false association has been broken down.

Assuming the above step of the treatment has been successfully carried out, we are now concerned only with cases, unilateral and alternating, in whom normal retinal correspondence exists. We have now to remove the amblyopia of the deviating eye in unilaterals and eliminate the suppression of the non-fixing eye in alternators.

(2) (i). Removal of Amblyopia (Unilateral Squint).

The necessity has already been mentioned for taking immediate steps to retard or remove amblyopia in the deviating eye of a child as soon as the squint has been noticed.* He should be kept under supervision until the time arrives when he is sufficiently intelligent to perform the exercises necessary to secure restoration of binocular vision.

Binocular vision may be encouraged in young children who are just changing from occasional to unilateral squinters by modifying the spherical portion of their refractive correction in such a way as to assist binocular fixation during near vision. For example: in divergent squinters a -1 D sphere, and in convergent squinters a $+2$ D sphere, may be added to the proper distance correction so that in near vision accommodation, and hence convergence, is stimulated in the divergent case and inhibited in the convergent case.

The child should not be allowed to remove the spectacles at any time during the day. With young children it may be necessary to tie them on. In some cases, where amblyopia has not seriously developed, the wearing of the correction is sufficient to remove the squint and provide binocular vision.

Steps are now taken to force the child to use the squinting eye in the hope that vision will be thereby restored. The good eye is completely and continuously occluded for one month, perhaps two months. For this purpose there are various kinds of occluders ranging from pads and wads

---

* §14.10.

of cotton wool to others which are better in fit and appearance. If there is no appreciable improvement in the vision of the squinting eye at the end of this period it is unlikely that further treatment will be successful and the case should be given over (at a later date) to operative treatment, so that the subject's appearance, at least, may be improved.

If, however, after the period of complete occlusion, the vision of the deviating eye shows improvement, or if vision is not below 6/36 or so on the first examination, further steps may be taken.

Medical practitioners frequently subject the child to a period of atropinisation of the good eye. When atropine is instilled into the good eye, which is emmetropic or corrected by glasses, distance vision with this eye may be somewhat blurred but near vision is impossible, since there is no accommodation. All near work must therefore be carried out with the squinting eye alone. This treatment, the atropine being instilled daily, is said to be continued for several months as long as any improvement in vision is observed at the monthly examinations.

Alternatively, partial occlusion of the good eye may be tried. This may be practised by using a total occluder for half the child's waking hours, or perhaps better, since this procedure may be neglected at home, by using some method of partial occlusion. There is, for example, a type of occluder which allows vision of the temporal field only, in the good eye. It consists of a piece of *Chavasse* glass, fixed behind the refractive correction of the better eye, and extending from the nasal side of the eyewire to the temporal corneal margin. A small rubber pad is also affixed so that no vision is possible between the frame and the nose. The Chavasse glass reduces central vision in the good eye to about 6/60. Thus whereas both eyes enjoy temporal vision, vision in all other parts of the field is denied to the good eye. The subject can thus move about comfortably, but is coerced into placing more reliance on the squinting eye. The occluder leaves the eye visible and is not unsightly.

Partial occlusion of the sound eye may also be practised by the subject at home by providing him with a special reading book in which some of the letters of the words are printed in black and others in a certain chosen colour. The sound eye is provided with a filter of the same colour, to be fixed to the spectacles. In this manner the whole of the subject matter of the book is free to be read by the amblyopic eye and only the black letters are visible to the good eye. The child cannot read the stories in the book except by using the amblyopic eye. The stories must be simple and interesting but not too familiar to the child or there is a danger of his reciting the gaps printed in colour from memory. The subject will not be able to use this reading book until there is a certain degree of useful vision in the amblyopic eye.

In order to raise the vision of the squinting eye to 6/18 and secure steady central fixation with it, at which stage (and not before) the next step in treatment may be undertaken, it may be necessary to continue the above-described processes for a long time, perhaps throughout the whole course of early childhood. Constant supervision is necessary, particularly to see that the deviation and amblyopia are not transferred to the better eye.

In the case of an older subject, a decision as to whether the case is to be proceeded with has to be made after a much shorter period. Generally, the steps taken to remove the amblyopia should produce some effect in four weeks or so or the case is not likely to progress.

As the vision in the squinting eye approaches equality to that of the good eye, the squint may become alternating, either eye being used for fixation.

During this attack on amblyopia it is a good plan to employ the cheiroscope (Fig. 14.8) at the sessions in the clinic and to supply a Pigeon-Cantonnet stereoscope (Fig. 14.7) for drawing exercises at home; the two halves HJ and HK lying flat and the partition HM vertical. The use of these instruments helps to develop correct binocular fixation and fusion by employing the hand and eye in combination. A brightly coloured picture is inserted in one side of the instrument, to be viewed by the squinting eye, and the subject is required to draw the picture on a piece of paper inserted on the other side of the instrument, the pencil he is using being observed and guided by the good eye. These instruments will be described subsequently.

(2) (ii). Breaking Down of Suppression (Alternating Squint).

The alternating squinter has to be made aware of the simultaneous existence of impressions from *two* eyes;

the image in the squinting eye has to be forced on his attention at the same time as the good eye is being used.

Slides of the bird and cage type (provided with suitable control marks to ensure that the vision is not merely alternating) may be used in the amblyoscope or similar device, for young children. The child wears his refractive correction ; the tubes of the instrument are set to correspond to the angle of squint and the intensity of illumination of the slide presented to the squinting eye is increased until this object is seen simultaneously with the other. In older subjects, unless signs of simultaneous macular vision (grade A.1) show within one or two weeks, success in the subsequent steps is unlikely, at least within a reasonable period.

The modern tendency is to stress the psychological aspect of the act of fusion and to take all possible steps, correspondingly to enlist the active mental co-operation of the subject. At first, unusual objects are presented to the subject, one to each eye, a septum* or " separator " restricting the view of each eye to its own object. The object for the squinting eye is brighter than that for the good eye, or of a strikingly bright colour. The good eye fixing steadily some ordinary object such as a copper coin, for example, the brightly coloured object is introduced into the field of the deviating eye and moved about, particularly from peripheral regions towards the macular region. The idea underlying this procedure is that strange combinations such as objects of different colours are less likely to be suppressed than similar objects. The coloured object may be a complicated coloured pattern capable of continuous movement as in the kaleidoscope.†

Sometimes the object presented to the squinting eye can be seen simultaneously with that presented to the good eye, but only when it is imaged on an extra-macular region of the squinting eye ; when moved inwards or outwards until its image falls on the fovea, the image is suppressed and, to the subject, the object disappears. There is simultaneous vision but not simultaneous *macular* vision. By variations of illumination and colour and by moving the object about in the neighbourhood of the foveal

---

* §12.5.

† Instruments have been produced to present this revolving coloured panorama to the squinting eye.

projection, simultaneous macular vision must be secured before proceeding to the next step.

As the subject gradually learns to attain simultaneous macular vision, the objects presented to the poorer eye are successively reduced in vividness and size. The objects may be introduced to the subject by means of a stereoscopic appliance such as the amblyoscope or synoptophore. The exercises are to be continued daily at home, for which purpose some comparatively inexpensive instrument such as the PIGEON-CANTONNET stereoscope may be serviceable. This consists essentially (Fig. 14.7) of two sheets of cardboard HJ and HK hinged together at H like the covers of a book and supported by a joining strip so that the angle between them is 135°. A third sheet midway between them carries a plane mirror M. A normal individual will view an object A″ directly with, say, the right eye and an object A′ by reflection at M with the left eye, the distances HA′ and HA″ being equal. The projections of the objects will be superposed at A″. If the objects are a stereoscopic pair, they will be seen as a single solid object at A″. A squinting person who possesses simultaneous macular vision and fixing A″ with the right eye will require the object A′ to be shifted in order that the two projections shall be superposed; the shift will be towards K in convergent squint. Thus scales with their zeros at A′ and A″ will serve to measure the angle of a squint and enable its progressive diminution with treatment to be followed. (To enable the moving object on the half sheet HK to be kept "square-on" to the corresponding object at A″, the sheet HK should be provided with some kind of guide rail.)

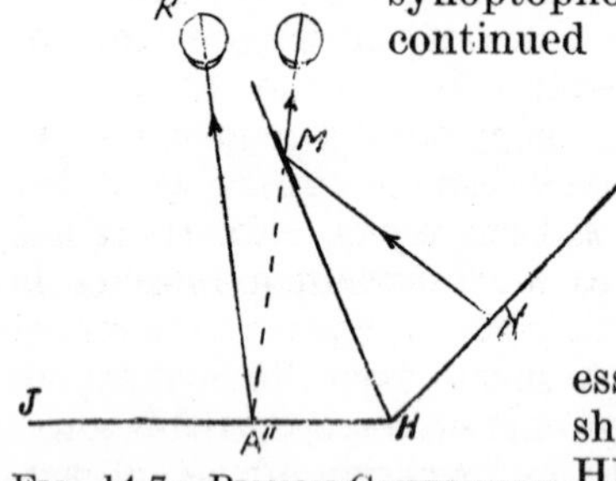

FIG. 14.7—PIGEON-CANTONNET STEREOSCOPE.

For the purpose at present under review, the eliciting of simultaneous vision, the instrument can be arranged with the two planes of cardboard lying horizontal and the intermediate partition HM vertical, the latter then merely acting as a septum or separator.

If persevered with, the process just outlined often proves successful in attaining simultaneous vision. It is persisted in until the subject can obtain such vision *at will* with ordinary objects.

In many cases of alternating squint it is found that the attack on suppression is assisted by covering, for alternate weeks, first one eye and then the other with a Chavasse glass occluder; to be worn at all times except when the above exercises are undertaken. In some cases this device is all that is required to break down suppression. It obviates the necessity on the part of the subject for continuing the habit of suppression.

When this step (2) has been successfully negotiated, the subject sees with both eyes simultaneously, but not necessarily with the *foveæ* of both eyes. It frequently happens that the two pictures in a stereoscope device are seen simultaneously, and in diplopia, so long as the images are not formed on the foveæ; but when the pictures are moved to correspond with the angle of squint, both images then falling on the foveæ, one or the other of the pictures disappears. In these cases simultaneous vision can be held except at the foveæ. The difficulty is central, in the brain.

(3). Establishment of Simultaneous Macular Vision and Examination of Power of Fusion.

The task now is to encourage simultaneous vision when the images are on the two foveæ. The procedure just described for eliminating suppression is continued in alternators and commenced in unilaterals until simultaneous *macular* vision is achieved in all cases. This can be checked on the synoptophore provided with slides of the type of Fig. 14.3 and with the tubes set at the angle of squint; it is observed that the two corneal reflexes are symmetrically disposed.

Up to this stage we have obtained no information concerning the fusion powers of the subject. The fact that he can see an object with both foveæ simultaneously does not necessarily mean that he is fusing the two uniocular impressions into a single mental percept. Some of the subjects who have survived the selective processes already described may now quickly acquire the power of fusion and be made to enjoy full binocular and stereoscopic vision. Others, who may have worked their way to this stage of simultaneous macular vision with reasonable despatch, are now found incapable of further progress.

And in others again, the progress is so slow and perhaps capricious, that to continue treatment is hardly a practicable proposition.

When the subject's fusion power is tested, in the manner described in §14.5, it is found that the cases fall broadly into the following groups :

(*a*) good fusion ability immediately and some stereopsis ;

(*b*) poor fusion at first, developing slowly during the first few visits for fusion training (see below) ; possibly rudiments of stereopsis ;

(*c*) subjects who attain simultaneous macular vision so long as the test objects are dissimilar, but who experience a confusing type of rivalry when two similar objects are presented. Neither image is suppressed but the fused percept bears little or no resemblance to the objects and may be an unrecognisable jumble ;

(*d*) subjects with no power of fusion and in whom no evidence of it appears after six visits or so.

It may be that as our knowledge of this subject of heterotropia progresses we may be able to relate such groups, as found in clinical practice, with the three tentative conditions of the fusion sense that emerged from the argument of §14.9 ; and still further, to the analysis of §13.15. Systematic comparison of this kind would provide better knowledge of the causation of the different groups, such as the above, that are encountered in practice ; and should lead to improved methods of treatment.

It may be tentatively suggested that group (*a*) includes cases where the onset of squint occurred in later childhood, ages 5 to 7 ; and those in whom a developed fusion sense was purposely inhibited. Possibly some form of psychological treatment will be found advantageous for the latter. Perhaps in group (*b*) the check in the development of fusion occurred earlier in life, due to illness. And in groups (*c*) and (*d*) may be found those individuals in whom the fusion sense did not develop due to congenital or inherited defects in the binocular apparatus.

Meanwhile, only cases of groups (*a*) and (*b*) are selected to proceed to the second stage of the treatment. Many of those in group (*a*) will require very little further attention.

14.13. Second Stage of Treatment.

The subjects we have selected to proceed to this stage of squint treatment, or orthoptic training, possess simultaneous macular vision and have given some evidence of fusion, but one eye still deviates. It is our purpose now to assist in strengthening the power of fusion and stereoscopic vision and to eliminate the deviation.

The processes described in step (2) (ii) for eliminating suppression in alternators are continued, on the synoptophore in the clinic and the Pigeon-Cantonnet stereoscope at home, using slides or objects of the type of Fig. 14.3. The subject is encouraged to see the pictures as a complete whole and to hold it so while one object is laterally displaced, as by moving the tubes of the synoptophore through small angles. In this way grade B.1 vision, under the special conditions as to illumination or vividness of the test objects, should be attained in two or three weeks—step (4).

The amplitude of movement (breadth of fusion*) of the slides or pictures is increased until the deviation is gradually reduced and binocular vision, grade B.2, obtained—step (5). It is claimed by some practitioners that the elimination of the deviation is expedited by encouraging a process of auto-suggestion in the subject, requiring him to make a strong " mental effort " concerning the distance of the test object. For example, in a case of convergent squint, the two pictures in the synoptophore, or diploscope or other device, are arranged so that the subject sees them in uncrossed diplopia. He is required to imagine them fused into a single picture situated very far away. It is claimed that if the subject can be made to concentrate on this suggestion of distance, the diplopia diminishes, the visual axes diverge and so the deviation is often rapidly lessened.

To encourage the subject to hold binocular vision in all parts of the field, exercises (step 7), aimed at stimulating the version and vergence movements of the eyes should be carried out at this stage, or after the next (stereoscopic) stage. Instruments, such as the kinetic stereoscope of MADDOX, are available for moving the two objects, set at any required stage of convergence, in all directions over the field. They may be employed in the clinic or at home.

The exercises are continued, now using objects or slides that are stereoscopic pairs (Figs. 14.2 and 14.4 illustrate the type and there is a large variety of such pairs available), and encouraging the subject to appreciate the sense of relief and solidity in the fused impression (step 6). If, up to this stage, it has been necessary to keep the object

---

* §5.5.

presented to the squinting eye more brightly illuminated than the other object, the intensity is now gradually equalised, the exercises being continued until ordinary pairs, of equal intensity, can be fused and seen in relief with the tubes of the stereoscope moved about over a considerable range on all sides of the orthophoric position. The subject then possesses stereoscopic vision—grade C.

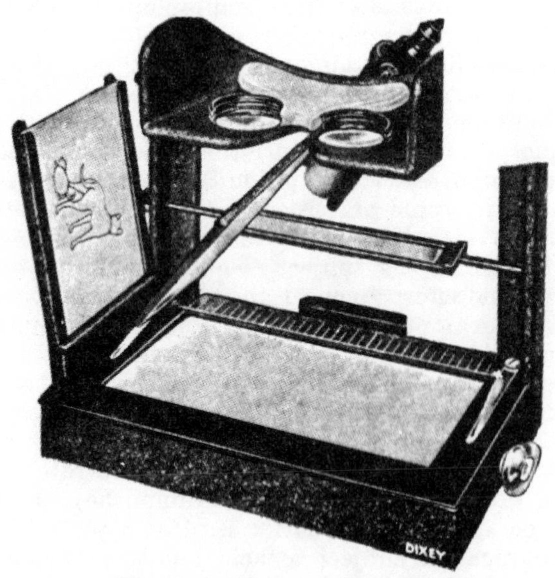

FIG. 14.8—MADDOX CHEIROSCOPE.

The exercises described may be supplemented at home by bar reading.* Another appliance deserving of mention, and preferred to other instruments by some practitioners, is the cheiroscope, introduced by MADDOX in 1928. This instrument is designed to employ the hand of the squinter to educate his squinting eye, imitating the natural process of infancy in which the hand and eye mutually perfect their training by trial and error. Briefly, one eye is allowed to see a certain object or picture and the other eye a pointer or pencil, which is moved about under the guidance of this eye to touch or draw the projection due to the first eye.* Thus, in Fig. 14.8, a picture inserted in the frame

* §14.6.

on the left is seen with the left eye by reflection at the inclined plane mirror. The right eye sees only the horizontal platform on which can be laid a sheet of paper. The subject traces on this paper the outline of the picture, the pencil being seen only by the right eye. Various modifications of the instrument are possible; the septum can be placed vertically and objects of interest to young children moved about with the hand on one side of the septum so as to appear to coincide with, or run after, corresponding objects in the other field of view. The relative illumination of the two sides can be varied.

14.14. Further Remarks on Treatment.

With some individuals the treatment described results in the elimination of the deviation and in the complete acquisition of stereoscopic vision, not only during the training periods, but also at all times during their everyday work. In other cases the subject still experiences difficulty in obtaining binocular vision when away from the training instruments; or there may even be some hesitation in decreasing his deviation below 5 or 6 prism dioptres or so. It may then be advisable to prescribe relieving prisms for constant wear, so that binocular vision is exercised throughout each day. As binocular vision becomes more firmly established, the prisms can be reduced in stages until binocular vision is comfortably achieved without prism aid.

Useful additional exercises may also be provided in such cases by the use of the series of stereoscopic cards designed by Dr. HEGG on the lines suggested earlier by JAVAL. These cards are to be viewed by the subject in a hand stereoscope. The series contains stereoscopic pairs of graded separations and graded depths of relief, intended to encourage stereoscopic vision in easy stages.

If these measures prove unsuccessful in completely eliminating the deviation, surgical operation may be decided upon. If orthoptic treatment is taken in hand as soon after the operation as practicable, binocular vision may be achieved, making the cure functional as well as cosmetic. It is not often that favourable results are achieved by treatment of post-operative cases, however; particularly if a period of more than a year of inactivity intervenes after the operation.

EXERCISES. CHAPTER XIV.

1. Describe the differences between the condition heterophoria and heterotropia.

Define the terms: fixing eye, deviating eye, angle of squint, amblyopia ex anopsia.

2. Define the terms: concomitant heterotropia and paralytic heterotropia.

Describe the differences between the two conditions in relation to (*a*) their subjective symptoms; (*b*) their cause; (*c*) the manner of determining which condition is present in a given case.

3. Give a classification of heterotropia according to the direction of the relative deviation of the eyes from the fixation position. Comment briefly on the relative frequency with which the different types in your table occur in practice.

Taking the type you consider the most common, give one good method of detecting its presence.

4. Define: concomitant, convergent, divergent, alternating and intermittent strabismus; perspective, fusion, secondary deviation. (B.O.A.)

5. Give a complete list of the varieties of heterotropia which may be classified under the heading "concomitant". Explain carefully the significance of each of the relevant words or terms that may be used in naming a given condition of heterotropia.

6. In a case of paralytic strabismus, why does the angle of squint vary with different directions of the gaze? How is it possible to distinguish between cases of paralytic and concomitant squint?

7. Describe briefly the following classes of concomitant heterotropia or squint: (A) intermittent: (1) occasional and (2) premonitory or incipient; (B) continuous or established: (1) unilateral and (2) alternating.

What will be the relationship between the primary deviation and the secondary deviation in L. convergent concomitant squint?

8. Explain what is meant by "suppression" of one of the two uniocular neural images. Give one or two examples of suppression as carried out in ordinary vision by normal people. Give a brief general account of its onset during the development of a squint and describe its association with amblyopia.

9. Give a brief account of amblyopia as acquired in conditions of heterotropia. In what varieties of heterotropia is amblyopia not encountered? When present what is its usual retinal extent?

10. Write a short account of the monocular and conjugate movements of the eyes in (*a*) convergent squint and (*b*) divergent squint.

It is sometimes found, when diplopia is by special means elicited in cases of heterotropia, that the diplopia is "incongruous". Explain the meaning of this term.

11. Explain how the presence of a squint and its variety may be determined (*a*) by the cover or exclusion test; (*b*) by the corneal reflex test. Briefly compare these two tests.

12. Explain carefully how to distinguish between conditions of orthophoria, heterophoria and heterotropia by means of occlusion or cover tests.

In what circumstances may these tests fail to indicate the actual condition ?

13. State the ocular movements that are concerned with obtaining and maintaining binocular single vision. Describe tests, connected with these movements, that it may be necessary to make in the course of an examination of the eyes and explain the significance of each of these tests.

14. How can you distinguish between a concomitant and paralytic strabismus by means of corneal images when using the ophthalmoscope or retinoscope ? What other points can be investigated by means of corneal reflected images ? What special precautions are necessary when making investigations with this method ? (B.O.A.)

15. Explain fully how to differentiate between heterotropia and heterophoria. What points are to be noted in investigating each of these conditions ?

16. What is meant by false macula ? In what condition is it found ? (S.M.C. Hons.)

17. What type of diplopia would be present in a case of divergent strabismus ? Distinguish between the primary and secondary deviations and explain why, in cases of paralytic strabismus, the secondary exceeds the primary deviation.

18. On looking straight forward the eyes of a person appear to be parallel, yet he is suffering from heterophoria or paralytic strabismus. Differentiate between these two conditions and enumerate the differences between them. Then state what tests you would apply to come to a definite decision of the condition. (S.M.C.)

19. Enumerate and classify the different grades of simultaneous macular vision. Explain how to determine, by means of the amblyoscope or the synoptophore, which grade a given subject possesses. In some cases such instruments could not be used for this purpose until certain preliminary steps have been taken. Explain this and state what these steps are.

20. Explain how the condition of the fusion sense of a subject may be determined by means of a stereoscope device such as the amblyoscope or synoptophore. Give diagrams of the slides that may be used, making clear how each pair of slides enables a conclusion to be drawn.

21. Describe three tests that are intended to determine whether a subject possesses binocular vision. Explain carefully just what conclusions can be drawn from each of the tests and state in what circumstances they may be unreliable.

22. What is stereoscopic vision ? Is it the same as binocular vision ? Explain exactly how you would prove that a person possessed true binocular and stereoscopic vision. (B.O.A.)

23. Describe carefully a reliable method for determining the angle of squint when the subject (*a*) possesses simultaneous macular vision; (*b*) does not possess simultaneous vision. In the latter case make quite clear how the angle of squint is determined from the observations made.

24. In making a rough determination of the angle of squint by Hirschberg's method, using a small light or ophthalmoscope lamp at 30 cm. as the fixation object, the deviation of the squinting eye is assessed at 40° to 45° when the corneal reflex is observed at the edge of the

cornea. With the aid of a diagram establish this approximate relationship; and find the angle of deviation when the reflex is observed 2 mm. from the pupil centre.

What account, if any, has to be made of the angle alpha ?

Describe briefly a more accurate method of measuring the angle of squint.

25. With the aid of a careful diagram, explain how to measure the angle of deviation, in a case of squint, by means of the perimeter. Explain any disadvantages or reasons for inaccuracy in the method you describe. Show clearly how the angle of deviation is obtained from the observations made.

26. Describe two methods of using the perimeter in order to measure the angle of deviation in a squint case. Give a careful diagram illustrating each method and state any disadvantages or cause of inaccuracy in each.

What is the significance, if any, of the angle alpha in measurements of this kind ?

27. Describe two pieces of apparatus by means of which a measure of the angle of deviation of a squinting eye is obtained, the principle in each case being that the subject observes with the fixing eye an object moved along some kind of tangent scale whilst the corneal reflection, in the squnting eye, of à light at the zero of the scale is observed.

Give a diagram in each case and explain clearly how the deviation is obtained from the observations made.

28. A person with right unilateral convergent squint is tested with a device of the type of the Priestley Smith tape. If the tape from subject's eye to ophthalmoscope is 60 cm. long and the corneal reflex in the right eye appears centrally in the pupil when the fixation object is 40 cm. from the ophthalmoscope; and if the angle alpha in the deviating eye is 4°, positive, find the angle of squint.

Outline briefly the further information you would require to obtain concerning the condition before deciding upon a course of treatment.

29. Describe carefully how to measure the angle of primary deviation in a case of R. exotropia. Explain why, in cases of paralytic squint, the primary and secondary deviations differ in degree.

30. Describe the theory advanced by Donders as to the refractive causation of heterotropia. Enumerate facts of observation that support the theory and others that are in opposition to it. Briefly compare with it the view that is held generally at present regarding the ætiology of heterotropia.

31. State the basic requirements for binocular vision; hence give a classification of the possible causes of heterotropia based upon the violation of these requirements. What appears to be the main general difference between the causation of heterotropia and of heterophoria ?

32. Give a classification of the varieties of heterotropia and also a classification of the possible causes. State the symptoms that may result from the condition.

33. Describe the instruments and the methods you would use in testing for the following: 'phorias, ductions, fusion, stereopsis, angle of squint. (B.O.A. Hons.)

34. Discuss the ætiology of convergent squint and the methods of investigating such a case. (S.M.C. Hons.)

35. Trace in detail the connection between hypermetropia and convergent strabismus and mention the remedial measures which should be adopted. (S.M.C. Hons.)

36. Explain carefully what is meant by L. convergent concomitant strabismus. Briefly outline the conditions which may predispose to or cause this type of strabismus.

37. Give an account of the possible causes of concomitant convergent strabismus. At what age does this condition usually commence and in what respects are the eyes and vision affected by it ?

38. Give an outline of the steps, in order, to be taken in treating a child, say four years old, with unilateral esotropia. Give a brief description of the purpose of each step and of any apparatus you suggest should be used.

39. What indications, in the case of an adult subject whose refraction you have determined, would prompt you to commence an investigation as to the presence of heterotropia ? How would you differentiate between heterotropia and heterophoria ? And how, assuming heterotropia is found, would you determine its variety and degree ? In what circumstances might non-operative treatment be useful and what, briefly, would such treatment consist of ?

40. Describe the steps that constitute what is described as fusion training or orthoptic exercises. In what variety or varieties of heterotropia is the training likely to be beneficial ? And what previous steps should have been taken ?

41. Describe, with a sketch of its construction, the cheiroscope of Maddox, the principles underlying its use and the kind of case in which its employment may be of benefit.

42. Enumerate the methods employed for the treatment of amblyopia in cases of unilateral convergent squint. State if, and how, it is possible to select cases which may be expected to benefit by treatment; and describe carefully the method of treatment that you would use.

43. State all you know about the usual treatment for convergent strabismus; indicate which cases are amenable to optical treatment and those in which an operation is necessary. What are the usual causes of divergent strabismus and what is the most successful treatment ? In what cases of strabismus can a favourable prognosis be given ? (B.O.A.)

44. Describe an instrument suitable for stereoscopic exercises and say when such exercises are likely to be of benefit. (B.O.A. Hons.)

45. How may glasses be used as an aid to correct squint in young children ? (B.O.A. Hons.)

46. Under what conditions would you consider it justifiable to order prismatic glasses ? Explain the principles on which they act. How would you prescribe them ? (S.M.C. Hons.)

47. Give a brief outline of methods which may be adopted in the non-operative treatment of convergent concomitant strabismus in a child seven years old. (S.M.C. Hons.)

48. What are the main objects and purposes involved in orthoptic training? Especially, what are the fundamental principles concerned in orthoptic training of phoria muscular imbalances? State the most reliable methods used in orthoptic treatment at the present time. (B.O.A.)

49. Give an account of the treatment to be accorded to a case of alternating esotropia. Explain the differences between this condition and unilateral esotropia. Would your remarks apply to cases of essentially alternating esotropia?

50. In what ways can a stereoscope be made use of by a sight-testing optician? (B.O.A.)

BINOCULAR VISION AND ITS ANOMALIES

CHAPTER XV

ANOMALIES OF SPACE PERCEPTION

15.1. Perception of Space.*

WE are born with a specialised retina and the quality of retinal local sign, giving us the faculty of localising objects in space. This is seen in the ability of the child, who can fix a light almost immediately after birth and in the immediate sense of direction of people born blind when their sight is restored later in life ; and it finds its counterpart in the chick, which pecks accurately at food immediately on emerging from the egg. It appears probable that retinal correspondence and the habits or reflex processes responsible for fusion of two monocular sensations and the power of the depth perception, are built up gradually by experience and integration in the higher levels of the brain during the first years of life. An essential physiological factor in our perception of depth is the presentation to the brain of slightly dissimilar impressions from the two eyes. It seems probable, however, that the factor of retinal disparity is always supplemented by, and sometimes dominated by, psychological factors. Changes of attention can quite easily shift the plane of an object. The appreciation of depth at distances beyond the few yards which is customary is the result of a gradual co-ordination of visual and muscular sensations, building up factors of experience. A marksman estimates a distance with fair accuracy by basing his judgment upon his experience of target distances : a cricketer uses his experience of distances learned on the cricket field and of the muscular effort required to throw a ball. When these factors of experience are eliminated our estimates of distance are fluctuating and sometimes quite poor, as in attempting, for example, to localise a flash of light in a dark room. Perception, that is the recognition and interpretation of the scene before us, results from the fusion of present stimuli from the two

* The student should revise §§1.4 (C) (D), 1.8, 1.13, 2.5, 2.6, 12.4, 12.6 12.17 and 12.19.

eyes with our memory of previous experiences and the sublimation of these into a single percept in the mind. How this is accomplished we do not know; it is presumably beyond the power of our minds to analyse since we do not possess faculties on a higher level with which to perform the analysis. What *is* mind and where is it located?

There is support for the view, from SHERRINGTON for example,* that the central nervous system on the one hand and the mind on the other play largely independent rôles. On this view the former is just a mechanism. It possesses certain capabilities, some of which are innate in the species and others are acquired during childhood and later experience; it reacts automatically to a given external set of conditions in a manner determined by these characteristics, being incapable of itself of reacting in any other way. In this manner are the subconscious and habitual acts of the body carried out. The mind, associated in some way with the central nervous system, may and frequently does, intervene, however. According as the attention of the mind is dispersed or is focused on this or that aspect of the scene, or on some external circumstances, so will the percept and the response of the individual vary. Thus a given scene may evoke different concepts and different experimental results in the same individual. The seemingly capricious results and "glimpsing" encountered at times by all experimenters are possibly due in some cases to uncontrollable waverings in attention.

Of the several monocular and binocular factors upon which our judgment of spatial relationship of objects is based, probably the two most important are perspective (monocular) and retinal correspondence or binocular parallax. Subsidiary factors are parallax, size, light and shade, colour, aerial perspective, and convergence of the eyes. It is possible, too, that the movements of the eyes as the gaze is shifted from one object to another in the field of view, or the estimation by the mind as the attention roams over the scene of the muscular efforts that would be needed to execute such movements, are also potent factors in our spatial estimation—a view that was strongly urged by STEVENS. The interpretation of a given scene will depend on the relative predominance of perspective features, colour, contrast, etc., in the scene itself and upon

* SHERRINGTON, C. S. 1940. *Man on His Nature* (Cambridge: The University Press).

the visual mechanism and the mind of the observer at the moment. Those visual characteristics of the observer that are acquired are learnt as a child during the early years of development; the normal sequence of learning is subject to variations as between one individual and another, due to illness and other causes. Hence some characteristics may be under- or over-developed and there may be, in consequence, antagonism between them. This may be smoothed out in ordinary vision, when all the factors are in normal operation, producing a certain spatial percept; but when the individual is confronted with unusual visual tasks his percept of the scene may be distorted. The task may be unusual in that some of the factors normally present (perspective in particular) are denied to him or factors are introduced in a confusing manner, as in some well-known optical illusions.*

Much less is generally known about these distortions or anomalies of space perception than about oculo-motor imbalance. It is a branch of the subject of binocular vision in which occur phenomena for which there is as yet no adequate explanation. It is likely that useful experience has been gained during the late war in connection with the examination and training of air pilots and users of binocular instruments of various kinds, but analyses of such information are not yet available. Meanwhile some simple examples of spatial anomalies and considerations bearing on them are described in the following sections, the matter of which has been largely taken from a paper by the author to the Physical Society, London.†

15.2. Effect of Size Lenses on Stereoscopy.

The term size lens, or iseikonic lens, has been applied to those lenses the form and thickness of which are modified in order to vary the size of the retinal image without affecting the refractive correction of the eye.‡

In particular a size lens is a thick bent lens of zero power, its surfaces being usually curved in the same sense (Fig. 15.1) so that it is, in effect, a Galilean telescope of very small magnifying power. If the back surface has power F_2 dioptres and assuming a refractive index of 1·50, a

---

* §§ 23.7 and 23.8.

† "Some Notes on Space Perception": *Proc. Phys. Soc.*, LVI, p. 293, 1944.

‡ §§ 15.6 and 10.19.

zero power size lens of thickness t mm. magnifies $tF_2/15$ per cent; i.e. with a back surface of power $-6 \cdot 0$ D the magnification is 2 per cent for 5 mm. thickness, 4 per cent for 10 mm. and so on.

If a person with perfect oculo-motor balance and space perception observes binocularly two isolated objects A and B (Fig. 15.2) lying in a horizontal plane through the eyes in a homogeneous field, A and B being placed so that they appear to lie in a frontal plane as indicated, then if a size lens be interposed before, say, the left eye, the object A on the left will appear to move backwards to some point C; i.e. the plane containing the mental projections of A and B is tilted about a vertical axis through an angle ϕ.

Before the interposition of the size lens the length AB subtends equal angles w at the eyes, the retinal images $a'b'$ and $a''b''$ are equal (assuming equal eyes) and the

FIG. 15.1—SIZE OR ISEIKONIC LENS.

physiological impressions $\alpha'\beta'$ and $\alpha''\beta''$ conveyed to the brain for fusion may be termed "equal". Out of these, which we may call cortical images, and the acquired experience of the individual, the final single mental percept is built up. The size lens increases the angle w under which the pencils from A and B enter the left eye, $a'b'$ is increased to $b'c'$ and the brain has to fuse the enlarged cortical image $\beta'\gamma'$ with the original $\alpha''\beta''$, as it would if presented with two objects C and B not lying in a frontal plane. The result is that A and B, which appear to be in a frontal plane in unaided vision, now appear to lie in or near the tilted plane CB.

If the fused perceptual image formed in consciousness were immediately *derived* from the retinal images and determined by their relative sizes, we might expect to be able to calculate the amount of stereoscopic effect or tilt ϕ caused by a size lens of given magnification from the geometry of figure 15.2. Experiment shows, however, that the tilt of field is not generally in accordance with such calculation. Psychological factors, arising probably from the unusual nature of the visual task and variations of attention, appear to falsify the retinal proportionality in forming the final mental image. Moreover, the amount of tilt obtained experimentally depends upon the nature of the scene AB; the tilt obtained when A and B are two isolated objects will not in general agree with the tilt that results when AB is a broken or continuous horizontal line.

However, there *is* some tilt of the field with all observers, provided that A and B are seen in a homogeneous field

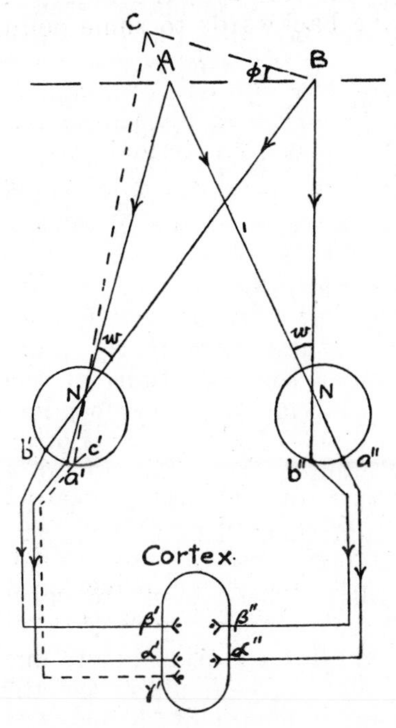

Fig. 15.2—Tilt of Frontal Plane AB through an Angle ϕ to an Apparent Projection Plane BC due to inequality in retinal or cortical images (Aniseikonia) or due to interposition of a size lens before left eye.

and the observation is not complicated by the presence of other factors such as perspective, etc.

If the objects A and B lie one *vertically* above the other in a frontal plane, the increase in the vertical dimension of the left retinal image produced by the size lens will not introduce any tilt of the field, but will make the binocular observation of the two objects uncomfortable. It is known that for any two objects to appear at different distances one of them must be seen in diplopia in a direction parallel to the interocular base line when the other is fixated and seen singly ; their parallactic angles must differ from one another. The size lens does not produce this condition when A and B are separated vertically ; it produces a diplopia of either A or B, depending on which one is being fixated at the given moment, in a *vertical* direction.

15.3. Distortion of the Frontal Plane in Stereoscopic Vision.

In a common laboratory experiment for determining the acuity of stereoscopic vision, two equal vertical rods or needles,* laterally separated, are viewed binocularly through an aperture so that their supports are invisible and they appear isolated in a homogeneous field. One rod, say the right, remains fixed in position and the other can be moved by the observer, with the help of a cord-and-pulley device, until it appears to lie at the same distance, i.e. in the same frontal plane, as the fixed rod. The precision with which this setting can be made is a measure of the observer's stereoscopic acuity. With a number of observers, it is found that not only do they vary in stereoscopic acuity, but some persistently place the left movable rod further away than the right, whereas others persistently place it nearer. In other words, under the conditions of the experiment in which the monocular factors of perspective, etc., are absent, the observer's plane of projection is often found to be tilted in one direction or the other about a vertical axis. The amount of this tilt is a function of the lateral separation of the rods and their distance from the observer. With knitting needles separated by 10 cm. and viewed at 4 metres, the tilt has been found to vary, for different observers, from zero to about $\pm$ 25°.

In the case of all observers, the interposition before one eye of a size lens magnifying one per cent alters the tilt of the frontal plane by an average amount of 15° or so at 4 metres. This figure is subject to wide variations, even with the same observer.

If experiments of the above type are continued, using as objects two equal black spots in a homogeneous white field, nothing else being visible, then when the spots are arranged with a horizontal separation, many observers show a tilt of the plane of projection, in one direction or the other about a vertical axis. And when the spots are arranged vertically one above the other, the observer's

* §12.22.

plane of projection will often be tilted about a horizontal axis, leaning so that the upper portion of this plane is towards or away from the observer. The author, for example, when set the task of placing the two spots so that they appear to him to be at the same distance away, lying one vertically above the other in a frontal plane, persistently places the upper spot farther away than the lower spot.

A size lens placed before one eye modifies the horizontal tilt but has no effect on the vertical tilt.

The above results are obtained from observations carried out in free space. For a given observer, tilts of the field in just the same sense are obtained when similar objects are viewed in a stereoscopic device such as a binocular measuring instrument, though the magnitudes of the effects are not generally the same as in free space.

It thus appears that when the eyes are given the unusual task of judging the relative positions of objects in space by using the stereoscopic sense only, factors of perspective, etc., being absent, one's impression of space is quite likely to be distorted in one direction or another. It would be

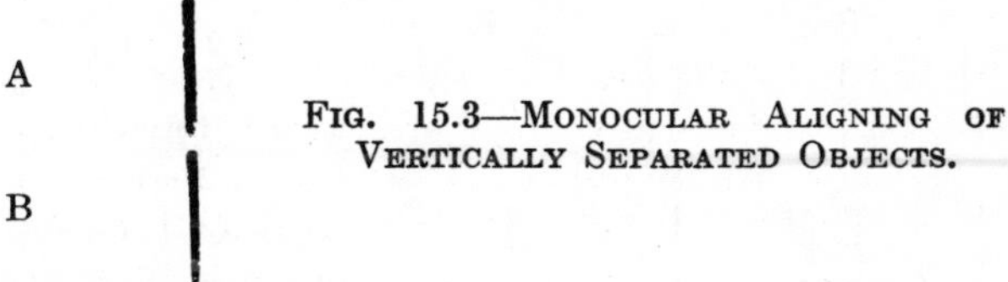

Fig. 15.3—Monocular Aligning of Vertically Separated Objects.

interesting to investigate whether this distortion is fixed for the individual or whether it can be modified by training or experience.

It should be remarked that the consistency of binocular observations of this kind is not very high ; individual settings may have a wide spread, due partly to the difficulty of maintaining the required degree of mental concentration and interest.

15.4. Monocular Aligning of Vertically Separated Objects.

Two black lines A and B of equal width are mounted vertically with a gap between their extremities, as indicated in Fig. 15.3, and are viewed monocularly against a white background. The line B is fixed and line A can be traversed horizontally, right and left by the observer : by using a scale and vernier the position of A can be determined to 0·01 mm.

With his head fixed in a head-rest the observer views the lines with one eye and traverses line A laterally until it appears to be directly above line B; its position is read off by a second observer; the mean of ten settings is taken. The settings are repeated for the other eye, the

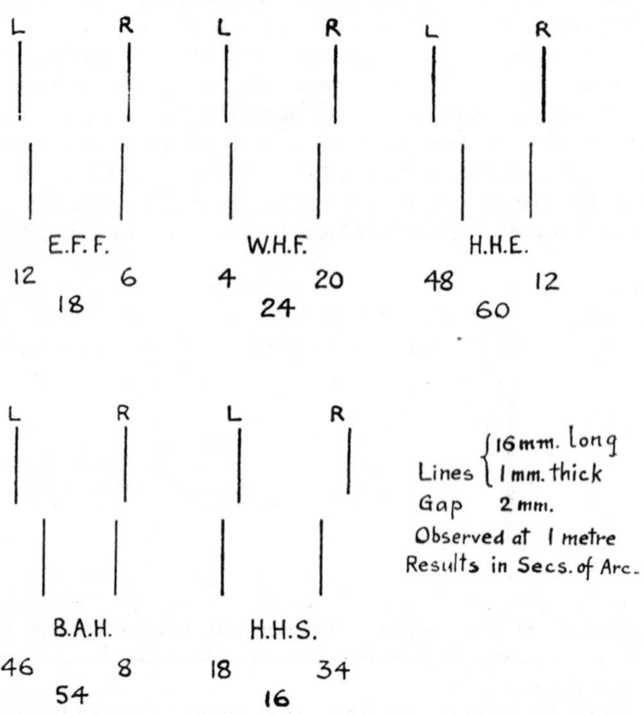

FIG. 15.4—MONOCULAR ALIGNING OF SEPARATED VERTICAL LINES. Actual positions when they appear in true vertical alignment.

head-rest being shifted sideways so that the second eye occupies the position previously occupied by the first. Figure 15.4 shows the results obtained for each eye with five observers. Each observer placed the upper line in the position indicated, and then pronounced them to be in vertical alignment.

This is an interesting phenomenon but no explanation of its bearing on the stereoscopic performance of the five observers has been forthcoming except that the fifth observer, H. H. S., who in this test is seen to have a bias in a sense different from the other observers, was also found to exhibit marked spatial distortion and at times peculiar hesitations in certain binocular experiments.

Similar results were obtained when the vertical lines were replaced by spots of length equal to their width.

The phenomenon would be expected to have some relation to the difference between the true and apparent vertical meridians of the retina described in §12.4.

15.5. Unequal Illumination of Stereograms.

Experience with stereoscopic instruments shows that if two stereograms are presented to the eyes so that they fuse in the usual way into a single projection in depth, then the stereoscopic sense of depth remains when the illumination

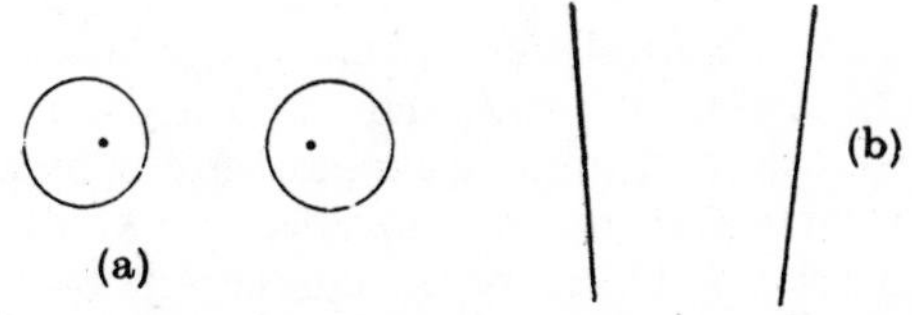

FIG. 15.5—STEREOGRAMS TO ILLUSTRATE DISTORTION CAUSED BY UNEQUAL ILLUMINATION.

of one of the stereograms is reduced to such an extent that it is only dimly discernible. Moreover, as the illumination is reduced, there occurs a lateral distortion of the field. The stereograms of Figure 15.5 (a) for example, are fused into a single spot standing out in front of a distant circle. When the right and left illuminations are equal, the spot appears centrally disposed with respect to the circle, but as the illumination of, say, the left stereogram is reduced, the spot moves laterally towards the left; that is to say, the fused projection assumes to an increasing extent the character of the brighter stereogram.

If the objects presented to the eyes are two nearly vertical lines, as in Figure 15.5 (b), they appear, under equal illuminations, as a single intermediate line with a vertical tilt, the lower end appearing near. If, now, the illumination for the left eye is reduced, the fused line leans over with its upper end towards the right.

VERHOEFF observed this phenomenon in 1933 and described a method of applying it as a test for stereoscopic vision which he classed as superior to the usual tests based on depth perception.*

15.6. Aniseikonia.

The fact that inequality of some kind—size, shape, sharpness, brightness, etc.—between the two retinal images may be one of the possible causes of motor imbalance or of faulty space perception has already been stated (§13.15).

Within recent years the view has been advanced† that appreciable derangements in the subject's stereoscopic projection and symptoms such as asthenopia may be caused, even with subjects with equal refractions in the two eyes, by small differences in size or shape, not necessarily between the retinal images but between the two neural patterns that are registered in the cortex and which we may call cortical images. It is on these cortical images as a basis that the final perceptual picture of the external field is built up and projected outwards. It is stated that symptoms that cannot be accounted for by the observed refractive errors and motor imbalance, symptoms which persist after these have been corrected or treated, are caused by these image size differences ; and that binocular vision is not possible when the image disparity reaches 4 per cent. AMES and his co-workers have essayed to measure these size differences and have prescribed lenses to modify the size of the retinal images without disturbing the refractive correction ; the image changes being produced, as explained in §§ 15.2 and 10.19, by what are called size lenses.

Although the phenomenon of aniseikonia, its effects and treatment, have not yet been adequately elucidated, the following account, which is taken from the author's paper,‡ will assist in understanding the import of the subject.

" The supposed nature of the condition known as *aniseikonia* (*an*, negative ; *isos*, equal ; *eikon*, image) may be explained with the aid of Figure 15.2. Objects A and B lying in a frontal plane, the distance AB therefore subtending equal angles at the two eyes, are observed binocularly. If the two eyes are equal, the retinal images

---

* *Am. Journ. Ophth.*, 3, 16, 7, July, 1933.

† By AMES and his colleagues at the Dartmouth Medical School, Hanover, U.S.A.

‡ *Loc. cit.*

$a'b'$ and $a''b''$ of the separation AB are equal. Nevertheless it may happen that the cortical images presented to the brain for fusion are unequal, the inequality arising during the process of transforming and transmitting the retinal images along the optical nerves to the cortex. The inequality may be caused, for example, by lack of symmetry in the distribution of the retinal receptors between the two eyes. However the difference arises, the brain and the mind have to contend with two unequal presentations. In consequence, the individual suffers from asthenopia, due to the strain of fusing the unequal images ; and further, his stereoscopic projection is distorted. This space distortion may not be evident in ordinary everyday vision, because we are seldom presented with objects isolated in space ; the field usually contains many objects and contours running in various directions and interconnected, in consequence of which we are continuously assisted in our spatial judgments by the monocular factors of perspective, and other factors. But it is claimed that the asthenopia and ocular distress may be serious when the disparity between the two images is only one or two per cent ; and further, that these symptoms disappear, in a high proportion of cases, when a size lens of suitable magnifying power is worn before the appropriate eye in order to equalise the two images.

Now there are undoubtedly people who, even after the most careful and skilled examination and treatment of their refraction and oculo-motor imbalance, continue to complain of ocular discomfort. (It is to be doubted whether there are many such people ; the complainants are often engaged in special occupation or are generally " nervy ".) Also, as we see from the experiments described above, many of us are afflicted with small spatial distortions which may conceivably contribute to the discomfort in ordinary vision and which would certainly affect the stereoscopic vision of a person who is called upon to perform some unusual visual task ; e.g. an aviator or the user of certain binocular measuring instruments, in playing certain games of skill, etc. If it can be shown that this condition called aniseikonia is responsible for such cases, then it is clearly of great importance, and aniseikonia treatment should be incorporated in all routine eye examinations.

But first it must be shown that the condition exists ; that it can be measured with a precision that is of practical value ; that a stable relationship can be established between its degree and the power of optical elements such as size lenses with which it is proposed to correct it. Moreover, before attempting to correct the condition optically, we require information as to whether the condition is of fixed degree in an individual or whether it is capable of alteration by training and experience.

Of these problems, only a short reference to attempts to detect and measure aniseikonia will be described.

The method that is now proposed by the Dartmouth School is somewhat as follows. Two targets are presented independently to the two eyes (Figure 15.6) ; the prominent central pattern is the same in each. One target is provided

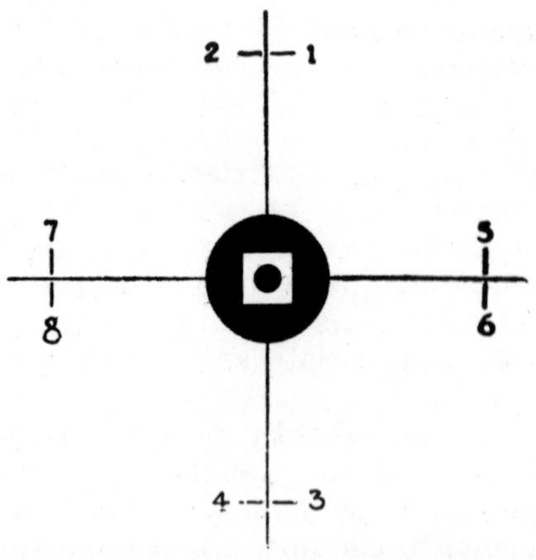

FIG. 15.6—TYPE OF TARGET USED FOR REVEALING ANISEIKONIA.

with short lines or dashes disposed on one side of the long radial lines and is seen by, say, the left eye ; these dashes are given odd numbers in the diagram. On the other target, presented to the right eye, the short dashes are on the opposite side of the long radial lines (even numbers). The dashes are at an angular distance of 4 degrees from the centre of the target. The arrangement is called an eikonometer. The eyes first observe and fuse the central patterns and then move out, say horizontally, to the short dashes 7 and 8 on the left. If the individual has no aniseikonia in the horizontal direction, the two dashes will be seen exactly opposite one another ; if horizontal aniseikonia is present, the dashes will be out of alignment. The degree of aniseikonia thus revealed is to be measured by interposing before the appropriate eye a size lens or telescopic system of such magnification as to enlarge the retinal image in that eye until the dashes are brought into alignment. The efficacy of the method depends on the assumption that the large central patterns remain fused even although they are now seen in peripheral vision. It is claimed that they do remain fused. If the central patterns are ineffective in holding the eyes in their original state of binocular fixation, then when turned to look at the dashes they are dissociated, and any observed lack of alignment of the dashes is a measure of heterophoria and not of aniseikonia.

With regard to the method of presenting the targets independently to the eyes, a polarization method is adopted by the Dartmouth School. The targets are projected on to a silvered screen by two projectors provided with polaroid screens placed perpendicularly to one another, and the observation is made through a second pair of crossed polaroids. In this way one target only is seen by each eye.

We* have tried several methods, including this polarization method, of presenting the independent targets, but have not succeeded in making any reliable measurements. In early attempts with the polarization method we could not obtain any relative displacement of the dashes with any observer. After a while certain observers reported occasional, but variable displacements. There were indications, we thought, that the outer vertical edges of the field, and perhaps even the ends of the long radial lines which are roughly equidistant from the dashes, were being unconsciously fused by the observer, thus locking the eyes for a while in a certain fixation position. Such fixation positions will vary according to the relative distances of the two target edges, or other pairs of marks in the field, from the dashes, and so will falsify the observed displacement of the dashes.

We accordingly made new targets in which the central patterns and all the markings are white on a black background, the radial lines running outwards to the extreme edge and, still using the polarization method, presented these targets in such a way that nothing was visible to the observer but the target marking. With these precautions

---

* At the Northampton Polytechnic, London.

some observers report varying degrees of displacement of the dashes on some, but not all, occasions.

Thus there is evidence that the central patterns of the targets sometimes remain fused when the eyes are directed towards the dashes, as claimed. But there appear to be other factors preventing reliable measurement.

If with a subject who observes no displacement of the dashes and possessing, therefore, no aniseikonia, a size lens is introduced before one eye, some displacement of the dashes must occur if the central patterns remain fused. We find that this does not always happen, however. After a momentary separation of the dashes as the size lens is introduced, the dashes frequently return to their original positions.

Let us assume that, in spite of the above failure to measure aniseikonia, the condition does in fact exist. Can it then be shown that it is the cause of cases of space distortion? We have seen that both horizontal and vertical tilts of the field are encountered in many individuals. It does not seem possible to establish any connection between magnification in the vertical direction and vertical tilt in the median plane; the latter can only arise as the result of *horizontal* diplopia of one of two vertically disposed objects. It would thus appear that vertical tilt is due to some cause other than aniseikonia. Even with regard to horizontal tilts of the field, the connection with aniseikonia is not too clear. It is true that magnification of one *retinal* image by a size lens produces a horizontal tilt, but there is a basic difference between this and unequal *cortical* images. In the former the angular subtenses of the object are different in the two eyes; in the latter the subtense angles are equal, and it would seem to follow from the known laws of binocular fusion (*vide* Sherrington, 1940) that the unequal cortical images would be projected to the one object in space, in which case no tilt of the field would result."

15.7. Summary.

The preceding sections describe but a few isolated characteristics of the psycho-physical processes of space perception and a few of the ways in which such perception may be distorted, even in individuals whose binocular vision is apparently normal as judged by the tests commonly applied. The causes of these and of other anomalies that further investigation will doubtless reveal are to be found among the broad classification given in §13.15, but much research is needed to relate cause and effect sufficiently clearly to be of service in practical clinical work. Such study bears directly on the work of the optical practitioner. It is needed in order to improve and rationalise the present somewhat crude empirical methods of diagnosis, measurement and treatment of squint and heterophoria and in dealing with the selection and training of those who are needed for visual tasks demanding a high standard of binocular vision.

Further observations on space perception will be found in §23.8. Reference should be made also to an important monograph by R. K. Luneburg entitled "Mathematical Analysis of Binocular Vision", Princeton Univ. Press, 1947; also to "An Essay on Binocular Vision" by Lord Charnwood, Hatton Press, 1950.

BINOCULAR VISION AND ITS ANOMALIES

CHAPTER XVI

ANISOMETROPIA

16.1. Definition. Varieties.

THE term anisometropia (a = not; iso = equal) is applied to that condition in which the refractive errors of the two eyes are unequal. Probably no two eyes are exactly equal if examined with sufficient precision; when carefully examined by clinical methods small amounts of anisometropia are extremely common and often cause little or no discomfort. In astigmatic eyes especially, differences in the magnitude of the cylinder components, or departures of their axis directions from the symmetrical position, occur frequently. In clinical practice the term anisometropia is usually restricted to differences of moderate and large degree, although a difference in refraction between the two eyes of, say, 3 dioptres or more may not interfere with reasonably comfortable binocular single vision. The likelihood and extent of such interference depends upon the nature of the refractive difference, the acuteness of vision of the eyes, the state of motor balance and the general nervous condition of the subject.

Evidently there are many possible varieties of anisometropia:

1. One eye emmetropic, the other hyperopic or myopic.
2. Both eyes hyperopic, to unequal degrees.
3. Both eyes myopic, to unequal degrees.
4. One eye hyperopic and the other myopic; a condition frequently described by the special term ANTIMETROPIA.

Astigmatism may be associated with the ametropia in any of the above combinations.

The condition is usually congenital, but may sometimes develop, e.g. the progress of myopia is sometimes unequal in the two eyes; or it may be the result of disease or operation. Aphakia in one eye is a special case of the latter.

16.2. Vision in Uncorrected Anisometropia.

Accommodation is exerted practically equally in both eyes, any difference there may be amounting to only a fraction of a dioptre ; hence a given object cannot be seen equally distinctly by both eyes in anisometropia. Nevertheless, the blurred image may be fused with the more distinct one and binocular and stereoscopic vision obtained, provided the anisometropic difference is not too marked. In some cases stereoscopic vision is said to be present with a difference of 5 dioptres between the refractions of the two eyes, but the stereoscopy attained can scarcely be good and the fusional efforts exerted in such cases frequently produce accommodative asthenopia.

Depending upon the degree of anisometropia, the visual acuity in the two eyes, and surrounding circumstances such as the motor balance, the vision obtained may be subdivided into four grades :

(*a*) *Binocular single vision* : usually the defect is of small degree in this case but, as remarked above, may amount to as much as 5 dioptres. The visual acuity must be reasonably good in both eyes. There may or may not be asthenopic symptoms.

(*b*) *Simultaneous macular perception* without fusion, the disparity between the retinal images being too great for fusion. If the visual acuity is good in both eyes there will probably be " antagonism "* between the right and left images and asthenopia in consequence.

(*c*) *Alternating vision*, one eye being used at a time. If, for example, both eyes having good acuity, one is emmetropic or hyperopic to a small degree and the other myopic, the subject may adopt the habit of using the former for distance vision and the latter for near vision, suppressing the image in the unused eye. Binocular vision is sacrificed but otherwise vision is comfortable.

(*d*) *Monocular vision* : this usually occurs when the defect is high, especially if the acuity is not good in the eye with the large refractive error. Only the better eye is used for both distance and near, the defective eye tending towards amblyopia ex anopsia and, possibly, to divergent squint.†

If this last condition were detected during childhood, the development of amblyopia could probably be prevented

---

* §12.6. † §13.15.

by suitable exercises, daily periods of occlusion of the good eye, and optical correction. The anisometropia is often unsuspected, however, when the subject has one reasonably good eye and achieves binocular fixation. If the condition persists undetected until adult life, exercises would be unsuccessful or at least so prolonged as to be impracticable; and a correcting lens will probably fail to affect the poor eye because of the amblyopia, or defective reception of visual stimuli.*

16.3. Treatment.

Except when attempting to arrest an amblyopia and restore single vision in a child, as mentioned above, and since accommodation does not assist one eye without affecting the other, the only treatment consists in the provision of suitable correcting lenses. The lens or lenses to be prescribed, and whether for distance or for near or both, depends upon the variety of anisometropia present, upon the visual acuity of the eyes, and upon other surrounding circumstances which will emerge as we proceed.

Broadly, the examiner should aim first at the ideal condition of full vision in each eye, both for distance and near, provided that this correction enables binocular single vision to be achieved, if not at once, after a few weeks' trial. If this is found to be impossible, either because of the nature of the case or because the subject will not persevere with a trial period, alternate use of the eyes should be attempted; one eye for distance and the other for near. Failing this second alternative, one eye having become definitely amblyopic, only the good eye needs attention and we try to provide that this eye may be used in both distance and near vision. We will consider each of these aims briefly.

(1) Attempt to attain binocular single vision:

In the case of children this attempt should be made with determination, even if one eye is amblyopic. Such measures as are necessary to deal with an amblyopia or a motor imbalance, if present, should be undertaken. The full correction for both eyes should be worn constantly. It may be that full binocular vision cannot be attained, but any definite improvement in the poor eye is of value.

---

* §13.15.

In the case of adults an attempt to leave the subject with binocular vision over a reasonable field of view can only be undertaken with any hope of success if the anisometropia is of tolerably small amount, say not more than 2 D to 3 D or so, and if some degree of binocular vision is already present. In such cases the full refractive correction should be worn constantly. Sometimes the symptoms of strain will disappear in a few weeks. If not, single vision may yet be obtained by modifying the refractive correction and so sacrificing distinct vision to some extent. Thus, whereas the full correction might be + 2 D and + 4 D, comfortable binocular vision may result by wearing + 2 D and + 3 D.

In many cases, however, including older adults with fixed habits and reluctance to try "experiments", the attempts to improve binocular vision will fail. Symptoms may arise that did not exist before. Whereas before correction one retinal image was blurred and could easily be neglected when required, correcting lenses produce two sharp images of different sizes which demand cortical attention, as it were. The subject, having grown accustomed to the anisometropic condition and being reasonably comfortable in so far as the anisometropia is concerned, is introduced to new and disturbing conditions. Such symptoms as existed previously were perhaps merely associated with the ametropia of one eye, or with the need for presbyopic addition, or with some degree of motor imbalance. In such cases it will usually not be worth while making the attempt to attain binocular vision.

It is to be borne in mind that the correcting lenses themselves, being of different powers, may introduce difficulties. The sharp unequal retinal images may be troublesome to fuse; the accommodation required for near objects is different in the two eyes; and whenever the eyes are rotated so as to observe a laterally placed object through peripheral portions of the lenses, they are subjected to different amounts of prismatic effect, which again may prevent fusion. This latter effect is of most importance in the vertical direction and arises therefore when the distance centred lenses are used in reading, when the eyes are depressed and their visual axes intersect the lenses at points approaching 1 cm. below the optical centres of the lenses. In cases of moderate and high anisometropia, a separate pair of spectacles should be used for near work, the lenses being decentred and the frame tilted so that the visual axes will pass normally through the optical centres when in the mean reading position. If, the subject being of an age requiring presbyopic addition, bifocals are worn, they must be very carefully centred.*

With regard to distance vision, the subject should be instructed to turn his head rather than his eyes when viewing laterally placed objects and so reduce these relative prismatic effects between the two eyes.

The effects of the correcting lenses, and the possibility of providing lenses of special design will be discussed in the next paragraph ; see also Chapter X.

(2) The attainment of alternating vision, one eye for distance and the other for near work :

Here again, in the case of adults, attempts to correct the refractive error, or to improve the vision, in one eye or the other, or both, may introduce disturbances that will not be tolerated. In general, if there are no symptoms of strain, the condition should be allowed to remain. If, the subject being not too old, symptoms are complained of, an attempt might be made to assist each eye to carry out its separate function in comfort. The lenses will, of course, depend upon the variety and extent of the anisometropia. If, for example, one eye is emmetropic and the other hyperopic, with good visual acuity in both eyes, the hyperopic eye may be corrected for distance and the emmetropic eye with the presbyopic addition, if such be required, in order to adapt this eye for near work. Generally, the more hyperopic eye will be fitted for distance vision and the more myopic eye for near vision.

(3) Correction for the good eye :

If any useful vision remains in the poorer eye, which is defective owing to amblyopia or to opacities in the media, and especially in children and young people, an attempt should be made by exercises and occlusion of the good eye to improve the vision in the poor eye, as already explained. Otherwise the good eye alone needs attention. In this latter event an opaque glass may be required before the poorer eye if the impressions it receives interfere with the vision of the good eye.

---

* *Ophthalmic Lenses ;* Ch. VIII.

16.4. Vision in Corrected Anisometropia. Anisometropia Spectacles.

Before correction, an individual with a small or even a moderate amount of anisometropia and with good visual acuity in both eyes may have binocular vision and some measure of stereoscopic vision, although at any given moment one retinal image will be blurred and different in size from the sharper image in the other eye. There is apparently sufficient adaptability in the fusion faculty to blend images that are formed on corresponding *areas* not merely points of the two retinæ.* The stereoscopic acuity is probably not high because of the lack of definition; and the binocular spatial projection may be faulty on account of the disparity in size of the images. But such stereoscopic vision as is present may be obtained without discomfort. The extent of the disparity in size of the retinal images depends not only upon the differential refractive error between the two eyes, but also upon the proportions of these errors that are respectively axial and refractive.†

The elasticity of the fusion mechanism does not extend so far as to allow of fusion of images with large differences of sharpness or size between them, so that a person with high anisometropia does not usually obtain binocular vision. He may, nevertheless, enjoy his alternating or monocular vision in comfort.

When lenses correcting the ametropia are worn the subject who, although with good visual acuity, had not previously obtained binocular vision and had neglected one image, may now experience trouble with his two sharp images. He may nevertheless attain binocular vision and *may* learn to do so with comfort. The subject who previously obtained some measure of binocular vision will also be presented with new conditions. The correcting lenses modify:

(*a*) The sharpness of the retinal images;

(*b*) The relative amounts of accommodation required of the eyes to view near objects;

(*c*) The rotations or vergence movements to be executed by the eyes in order to obtain single vision of laterally situated objects, or near objects, through the distance correction.

(*d*) The sizes of the retinal images.

---

* §12.4. † §§ 3.13 and 10.12.

With regard to the last two effects, consider the rather extreme case of a subject emmetropic in the left eye and aphakic in the right eye, which was previously emmetropic. Assuming the distance correcting lens to be thin and to be worn in our standard position $12\frac{1}{3}$ mm. from the cornea, its power is 11·25 D, and the right retinal image is 25 per cent larger than the left.* This amount of disparity will almost certainly prevent binocular vision. Further, suppose the subject to be engaged in close work such as reading, the visual axis of the left eye being depressed below the primary direction by, say, $15\frac{1}{2}°$ or 27·75△, which is equivalent to 10 cm. at a distance of 33·33 cm. beyond the correcting lens.† The visual axis of the right eye intersects

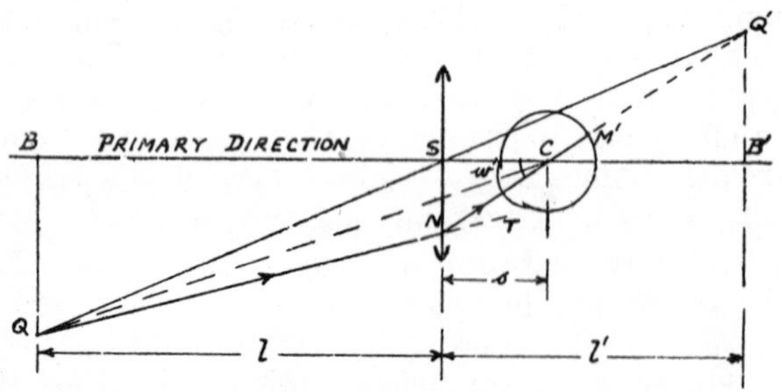

Fig. 16.1—Rotation of Eye to observe object Q through correcting lens at S.

the lens at a point N (the near visual point) several millimetres below its optical centre, so that there is a base-up prismatic effect equal to angle CNT (Fig. 16.1). Thus whereas the left eye, without a correcting lens or provided merely with a plane glass, observes the object Q along the direction CQ, the right eye must rotate downwards until its visual axis occupies the position CN. It is easy to prove that the angle SCN $= w'$ is equal to 38·62△, on the assumption of a thin lens; the method of calculation will be indicated in the next paragraph. Thus to obtain single vision of a point Q the eyes would have to be placed in a position of left supravergence amounting to 38·62 − 27·75 = 10·87△, which is more than they can accomplish. Hence binocular vision of objects situated 15 degrees

* §3.14.

† Although the head will be lowered the eyes will, in addition, rotate downwards below the primary direction.

vertically, up or down, from the primary direction would be prevented by this relative prismatic effect. More latitude is possible in the horizontal direction, but it will be clear that these prismatic effects will limit binocular vision to a considerably restricted field of vision, particularly in the vertical direction. Outside this region diplopia will arise and vision will be extremely uncomfortable.

(This upsetting of the normal vergence relationship between the eyes, in the horizontal or vertical direction, by the lenses correcting anisometropia—or by decentred lenses in isometropic cases—is sometimes referred to as a condition of *false* or *artificial heterophoria* ; see Ex. 21 of Chapter XIII.)

In small to moderate amounts of anisometropia, the rotations required of the eyes to obtain single vision of laterally situated objects can be made more nearly equal by appropriately bending the correcting lenses ; and a similar effect can to some extent be obtained by adjusting their relative thicknesses. The forms of the lenses should be such that, in general, the back surface of the more positive or less negative of the two lenses should approximate to plano and that of the less positive or more negative should be strongly negative.*

The bending of the correcting lenses to secure this equalisation of prismatic effects also tends to reduce the disparity between the sizes of the retinal images in hyperopic anisometropia when the stronger of the two lenses is of appreciable power. In lower degrees of hyperopia and in myopic anisometropia, on the other hand, the bending required to reduce relative prismatic effect increases the retinal disparity (see §10.19).

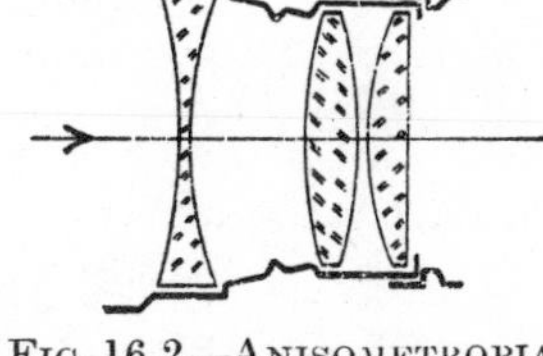

FIG. 16.2—ANISOMETROPIA CORRECTING LENS.

If an attempt is made to provide the subject with binocular vision in cases of large amounts of aniso metropia, single lenses are inadequate ; compound lens systems are necessary. Fig. 16.2 shows such a spectacle lens combination, designed by von ROHR. They are designed primarily to reduce the inequality in the rotations required of the eyes and secondarily to reduce the disparity between the

* See also : *Ophthalmic Lenses ;* Ch. XVI.

sizes of the two retinal images. Although similar in external appearance to telescopic spectacles, their construction is different in principle. By means of such anisometropic spectacles, subjects with an anisometropic difference as high as 20 dioptres have been provided with stereoscopic vision over a moderate field. Thus many anisometropic subjects who will not tolerate the discomfort (diplopia, etc.) introduced by ordinary single spectacle lenses could be provided with binocular vision if they could be persuaded to wear these compound systems. But many people object to their conspicuous appearance and will not wear them unless their livelihood demands binocular vision.

The prismatic effects are eliminated in contact glasses, which move with the eyes, but the retinal image disparity (the ametropia being axial) is increased by them.*

Lenses designed for the sole purpose of equalising the retinal images, for subjects who are not anisometropic but whose ocular images may be unequal, are described in §10.19.

16.5. Accommodation and Eye Movements in Corrected Anisometropia.

The accommodations and vergence movements the eyes are called upon to execute can be calculated with the aid of expressions (12.5) and (12.6) of §12.23. With only one lens before each eye, the distance correcting lens of power $\boldsymbol{F}$, assumed in the general case to be decentred c cm., these expressions become

$$\theta = -\frac{(h\,L - c\,F)\,S}{(S - L - F)} \qquad (16.1)$$

$$\text{and } A = \frac{-\,L\,D^2}{(D - F)\,(D - L - F)} \qquad (16.2)$$

The quantity $(-\,\boldsymbol{hL})$ is the angle w subtended by the object with the primary line. In the case of a distant object we have consequently

$$\theta = \frac{(w + c\,F)\,S}{(S - F)} \qquad \text{and } A = 0 \qquad (16.3)$$

and when the lenses are centred for distance, so that $c = 0$,

$$\theta = \frac{w.S.}{(S - F)}$$

We will illustrate these effects of the distance correction, centred or decentred, on the accommodation and vergence movements of the eyes by one or two examples.

* §§ 10.12, 10.13 and 3.14.

Example : A person wearing R. and L. + 12·0 D sph., each lens being decentred out by 1 cm., observes a distant object straight ahead. The correcting lenses (assumed thin) lie in a plane 27 mm. in front of the centres of rotation. Find the extent of rotation required of each eye.

Answer : We will solve this from first principles and then check by means of the above expressions.

We need only consider one (say the right) eye since the conditions are symmetrical. In Fig. 16.3 the optical centre of the + 12 D

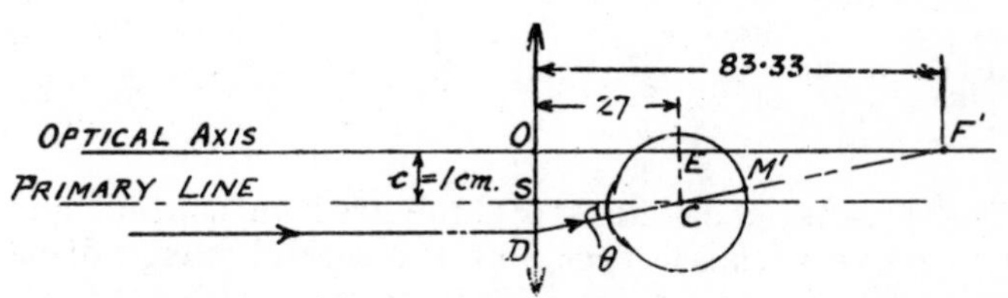

FIG. 16.3—ROTATION OF EYE TO OBSERVE DISTANT OBJECT THROUGH DECENTRED CORRECTING LENS. EXAMPLE OF §16.5.

lens is at O and its second focal point at F′, where OF′ = 8·33 cm. The eye's centre of projection is at C, its primary line is SC and SC = 27 mm. Rays parallel to the primary line from the distant object all unite in F. The particular ray through the centre of projection is DCF′ and the eye has to rotate (converge) through the angle SCD = θ to receive the image on the fovea M′. If the diagram be drawn carefully to scale the angle θ may be measured; it will be found to be rather more than 10° or 17·5Δ.

Or from the geometry of the diagram:

$$\tan\theta = \frac{\text{CE}}{\text{EF}'} = \frac{10}{56\cdot 33} = \cdot 1775 \quad \text{or } \theta = 17\cdot 75\Delta$$

The result could be obtained at once from expression (16.3,) in which, since the object is straight ahead, w = 0. Thus

$$\theta = \frac{(w + c\,F)\,S}{S - F} = \frac{1\cdot 12\cdot 37}{37 - 12} = 17\cdot 75\Delta$$

It is observed from the diagram that although the lens is decentred the distance SO = 1 cm., the portion of the lens concerned in the refraction of the significant ray is at D, which is removed more than 1 cm. from the optical centre of the lens. Thus, because of the forward position of the lens relative to the eye's centre of projection its prismatic effect is actually greater than the product $F \times c$ (= 12Δ) which is roughly taken to be the effect in clinical work. With lenses of more moderate power the difference between the exact and rough results is much smaller.

Example : An anisometrope with P.D. = 60 mm. wears centred distance corrections of – 2 D and – 12 D for the left and right eyes respectively. Find the convergence and accommodation required when he looks straight ahead at an object on the median line 25 cm. beyond the lens plane.

Answer : Here $h = 3$ cm. $L = -4$ D. $c = 0$

Left Eye. $\theta = -\frac{3(-4)\,37}{(37+4+2)} = +\,10 \cdot 33\triangle$ convergence

$$A = \frac{4 \times 71\cdot4 \times 71\cdot4}{73\cdot4 \times 77\cdot4} = 3\cdot59 \text{ D}$$

Right Eye $\theta = -\frac{3(-4)\,37}{53} = +\,8\cdot38\triangle$ convergence

$$A = \frac{4 \times 71\cdot4 \times 71\cdot4}{83\cdot4 \times 87\cdot4} = 2\cdot80 \text{ D}$$

The mean convergence of each eye is 3·1 M.A.; one eye is called upon to accommodate 0·79 D more than the other.

Suppose a distant object at an elevation of 10° is to be observed. We have $w = 10° = 17\cdot63\triangle$.

Left Eye. $\theta = \frac{wS}{S-F} = \frac{17\cdot63 \times 37}{39} = 16\cdot72\triangle$

Right Eye. $\theta = \frac{17\cdot63 \times 37}{49} = 13\cdot31\triangle$.

The relative rotation (left supravergence) required is 3·4△, which will cause trouble.

Calculations on the effect of the anisometropic correction on the sizes of the retinal images are considered in §10.12. It is to be noted that the lenses have been assumed thin in the above.

CHAPTER XVI. EXERCISES.

1. Explain the meaning of the term anisometropia and write a short account of the quality of vision obtained in different degrees of anisometropia and varying surrounding conditions.

Without going into detail, indicate briefly the general course of treatment that might be attempted.

2. A subject requires: R. + 3·0 D sph.; L. − 3·0 D sph. Discuss the difficulties of providing such a case with a comfortable correction. What comfort tests would you apply ? (S.M.C.)

3. Why is anisometropia more awkward to correct in the vertical than in the horizontal meridian ? (B.O.A.)

4. What are the difficulties attending the measurement and correction of anisometropia ? Illustrate your answer with reference to the case :—

R. − 5·00 D cyl. ax. 45°. L. + 5·00 D cyl. ax. 135°. Age 20 years. Monocular corrected acuity 6/6 in each eye. No previous correction worn. (S.M.C.)

5. Discuss briefly why asthenopia is a marked symptom in certain cases of anisometropia and not in others. Is it possible for asthenopia to occur in anisometropia only as the result of wearing lenses which correct the error ? Give reasons.

6. Give an account of the new conditions to which an anisometrope, who had not previously enjoyed binocular vision, is subjected when he is provided with lenses correcting his ametropia. For what reasons may binocular vision still be unattainable ? Describe briefly steps that might be taken to render vision comfortable.

7. What are anisometropia spectacles? Explain the difficulties they are intended to surmount and the principles of their design and construction.

8. What two main optical causes of binocular discomfort arise when a case of anisometropia is corrected by ordinary spectacle lenses? Give a brief description of types of lenses for correcting anisometropia and making binocular vision possible (*a*) when the anisometropia is of low degree; (*b*) when it is of high degree.

A person is corrected for distance by R. + 2·50 D sph. and L. + 15·0 D sph. What is the condition of the subject when using these glasses for reading?

9. A person wears the following lenses, each decentred 4 mm. out; R. − 12·0 D sph. and L. − 12·0 D sph. The lenses are 27 mm. in front of the centres of rotation of the eyes. Find graphically and by calculation, based on the construction, the angle between the right and left visual axes when a distant object is observed straight ahead. Confirm your result by the expression (16·3).

10. A spectacle frame is glazed with a centred distance correction of − 8·0 D sphere before each eye, the plane of the lenses being 25 mm. in front of the centres of rotation. A distant point object directly in front is viewed through the lenses, whilst the frame is laterally displaced 5 mm. in its own plane. By how much must the eyes rotate and through what portions of the lenses will the eyes be looking? What extra rotation will be necessary for an additional displacement of 5 mm. forward of the whole frame? (S.M.C.)

11. A pair of eyes wearing R. and L. + 4·00 D sph. centred for distance observes a distant object straight ahead on the median line. The P.D. is 60 mm. If the lenses are both decentred 5 mm. out, by how much must each eye rotate to maintain clear single vision of the object? Assume distance from lens to centre of rotation of eye = 25 mm. Express your result in Δ and in M.A.

Give a clear diagram and obtain your result from it. If any formula is used, prove it.

12. An anisometrope with P.D. = 68 mm. wears centred distance corrections of R. − 4·0 D.S. and L. − 16·00 D.S. Find the convergence and accommodation required of each eye in order to view an object lying on the primary line of the right eye and 33⅓ cm. beyond the lens. The lenses are 14 mm. in front of the principal points and 27 mm. in front of the centres of rotation of the eyes.

To what condition will the eyes be subjected when reading?

13. A person has ocular refractions R. − 10·0 D and L. − 3·0 D, the ametropia in both eyes being axial. If each eye is fully corrected by a lens placed 12 mm. from the cornea, compare the sizes of the R. and L. retinal images. (N.B. Refer to §3.12.)

What effect might this disparity between the images have on the person's vision; and what other difficulties will probably arise?

14. Explain, with the aid of diagrams, why the correction required by a patient with marked anisometropia must necessarily cause discomfort at first. (B.O.A.)

THE STIMULUS

CHAPTER XVII

RADIATION

17.1. The Electromagnetic Spectrum

RADIATION is electromagnetic in character and varies in frequency, and so in wavelength, over an enormous range according to the manner in which it is produced. The complete range, in other words the complete electromagnetic spectrum, is indicated in Fig. 17.1. Of the total of seventy octaves or so explored to date the range to

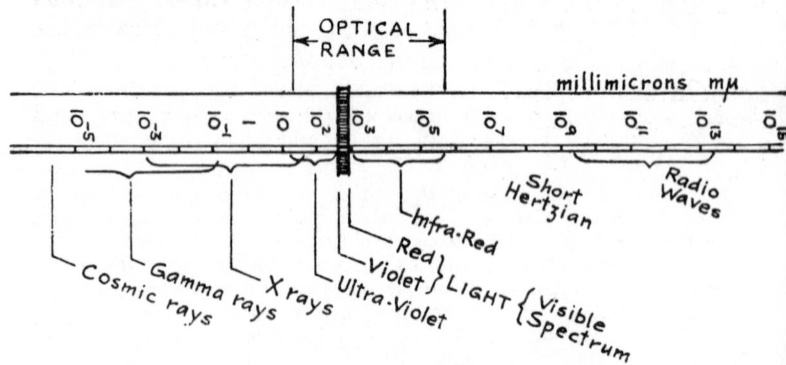

FIG. 17.1—THE SPECTRUM OF RADIANT ENERGY OR ELECTROMAGNETIC SPECTRUM.

which the human eye has become adapted, i.e. the VISIBLE SPECTRUM or light, occupies rather less than one octave. As would be expected, different mechanisms are needed to produce radiations with such enormous variations in frequency. The electrical waves of relatively low frequency used in radio communication are generated by the oscillation of electrical circuits. Also by electrical means, but using apparatus of smaller dimensions, waves have been produced with wavelength as low as 0·1 mm. or 10^5 *mμ*.* To produce those radiations of higher frequency falling within the infra-red, visible and ultra-violet regions which make up what is called the *optical range*, the requisite energy is

* 1 *mμ* = 1 millimicron = 10^{-6} mm. For definitions of units see Appendix.

obtained from actions set up within the material of the generating body. In some manner the constituent atoms of the material have to be energised. By using luminous sources of energy such as flames, arcs and lamps, radiations extending from wavelength $\lambda = 0 \cdot 4$ mm. in the infra-red to the region of 10 $m\mu$ in the ultra-violet have been produced.

The higher frequency regions of the electromagnetic spectrum include X-rays, gamma rays and the so-called cosmic rays. X-rays may be produced by bombarding a metal with fast-moving electrons ejected from an incandescent filament in a highly exhausted vacuum tube, a high potential difference being maintained between the filament and the metal target. They extend from 27 $m\mu$ to about one thousandth $m\mu$; the production of these short or "hard" X-rays requires a pressure of the order of a million volts and large and special tubes. Gamma rays, which may be considered as very hard X-rays, are one of the three distinct forms of emanation (α, β and γ) spontaneously emitted by radium and other radio-active substances. Cosmic rays have the highest frequency and are the most penetrating. They reach the earth from outer sources and are believed to originate during atomic formation in other parts of the universe.

The effects produced by these various radiations will be considered below. Although they vary so enormously in wavelength, are produced by such different methods—electrical oscillations, luminous sources, electronic bombardment, radio-active emanation—and exhibit such diverse effects, they are all physically the same thing. It is because of the properties of the human eye that a certain range of these radiations, extending from about 390$m\mu$ to 750$m\mu$ (400 to 700 $m\mu$ in normal daylight conditions), arouses in us the sensation of vision; the retina of our eye has developed to utilise this range.

17.2. The Structure of Matter.

Towards the end of the nineteenth century new discoveries by leading physicists started a revolution in our conception of matter and energy. Were it not for such obvious practical evidence as radar and the atomic bomb the uninitiated would be inclined to dismiss the complexities of the modern atom, not long ago thought to be indivisible, as a physicist's fanciful dream. Only the barest outline of this complicated subject can be given here.

All matter, solid, liquid and gaseous, consists of atoms. The atom consists of a compact central core or nucleus in which practically the whole mass of the atom is concentrated and which carries a positive charge E. Around the nucleus are electrons which are negatively charged. The modern physicist will be chary of stating how these electrons move around the nucleus, but a useful picture of the arrangement is obtained by supposing them to revolve around the nucleus. On this view the atom is a small planetary system. The nucleus may itself be a composite structure with proton, neutron, positron, etc., but this complexity we shall largely ignore. The electrons revolve at enormous speed and the atom is a tiny reservoir of energy. In its normal state an atom is electrically neutral, the sum of the negative charges on its revolving electrons balancing the positive charge on the nucleus. The electrons may be ejected from the atom, spontaneously as in radio-active substances, or under some kind of stimulation such as heat, electronic bombardment, etc.

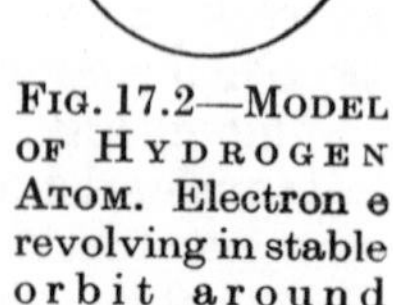

FIG. 17.2—MODEL OF HYDROGEN ATOM. Electron e revolving in stable orbit around Nucleus N.

The simplest of all atoms is that of hydrogen (Fig. 17.2). Its nucleus consists of one proton and it has one revolving electron.* The mass of the proton is 1,846 times the mass (m) of the electron. The diameter of the atom, that is the diameter of the electron's orbit, is many thousands of times the diameter of the electron. Thus the atom, though so small, is mostly empty space.

In all the known elements the heavier they are the more complex become their atoms ; they possess more electrons and more complicated nuclei. The number of electrons in an atom is its ATOMIC NUMBER, which is to be distinguished from atomic weight. The atomic number of hydrogen is 1 and its atomic weight is 1 (very nearly). Helium, the second element in the periodic table, has atomic number 2 and atomic weight 4. Its nucleus contains 2 protons and 2 neutrons firmly bound together and it has 2 revolving electrons. If the nucleus of an atom of some substance contains Z protons and N neutrons, there will be Z electrons

* The electron charge (e) is $4 \cdot 80 \times 10^{-10}$ electrostatic units (E.S.U.) or $1 \cdot 6 \times 10^{-20}$ electromagnetic units (E.M.U.). The mass of the proton is $1 \cdot 66 \times 10^{-24}$ gramme. The diameter of the atom is about $1 \cdot 0 \times 10^{-8}$ cm.

circulating about this nucleus in the normal atom and its mass will be very closely (N + Z) times that of the hydrogen atom. The atomic weight of the heaviest known substance, uranium, is 235 or 238 depending upon whether we are dealing with one so-called isotope or the other; in both cases the atomic number is 92 so that there are 92 protons and 92 electrons.

If a neutral atom loses an electron, it then possesses a positive charge and is called an ion; it is said to be *ionised.* A hydrogen atom can show one positive charge and no more; a helium atom can show one positive charge or two, but no more.

The emanations given off spontaneously by radium, etc. have been found to be of three distinct kinds. The alpha rays are the nuclei of helium atoms and so comparatively heavy; the beta rays are electrons; the gamma rays are electromagnetic waves. They all come from the nucleus of the radio-active substance, which becomes gradually transmuted, through intermediate stages, to different substances and finally to lead.

The electrons of any atom can exist only in orbits of certain definite radii, each orbit representing a definite level of energy W_1, W_2, W_3, etc. The innermost orbit is number one. The chemical properties of an atom are determined by the number of atomic electrons. In chemical actions rearrangement of electron orbits round the nuclei take place without any change in the nuclei.

17.3. The Origin of Radiation. Spectra.

Radiations falling within the infra-red, visible and ultra-violet regions and the regions of still higher frequency are due to oscillations of the molecules or of the atoms of the radiating source, or to changes taking place within the atoms themselves. Broadly, in the case of solids and liquids and, in special circumstances, dense gases, made incandescent by the application of heat, the radiation is caused by the increased agitation of the molecules and when the radiation is analysed, a *continuous* spectrum results. When the exciting agency produces vibrations of the atoms within the molecules, *band* spectra are produced. *Line* spectra are obtained when the radiation involves changes within the atom. The greater the energy used to excite the atom, the more are the inner orbital electrons affected and the higher is the frequency of the resulting radiation.

When a given atom of a gas or vapour is in its so-called stationary state, its electrons revolve steadily in their several innermost or stable orbits and no absorption or emission of energy by this atom takes place. When a sufficiently powerful external agency acts upon the gas or vapour the atom will become "excited", in which case a given electron will move away from the nucleus to an outer orbit. The atom will remain in this excited state for only a very short time, about 10^{-8} second; it will then return to its stationary state: that is, each electron returns to its stable inner orbit, emitting a single quantum of energy as it does so. It delivers a kick, as it were, to the "ether" and sets up a train of waves carrying the energy. The quantum is the smallest amount of energy that an atom can emit. Each quantum of energy has the value hf where f is the frequency of the electron concerned and h is called PLANK'S universal constant of action. By various methods h has been found to have the value $6 \cdot 6 \times 10^{-27}$ erg-second. If an excited electron falls from an outer orbit of energy level W_m to its inner orbit of energy level W_n, the emission of the quantum of energy takes place according to the fundamental law

$$W_m - W_n = hf = h\frac{c}{\lambda} \tag{17.1}$$

and the radiation due to this electron is of a single frequency f or wavelength λ; a *single line* spectrum is produced. Taking the velocity of light (c) as $299 \cdot 8 \times 10^6$ metres per second, then if λ be expressed in $m\mu$

$$W_m - W_n = \frac{6 \cdot 6 \times 10^{-27} \times 299 \cdot 8 \times 10^{15}}{\lambda}$$

$$= \frac{1979 \times 10^{-12}}{\lambda} \text{ erg} \tag{17.2}$$

It is to be noted that whereas PLANCK'S constant is an absolute constant of nature, the quantum is a variable quantity; it varies with the frequency of the radiation. For X-rays and gamma rays it is large; for infra-red it is small.

Commencing with the enquiry by the Swiss schoolmaster BALMER (1885) it has been shown that the complete spectrum of hydrogen consists of five groups of lines and that the wavelength λ of any line of any group is given by the relation

$$\frac{1}{\lambda} = N\left(\frac{1}{n^2} - \frac{1}{m^2}\right) \tag{17.3}$$

in which m and n are the numbers of the electron orbits concerned in the emission of radiation of wavelength λ. The quantity N is known as the Rydberg constant; it depends upon PLANCK'S constant h and on the electron properties of the particular substance. The wavelengths of the lines in the spectra of many elements have been investigated in this way and the predictions of the quantum theory concerning the emission of radiation have been substantially confirmed by experiment. Equation (17.2) shows that the shorter the wavelength of the radiation the greater is the energy involved. The very short gamma and cosmic rays are associated with changes occurring within the nucleus, for which enormous disruptive forces are required.

According to the quantum theory, therefore, energy is radiated from a source in separate discrete corpuscles or quanta and is not emitted continuously as was believed on the wave theory. Moreover, these quanta are emitted in successive bursts even by a source which is ordinarily described as a steady or a constant source. If apparatus is set up to produce flashes of light, flashes delivered at one setting of the apparatus will not all contain the same number of quanta.

17.4. Emission of Light.

We see that atoms are normally unexcited and that energy must be supplied to them in some way in order to raise the electrons to orbits of higher energy level so that the radiation of this energy may follow. The exciting energy may be supplied by various thermal, electrical and chemical processes. When the wavelength of the resulting radiation falls within the limits of the visible spectrum the radiating body is said to be luminous and the emission of such luminous radiation is called LUMINESCENCE or INCANDESCENCE according to the manner in which the exciting energy is supplied. Thus we may subdivide the emission of light into:

(1) INCANDESCENCE OR TEMPERATURE RADIATION OR THERMOLUMINESCENCE: the energy is supplied as heat and the radiation is due to the increased temperature of the body. Examples: the sun, incandescent lamps, common arc, gas flame.

(2) ELECTROLUMINESCENCE: from all kinds of electrical discharges through gases. Examples: electric discharge or gaseous conduction lamps, sparks.

(3) CHEMILUMINESCENCE: from the energy set free in a chemical reaction. Examples: some flames, oxidisation of phosphorous, decaying matter, fungi, the firefly (probably).

(4) PHOTOLUMINESCENCE OR FLUORESCENCE: the energy is supplied as radiation, ultra-violet or visible, is stored up for a certain period and then emitted at a different, usually longer, wavelength.

All sources of light fall into one or other of the above classes: practical light sources belong almost exclusively to the first two classes. Temperature radiation, as from an

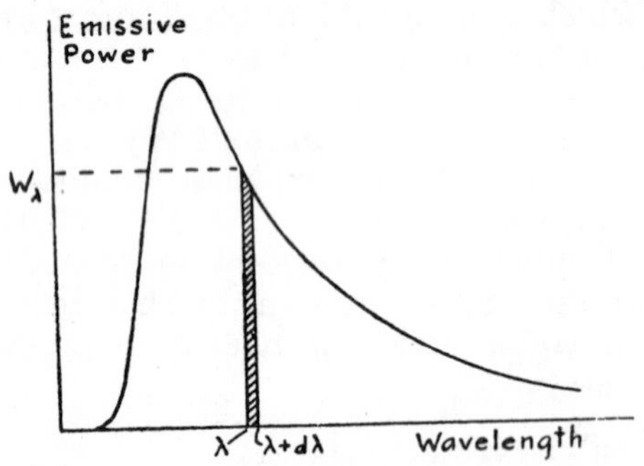

FIG. 17.3—TYPICAL RADIATION CURVE OF BLACK BODY OR FULL RADIATOR.

ordinary incandescent lamp, may extend over a range embracing the ultra-violet, the visible spectrum and the infra-red range as far as $\lambda = 0{\cdot}4$ mm. or so. The temperature of the lamp filament is raised by the passage of a stream of electrons which we call an electric current. On the other hand, the radiation from gaseous discharge lamps is not due to a rise in temperature.

17.5. Temperature Radiation. Incandescence.

When a liquid or solid is heated sufficiently to emit copious radiation, if this is examined by heat-registering instruments for the infra-red range and by a spectroscope within the visible range, it is found that radiations of *all* frequencies between the upper and lower limits are present; the spectrum is continuous, as represented in Fig. 17.3. All bodies are continually exchanging radiant energy and a given body is in thermal equilibrium when it receives and absorbs as much energy as it radiates. The amount of energy emitted per unit area of the surface of a body per second is called the *emissive power* of the surface and may be represented by W. The proportion of incident energy absorbed by a body per unit area per second is its *absorptive power*, A. Both W and A can be measured; W may be expressed in ergs per second or in watts. If S is the area of the surface, the total power radiated is WS watts.

Experiment shows that different substances at the same temperature radiate different total quantities of energy; moreover, they do not radiate the different wavelengths in the same relative proportions. One substance may emit a larger proportion of long wave (red) radiation than another; that is, their radiations possess different *spectral distributions*, or different qualities. It is found that surfaces which emit strongly when heated also absorb radiation strongly when cool and that weak emitters are weak absorbers. In a house provided with central heating one radiator may be painted black and another with, say, aluminium paint. When they are cold the latter reflects more light than the former and so appears bright; it is absorbing less light than the black radiator. When they are hot the black radiator will emit more radiation (heat) than the aluminium one.

A body capable of absorbing *all* the energy falling on it, reflecting and transmitting none, is called a BLACK BODY. It follows from the above that such a body is the best possible radiator; that the thermal radiation from it is greater, at every wavelength, than that from any other body at the same temperature. Hence a black body may also be described as a FULL RADIATOR. A tungsten lamp radiates less than half as much power per unit area of filament surface as the same area of a full radiator at the same temperature. No known substance has the ideal black body properties; even lamp-black reflects about one per cent; but it is possible to achieve full radiation very closely by means of an enclosed furnace provided with a small opening. The radiation from such an enclosure, both the total amount and the spectral distribution of it, is found to depend *only* on its temperature and to follow the black body laws very approximately. Indeed the temperatures of furnaces in practice are determined with an optical pyrometer. The full radiator is extremely useful as the standard radiator against which to compare the performances of other sources ; it represents the upper limit which they may approach but can never exceed. The properties of the full radiator have therefore been the subject of much careful study, particularly by PLANCK.

When the energy radiated by a full radiator furnace at a certain temperature is spread out into a spectrum and the energy contained in successive narrow wavelength bands is measured, a curve of the form shown in Fig. 17.3 is obtained, connecting emissive power and wavelength. The narrow shaded area represents the energy radiated per second between wavelengths λ and $\lambda + d\lambda$, where $d\lambda$ is a very small increment of wavelength. We will refer to the energy represented by the shaded area when the interval $d\lambda$ is one millimicron ($m\mu$) as the energy at wavelength λ and the emissive power at this wavelength as W_λ ergs per second (or watts) per square cm. of radiating surface per $m\mu$. The total area under the curve gives the total energy of all wavelengths radiated per second by unit area of the body at the particular temperature.

The curves of Fig. 17.4 show how the emissive power of a full radiator varies with its temperature. From them two main conclusions may be drawn, one concerning the total quantity of the emitted radiation and the other its quality, namely :

1. As the temperature rises, the total quantity of radiation rapidly increases.
2. As the temperature rises, the wavelength at which the radiation is a maximum, i.e. the *dominant wavelength*, is displaced steadily towards the short wavelength end of the spectrum ; and consequently the proportion of short wave (blue) radiation increases. At a certain temperature (about 6500° K) the proportion of radiation lying within the visible spectrum reaches a maximum.

The first of these conclusions is contained in the STEFAN-BOLTZMAN law (1879) that the total emissive power is proportional to the fourth power of the absolute temperature of the body

$$\text{i.e.} \quad W = \sigma T^4 \qquad (17.4)$$

where T is the temperature on the absolute or Kelvin scale (found by adding 273 to the temperature on the centigrade scale) and $\sigma = 5 \cdot 72 \times 10^{-5}$ erg per cm.^{2} per second. At a temperature of 2000° K (about the melting point of platinum) the emissive power is thus $5 \cdot 72 \times 10^{-5} \times (2000)^4$ ergs/cm.²/sec. $= 91 \cdot 5$ watts/cm.²; whilst at 5000° K, approaching the effective temperature of the sun, it is 3575 watts/cm.² or $4 \cdot 79$ horsepower/cm.² It is to be noted that the law applies to the total radiation from the source, not to the amount of *light* emitted by it.

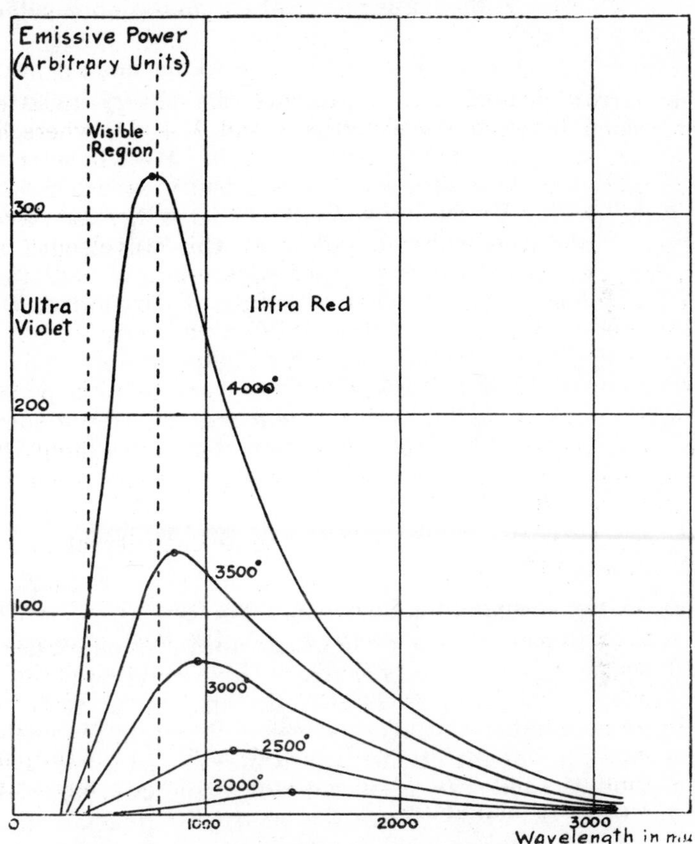

FIG. 17.4—BLACK BODY RADIATION CURVES, IN APPROXIMATELY CORRECT RELATIVE PROPORTIONS. CIRCLES MARK DOMINANT WAVELENGTHS AT VARIOUS TEMPERATURES

With regard to the second conclusion, the dominant wavelength λ_m is given by WIEN'S displacement law

$$\lambda_m T = 2 \cdot 884 \times 10^6 \qquad (17.5)$$

in which λ_m is expressed in $m\mu$.

The human eye in daylight is most sensitive to yellow-green light of wavelength 555 $m\mu$ which is the dominant wavelength of a black body at temperature 5200° K; and solar radiation, allowing for the absorptive effects of the earth's atmosphere, corresponds approximately to this temperature. The human eye thus appears to have adapted itself very well to the main source of the radiation to which it is subjected.

The curves of Fig. 17.4 show in a striking manner what a very large proportion of the radiation emitted even by a full radiator, lies within the infra-red region and is consequently of no use as light. Incandescence is a most inefficient method of producing light. An ordinary 100 watt tungsten lamp, for example, would emit forty times more light if all the emitted radiation were confined to a narrow band at $\lambda = 555\ m\mu$ instead of being spread out over such a wide range of wavelengths; that is, in this sense, the efficiency of the lamp is only 2·5 per cent.

It was the investigation of these radiation phenomena that induced PLANCK to propose his quantum hypothesis in 1900. At low temperatures long waves predominate; at very high temperature the radiation is predominately of short wavelength, and the body appears bluish in colour. Information concerning the quality of the radiation, which we appreciate as colour, is provided by the shape of the radiation curve.

17.6. Gray and Selective Radiators.

Most artificial sources of light are incandescent sources and so give continuous spectra. They may be divided into gray bodies and selective radiators. A GRAY BODY is one which radiates at every wavelength within the visible spectrum an amount of energy bearing a constant ratio to the amount radiated by a full radiator at the same temperature. Over the visible range the energy distribution curve (Fig. 17.4) of such a body has the same shape as the full radiator curve for the same temperature; but each ordinate is less by a constant factor than the corresponding ordinate of the full radiator curve. Hence the quality (colour) of the light it emits is the same as that emitted by the full radiator at that temperature, although the quantity (brightness) is less, being equal to that emitted by a full radiator at some lower temperature. This lower temperature is called the black body or *brightness temperature* of the gray body.

For example: at 3000° K a full radiator emits $5 \cdot 72 \times 10^{-5} \times (3000)^4$ ergs per cm.^{2} per second = 464 watts per cm.^{2} At the same temperature it is found that the metal tungsten (which approximates to a gray body) emits only 154 watts per cm.^{2}, which is the rate of emission of a full radiator at 2280° K; this is its brightness temperature. The ratio $154 \div 464 = 0 \cdot 34$ is called the *emissivity* of tungsten at 3000° K. The emissivity of practical sources is always less than unity. Carbon, platinum and iron are very nearly gray bodies.

In addition to black and gray bodies there are SELECTIVE RADIATORS. The spectral distribution of the energy from such a radiator differs from that of a full radiator at the same temperature; its curve is not of the same shape as the full radiator curve, and so it emits light which appears different in colour, being too blue or too red. The curve may, however, be of almost the same shape, within the visible spectrum, as that of a full radiator at some higher or lower temperature, so that the two sources will appear the same in colour. The temperature of a full radiator that emits light of the same colour is called the COLOUR TEMPERATURE of the body in question. Whereas the brightness temperature of a body must always be less than its true temperature, since no radiator can emit more fully than the ideal full radiator, the colour temperature may be higher (blue radiator) or lower (red) than the true temperature. The clear sky is said to have a colour temperature of about 25000° K even though its blue colour is due to scattering and not to temperature.

The colour temperature of a gray body is the same as its true temperature. The brightness temperature of any thermal radiator must be less than its true temperature. The emissivity of a gray body is independent of wavelength; of a selective radiator it is a function of wavelength.

A method of transforming the infra-red output of incandescent light sources into useful light would be of great benefit, but no method has yet been discovered.

17.7. Electroluminiscence.

The energy required to excite the atoms of a body to radiation can be supplied by various electrical means. One method consists in bombarding the atoms of a gas or vapour at low pressure with electrons. If the electrons are made to acquire sufficient velocity and therefore kinetic energy, they will repel electrons in the gas atoms to outer orbits or even cause them to be ejected from the atoms, which consequently become ionised. The resulting radiation possesses certain definite frequencies that are characteristic of the gas or vapour being used and the spectrum is a line spectrum as distinct from the continuous spectrum obtained from a temperature radiator.

One way in which this electronic bombardment can be achieved is illustrated in Fig. 17.5. A metallic filament F, a spiral or grid G and an electrode P are held in a glass tube containing a gas or metallic vapour at very low pressure. When the filament is heated to incandescence by a battery B, it emits electrons. These are accelerated across the space FG by the voltage V which maintains

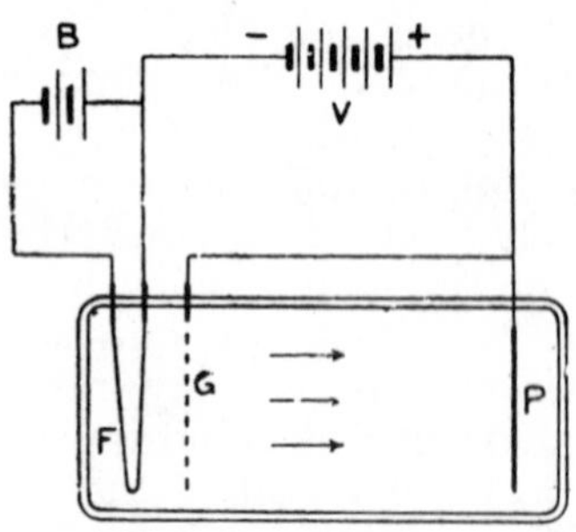

FIG. 17.5—GASEOUS DISCHARGE LAMP.

G at a positive potential relative to F. The stream of electrons passes through the grid and travels to P with a velocity controlled by the potential difference between F and G, colliding with the gaseous atoms on the way. At a low voltage no radiation takes place since the bombarding electrons have insufficient velocity. If the voltage is gradually raised, a critical value V_r is reached at which radiation of a definite single frequency is suddenly emitted; the energy of the bombarding electrons has now increased to a value, $W_m - W_n$ of equation 17.2, which is sufficient to force gaseous electrons from one orbit to the next, so that radiation is emitted as the displaced electron falls back to the first orbit. When $(W_m - W_n)$ is expressed in ergs, the wavelength of this radiation is given by

$$\lambda = \frac{1979 \times 10^{-12}}{W_m - W_n} \text{ m}\mu \quad \text{from equation (17.2)}$$

This critical value of the potential (V_r) is the first radiating or *excitation potential* of the gas. It can be calculated from the above equation and the fact that an electron carrying a charge e and falling through a potential difference V acquires energy equal to $W_m - W_n$. In the case of mercury vapour, experiment shows that the first excitation potential is about 4·9 volts, the radiation being of the single wavelength 253·7 $m\mu$. For sodium vapour the corresponding figures are 2·1 volts and 589·3 $m\mu$, this being the well-known yellow doublet of the sodium spectrum.

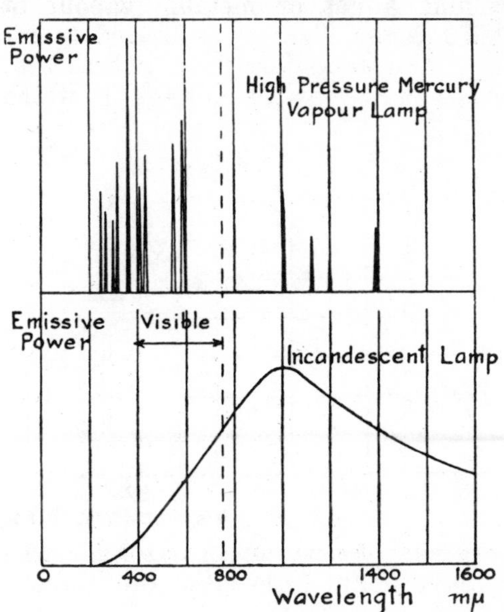

FIG. 17.6—DISTRIBUTION OF ENERGY IN LINE AND CONTINUOUS SPECTRA (NOT TO SCALE.)

If the voltage is further increased, other single line radiations are emitted until the *ionisation potential* is reached at which the complete arc spectrum of the gas or vapour is produced. The ionisation potential (volts) of a few substances are approximately: caesium 3·9, sodium 5·1, mercury 10·4, argon 15·7, neon 21·5, helium 24·5.

Gaseous discharge lamps are historically older than the more familiar incandescent lamps but have come into active commercial use only during the last few years. In Fig. 17.6 the radiation from a high pressure mercury vapour lamp, giving a line spectrum, is exhibited in comparison with that from an incandescent lamp at temperature 3000° K or so, giving a continuous spectrum. As a source of light, apart from its subsidiary equipment, the former is more efficient than the latter since a much greater proportion of the total energy is emitted within the visible region. Moreover, the powerful ultra-violet lines in the mercury spectrum may be transformed into light by coating the inside surface of the lamp (or of an outer bulb) with a fluorescent material such as zinc sulphide. In practice, the losses arising in the subsidiary equipment of these lamps reduce the efficiency.

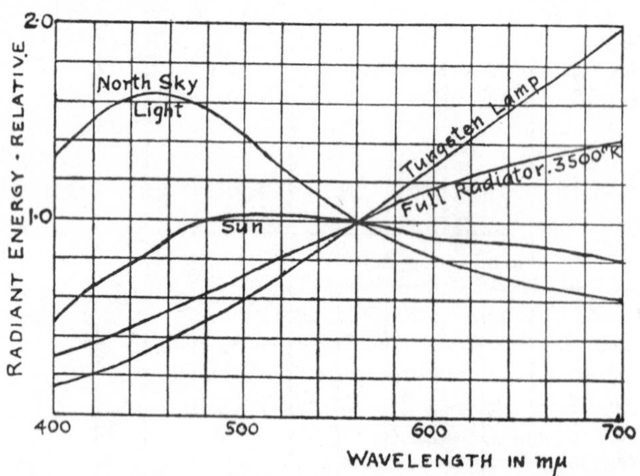

Fig. 17.7—Energy Distribution Curves for certain sources within the Visible Spectrum.

Fig. 17.7 shows the spectral energy distribution curves for a full radiator and a number of common light sources. They give relative values only and, for convenience in showing up the relative performance of such sources, are all made to pass through unity at wavelength 560 $m\mu$.

17.8. The Effects of Radiation.

Radiant energy reaching our planet is essential to our existence. We have learnt to harness most regions of the total spectrum in special ways to serve our needs. From the high frequency gamma and X rays to the low frequency electrical oscillations we utilise radiation in hundreds of ways in medicine, scientific research, industry, navigation, amusements, and so on. It is possible also that some of the radiations, e.g. cosmic rays, affect the ecology of human life in ways of which we are as yet unaware. Any body on which radiation falls is said to be *irradiated.*

In whatever manner a given stream of electromagnetic radiation may have been produced, it is energy capable of setting up some kind of action in any body by which it is absorbed. Of the radiation incident on a body it is only that which is absorbed which can exert any effect on the body (DRAPER, 1879). As a result of such action the energy reappears in some other form. When we seek to investigate the nature of these actions we are to picture the radiation (except at least when dealing with the low frequency electrical regions) as consisting of streams of quanta,* all of the same nature and travelling at the same speed and differing from one another only in their energy content, according to their frequency. The energy of a quantum is given in ergs by the product hf. A quantum of near infra-red radiation of wavelength 1000 $m\mu$ has energy of about 2×10^{-12} erg; a quantum of ultra-violet of wavelength 200 $m\mu$ has five times as much energy. A given stream of radiation may consist of a mixture of quanta of all energy values between certain limits. What will happen when they suddenly impinge on an object and find themselves amongst the whirling atoms near the surface of the object? Clearly this will depend upon the complexity of the atoms, i.e. upon the nature of the irradiated substance. The fate of an infra-red quantum will generally be different from that of an ultra-violet or a visible quantum. Some quanta are reflected, some are absorbed, i.e. they give up their energy to reappear in another form; some pass through the medium, which we say is transparent to such radiation.

A wide variety of effects is to be expected. They may be subdivided thus:

1. Thermal Effects.
2. Electrical Effects:
   (*a*) change in electrical conductivity; e.g. selenium;
   (*b*) the photoelectric effect;
   (*c*) "radio" reception.

* When the radiation lies within the optical range, the quantum is sometimes called the light-quant. The earlier word "photon" should be discarded as this has been given another meaning; see §18.10.

3. Chemical Effects:
   (*a*) photographic;
   (*b*) fading of dyes, hardening of substances, etc.
   (*c*) biological: (i) erythemal effect (sunburn); (ii) breakdown of tissues; (iii) retinal actions leading to visual effect.
4. Fluorescence and phosphorescence.
5. Mechanical pressure.

An irradiated body that can be adapted to measure the incident radiation or put it to some useful purpose may be called a detector of radiation. The detector records

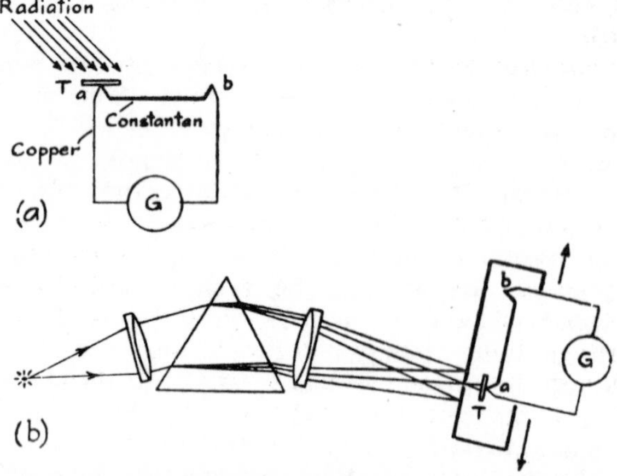

FIG. 17.8—RADIOMETER AND SPECTRORADIOMETER. G. Galvanometer.

only that proportion of the radiation that is converted into the form of energy to which it responds. With some detectors, called *non-selective*, all the energy of all the quanta is converted into heat; they treat quanta of all frequencies alike. The resulting rise in temperature can be measured by such non-selective detectors as the radiometer, the radio-micrometer, the thermopile and the bolometer; the process is called RADIOMETRY. In these instruments the radiation to be measured is directed on to a narrow vane or thermo-junction, the rise in temperature of which produces a rotation of the mechanism carrying the vane, or an electric current, either of which is a measure of the radiation. Fig. 17.8 (a) diagrammatically shows radiation incident on a blackened target T attached to one junction of a thermo-couple made by joining two wires of, say, copper and constantan, at the junctions *a* and *b*. When the temperature of *a* is raised by the absorption of the radiation, an E.M.F. is produced and a current will flow which is directly proportional to the watts per unit area of radiant energy falling on the target. Thus the total irradiation, irrespective of wavelength, is measured.

If it be desired to study the distribution of energy amongst the wavelengths comprised in the radiation, i.e. *spectro-radiometry*, the radiation is first spread out into a spectrum by a suitable prism or a calibrated filter so that isolated bands can be successively explored as indicated in Fig. 17.8 (b).

Instruments of this non-selective type are sensitive to about 10^{-11} watts per mm.^{2}. Is is by their use that the full radiator energy distribution curves of Fig. 17.4 were determined.

Most bodies on which radiation falls are, however, *selective* detectors. They do not treat all quanta alike but respond only to quanta of certain frequencies. Light-sensitive cells, the photographic plate and the human retina are selective detectors. In the photographic plate, quanta of a range lying within certain limits, striking the silver bromide grains, affect them in such a way that the subsequent developing process changes the grains into metallic silver; and the density of the silver deposit is a measure of the energy reaching the plate. Each type of detector exhibits its characteristic effect. If we expose a detector to successive narrow bands of radiation, somewhat as illustrated in Fig. 17.8 (b), and adjust the source for each band so that the quantity of energy is kept constant, at say 1 watt per cm.^{2}, and if we measure the effect produced in the detector for each band, we obtain its *response curve*, connecting response with wavelength. The forms of such curves for a few types of detector are illustrated in Fig. 17.9. Curve (b) shows that a certain photographic plate responds between λ 220 and λ 740, radiation of λ 375 producing the maximum effect. Curve (d) shows that the eye responds maximally to wavelength 555 $m\mu$ and does not respond at all below 400 $m\mu$ or above 700 $m\mu$ or so.

An arrangement for producing a constant quantity of energy at all wavelengths throughout the visible spectrum, as above, we speak of as an *equal energy source*; its radiation curve is a straight line parallel to the x axis. There is no single source which satisfies this condition, even the ideal black body falls short of it, but we can obtain the effect by experimental manipulation; by using a filter, for example.

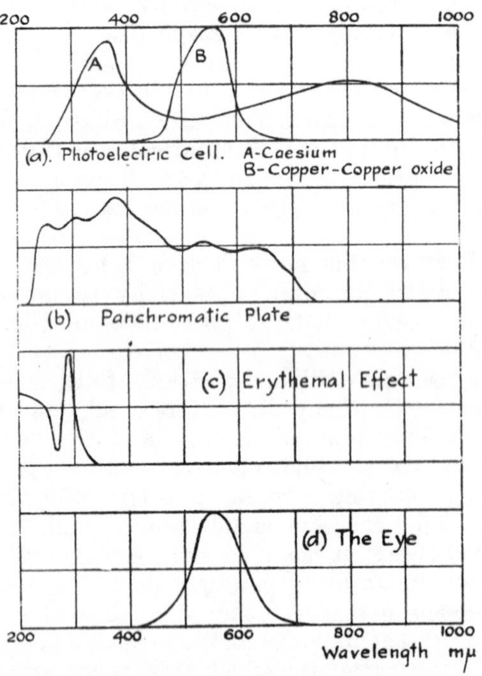

FIG. 17.9—RESPONSE CURVES OF SELECTIVE DETECTORS OF RADIATION SHOWING RELATIVE SENSITIVITY FOR AN AMOUNT OF INCIDENT ENERGY THAT IS CONSTANT AT ALL WAVELENGTHS. (EQUAL ENERGY SOURCE).

17.9. Light Sensitive Cells.

Light sensitive cells deserve mention since they are employed in photometry and in colour work. There are two main classes of such cells: photo-conductive and photo-emissive. The former depend upon the change in electrical resistance of certain substances, such as selenium, when illuminated. Selenium cells find application in television.

The basis of the photo-emissive or photoelectric class is the so-called photoelectric effect; i.e. when light is incident on certain metals, electrons are ejected. These cells are of two main types: (a) vacuum or gas-filled cells, and (b) copper-copper oxide or barrier layer cells. Many of the former resemble wireless valves and contain two electrodes, the cathode consisting of a film of potassium, caesium, rubidium, etc., deposited over an extended area inside the bulb, the anode being a thin wire projecting to the centre of the bulb as represented diagrammatically in Fig. 17.10. The anode is maintained positive relative to the cathode by an external battery. When light is directed on to the cell as indicated by the arrow, the ejected electrons cross the bulb to the anode, this current depending upon the number of such electrons per second and being, therefore, proportional to the intensity of the incident light. When the current reaches its "saturation" value, which depends upon the applied voltage, it is of the order of a few microamperes per lumen.

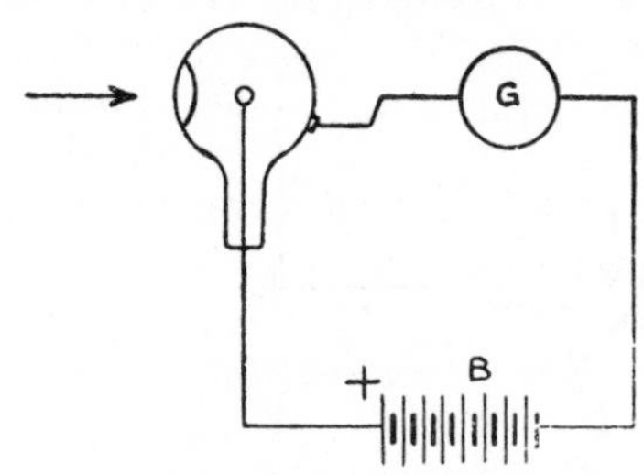

FIG. 17.10—PHOTOELECTRIC CELL. B. Battery. G. Galvanometer.

The gas-filled type of cell contains an inert gas such as argon at very low pressure. The sensitivity is thereby increased due to ionisation of this gas. The electrons on their way from the cathode collide with gas atoms; if the applied voltage is sufficient, the electrons possess the requisite energy to eject electrons from the atoms and so th number of electrons reaching the anode for a given amount of light is increased.

These vacuum and gas-filled cells are used largely in connection with sound-recording from motion-picture film; the response curve A in Fig. 17.9 (a) refers to one of these. Since the curve extends throughout the visible spectrum, it can be made similar to the response curve of the eye by using suitable filters and may then be employed for photometric purposes

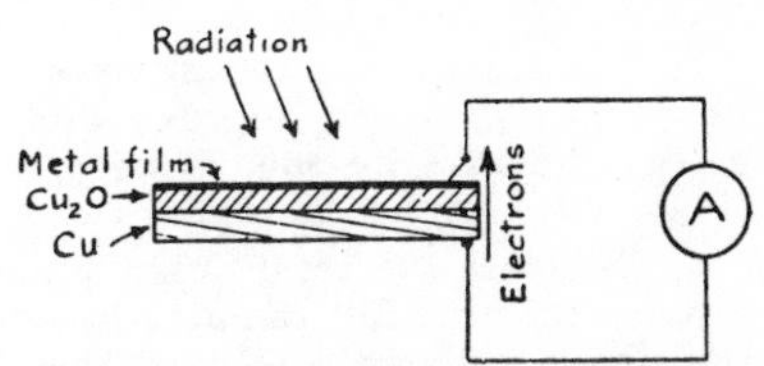

FIG. 17.11—COPPER—COPPER OXIDE OR BARRIER LAYER CELL.

A great advantage of the copper-copper oxide type of cell is that no external electromotive force is needed. As sketched in Fig. 17.11 the cell consists of a purified copper plate coated with cuprous oxide, on which is deposited by sputtering a transparent film of gold or aluminium. On illuminating the cell, electrons are ejected from the cuprous oxide layer to the gold, the current thus generated being of the order of 10^{-4} ampere per lumen. It can be connected up to a moving coil galvanometer calibrated directly in foot-candles and so used as an efficient illumination photometer; it is also used by photographers as an exposure meter. It can be made so that its response curve approximates to that of the eye; compare curve B in Fig. 17.9 (a) with curve (d).

EXERCISES. CHAPTER XVII.

1. Show in their proper sequence on a diagram the various ranges of radiation that are comprised within the electromagnetic spectrum. Indicate on the diagram the approximate wavelength limits of each range, marking particularly the extents of the optical range and the visible spectrum.

Give a brief account of the means that may be adopted to produce these different ranges of the total spectrum.

2. Write a short account of the structure of the atom and of the manner in which radiation is emitted from it. What is a quantum of energy ?

3. In the hydrogen spectrum the Balmer group of lines lies within the visible spectrum, and for this group the innermost orbit to which the electron falls is number 2 (i.e. $n = 2$). Show that if the electron falls from orbit number 3 (i.e. $m = 3$) to orbit number 2, the wavelength of the radiation emitted is $656 \cdot 5\ m\mu$ which is, very approximately, the wavelength of the red (C) line of the hydrogen spectrum. The Rydberg constant for hydrogen is $109677 \cdot 6$ cm.$^{-1}$. Find also the wavelength of the radiation emitted when the electron orbits concerned are the second and the fifth.

4. Explain what is meant by a black body or full radiator. Draw two curves showing approximately the spectral distribution of the energy radiated by such a body at absolute temperature 1000° and 3000°, marking the limits of the visible spectrum on the diagram.

5. Calculate the total quantity of energy in watts radiated by each square cm. of a full radiator at temperature 2848° K; calculate also the dominant wavelength of this emitted radiation. Explain what would happen to these two quantities if the temperature were to rise to 4000° K.

6. Write a short essay on temperature radiation, or thermo-luminescence, and electroluminescence. Give examples of practical sources which emit light in these two ways. What is the characteristic difference between the spectra of the light they emit ?

7. With the aid of a diagram showing their energy distribution curves, explain the differences between a black body, a gray body and a selective radiator. Explain also what is meant by colour temperature.

8. Give diagrams showing the form of the energy distribution of the radiation with reference to wavelength of the two following lamps when operating under normal conditions:

(*a*) a gas-filled tungsten lamp;
(*b*) a mercury vapour discharge lamp.

Explain why the luminous efficiency of one should be higher than that of the other.

9. Explain the meanings of the terms selective detector and non-selective detector, of radiation. Give examples of each. Give a diagram showing the approximate forms of the response curves of a few selective detectors.

10. Write a short account of the complete radiation spectrum extending from the long electrical waves at one end to the short gamma and cosmic rays at the other end. Indicate by name the various regions of radiation in their order on a diagram, inserting figures giving their approximate wavelengths.

Why is the spectrum sometimes called the electromagnetic spectrum? Make a brief mention in your essay of the work of HERTZ and RÖNTGEN in developing our knowledge of radiation. (S.M.C.)

11. Explain what is meant by a full radiator, or black body, and a gray body. Explain also the terms brightness temperature and emissivity as applied to a gray body. Give examples of gray bodies and state briefly how a full radiator can be achieved in practice.

12. Explain the terms colour temperature and brightness temperature and their relations to the true temperature of a body.

13. Explain the terms quantum and light-quant. Give a short account of the quantum theory of radiation and its main difference from the wave theory.

14. Write a short account of the emission of radiation from the atom. In what ways can radiation of wavelength 0·25 mm. be produced? What are the properties of this radiation?

15. Write a short essay on the different types of luminous radiation, stating ways in which they may be produced. To which types do practical sources of light belong?

THE STIMULUS

CHAPTER XVIII

LIGHT

18.1. The Visibility of Radiation. Luminosity Curve.

THE eye* is a selective detector which selects and uses the 390—750 $m\mu$ range of radiation. The magnitude of the effects produced on the eye by the different wavelengths, or in other words the response of the eye to different wavelengths, was illustrated in Fig. 17.9 (d). This important curve requires further discussion.

The eye differs from other selective detectors, particularly in one important respect.† In the case of the photographic plate, for example, although radiation of λ 530 produces a smaller effect than radiation of λ 450, as shown in Fig. 17.9 (b), both radiations produce the same *kind* of effect, a deposition of silver. In the eye, the λ 530 radiation arouses a much greater visual effect than an equal quantity of λ 450 radiation; the former appears much brighter. But apart from this difference in *magnitude*, the effects are different in kind, in *quality*; the former is a green sensation and the latter blue.

Leaving the quality (colour) difference to be discussed later, we are concerned at present with the difference in magnitude of the visual effects. We say the apparent brightness or luminosity of λ 530 radiation is greater than that of λ 450 radiation. If we were to introduce the λ 450 light into the left-hand half of a photometer head and the λ 530 light into the other half, keeping the amounts of *energy* equal in the two halves, it would be observed at once that the right-hand half was the brighter. To determine how much brighter, however, is not so easy, because

* The term eye is often used for brevity to connote the whole of the visual mechanism; it will usually be evident from the context whether the eye alone or the whole mechanism is intended.

† It differs also in that we cannot measure the response of the eye, which is a sensation, in physical units; and again, whereas the effect of radiation on a photographic plate will accumulate for a long time so long as the exposure to light continues, the response of the eye is not cumulative except over a fraction of a second—a regenerative process arises in the retina. These matters are discussed later; e.g. §§ 20.3 and 21.2.

of the difference in colour. It might be suggested that we could increase the energy in the left half-field until the two halves appeared equally bright; if W_1 (watts) were the energy in the left half and W_2 in the right half when equal luminosity is obtained, we could say that the relative luminosities of these two wavelengths for equal amounts of energy are in the ratio

$$\frac{\text{luminosity of } \lambda 450}{\text{luminosity of } \lambda 530} = \frac{W_2}{W_1}$$

With two lights differing so much in colour, however, it would not be easy to determine when they appear equally bright; but we could adjust the energies until the left half-field was perceptibly less bright than the right half and adjust again until it was perceptibly brighter and take the mean of the two energy ratios. The result would probably not be accurate, however. The accuracy can be improved by using what is called the step-by-step method.* Starting at one end of the spectrum we find the relative amounts of energy to produce equality of luminosity for two closely adjacent wavelengths, such that there is very little colour difference in the two halves of the field. We repeat, using the second of these two wavelengths and a third a little further along the spectrum. In this way we obtain the relative luminosities of all wavelengths in the spectrum for equal amounts of energy, i.e. for an equal energy source (§17.8). When the results are plotted against wavelength we obtain the so-called LUMINOSITY CURVE for an equal energy source. It shows how the light sense of the eye varies with wavelength.

Fig. 18.1 depicts what is called the photopic luminosity curve for the normal human eye. It applies to foveal (cone) vision under bright or photopic conditions; i.e. the experiments were carried out under conditions where the brightness of the field did not fall below 10^{-1} to 1 foot-lambert and the eye had been " adapted " to these relatively bright conditions. We see that under such conditions the eye is most sensitive to light of wavelength 555 $m\mu$; the colour of the sensation is greenish-yellow. The visual effectiveness of wavelengths 510 $m\mu$ and 610 $m\mu$ is seen to be only half as great; the *luminosity factor* (v) is 1 at λ 555, 0·5 at λ 510 and λ 610, 0·1 at λ 470 and λ 650, and

* The flicker method could also be used; see §18.9.

so on. The luminosity factors from which Fig. 18.1 has been plotted are given in Table V, Appendix.

Although Fig. 18.1 has been agreed as the standard photopic luminosity curve, there are fairly wide variations from it amongst any group of observers, due to variations in macular pigment which absorbs the light selectively, and to other causes. The individual curves are all of the same general shape, however. Moreover, for any one

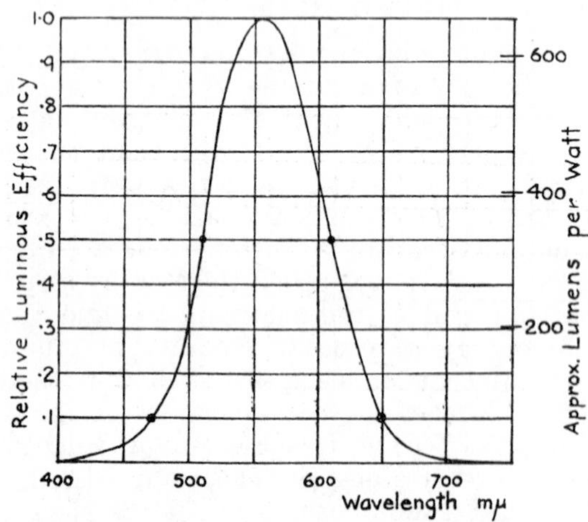

FIG. 18.1—LUMINOSITY CURVE OR CURVE OF RELATIVE LUMINOUS EFFICIENCY FOR NORMAL (PHOTOPIC) EYE; EQUAL ENERGY SOURCE.

individual the curve may vary according to the time of year and diet, maybe because of changes in vitamin A content.

The curve does not apply under conditions of low illumination; under these conditions we obtain what is called the *scotopic* luminosity curve, which will be discussed later (§20.9).

18.2. Luminous Flux.

No actual source of light, not even the full radiator, is an equal energy source. Curve A, Fig. 18.2, gives the distribution of the energy radiated by an incandescent lamp at temperature about 2500° K*; the area under the curve, extending into the ultra-violet and infra-red, gives

* Compare Fig. 17.4.

the total flow or flux of *energy* from the lamp, most of which is useless for vision. To represent the sensation response of the normal eye receiving radiation from such a lamp the ordinates of the luminosity curve P, which applies to a source giving *equal* amounts of energy at all wave-lengths, would have to be reduced in the proportions given by the ordinates of curve A. The area under the resulting curve B, the light distribution curve for the particular

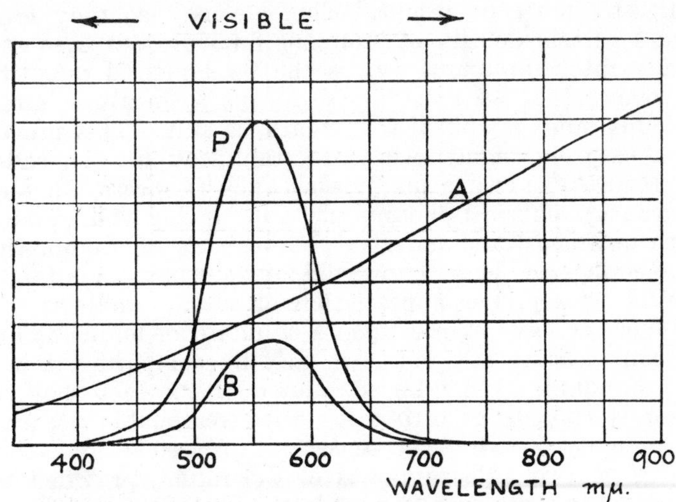

FIG. 18.2—LIGHT DISTRIBUTION CURVE (B) OF INCANDESCENT LAMP. A, ENERGY DISTRIBUTION CURVE OF LAMP; P, LUMINOSITY CURVE OF EYE.

lamp, represents the *light*-giving performance of the lamp or the LUMINOUS FLUX issuing from it. Its shape depends upon the performance of the eye as well as the lamp. We cannot measure luminous flux in units of energy; we have to adopt a unit of light or flux; this is called the LUMEN.

Luminous flux is not just energy; it is a flow of energy weighted according to its capacity to stimulate the eye; it is the rate of flow of *light*. If the luminous source S in Fig. 18.3 is a powerful source such as the crater of an electric arc, there is a heavy concentration of energy flux and therefore also of luminous flux within a cone such as SAB and a surface at A receiving it will be well illuminated. We would say that the *luminous flux density* across the section of the cone is high.

18.3. The Measurement of Light. Photometry.

In our daily tasks it is seldom that we look directly at a primary luminous source* ; practically all the objects around us are seen by means of light which they reflect or transmit to our eyes ; i.e. they are secondary sources. In order that we shall perform our visual tasks accurately and with reasonable comfort the objects we are looking at, especially if they contain fine detail or are poor in contrast,† must be bright. This means that they must send a certain density of luminous flux into our eyes at a steady rate ; luminous flux is the fundamental quantity. It follows that we must devise means to measure luminous flux and establish a standard, a unit. This process of measuring light, with its ramifications, is called PHOTOMETRY. It has subdivisions such as spectro-, heterochromatic-, physical photometry, etc. It has wide applications in science and industry, is the basis of illuminating engineering, and some knowledge of its principles is fundamental to a proper appreciation of visual problems.

When we have agreed upon a standard of luminous flux we can measure any unknown flux by comparing it with this standard. We take advantage of the fact that the brain is capable of estimating with reasonable accuracy the equality of two visual sensations aroused by radiations falling on two adjacent areas of the retina, provided the sensations are not too different in colour. The arrangement used to bring the two lights into juxtaposition for comparison is a PHOTOMETER.

A luminous flux of standard density and quality (colour) could be produced in several ways. The most convenient procedure in practice is to set up and maintain a standard source ; but even so, we define it in terms of luminous flux, as below.

18.4. Luminous Flux and Luminous Intensity.

Fig. 18.3 may help in reaching an understanding of the four main concepts that arise in photometry ; these are luminous flux, luminous intensity, brightness‡ and illumination.

---

* I.e. a body or object emitting light by virtue of a transformation of energy into radiant energy within itself ; e.g. the sun, electric lamp.

† §2.9.

‡ The term now recommended is *luminance* ; we will use either of these terms.

The account given here will be brief; a full discussion would be lengthy as there is controversy over the terminology of the subject; and in any case is not possible until the properties of the eye and visual mechanism have been more fully considered.

At S is a luminous surface (e.g. a portion of a lamp filament) radiating energy, and therefore luminous flux, in all directions. SA is the normal to the surface. At

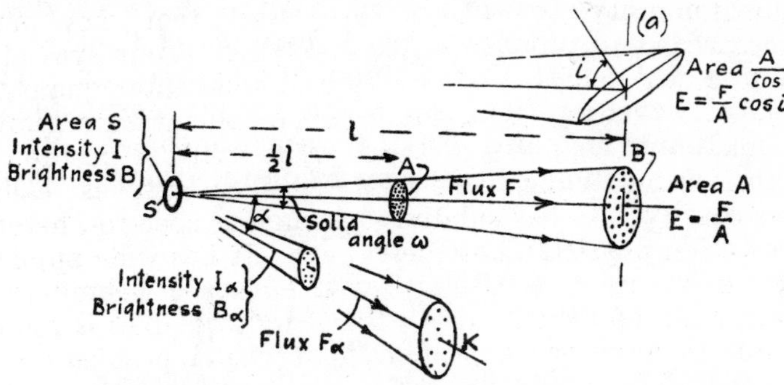

FIG. 18.3—SMALL SURFACE SOURCE AT S RADIATING LUMINOUS FLUX F WITHIN SOLID ANGLE ω ALONG NORMAL SAB AND FLUX $F\alpha$ WITHIN SOLID ANGLE ω ALONG OBLIQUE DIRECTION SK. IF SURFACE IS A PERFECT DIFFUSER, THEN $B\alpha = B$.

first we will suppose the surface to be of negligible area so that we may call it a *point source.* If this were radiating equally in all directions it would be called a uniform point source. In practice the surface will not radiate uniformly in all directions; the flux will be packed more densely in a cone surrounding the normal SA than within an equal cone in an oblique direction such as SK—the dots shown in the cross sections may be conceived as representing light quanta. The concentration of flux in any direction will depend upon the luminous intensity (or candle power) of the source in that direction.

If F is the luminous flux within a narrow cone of solid angle ω surrounding a certain direction, then the LUMINOUS INTENSITY of the source in that direction is given by I where

$$I = \frac{F}{\omega} \tag{18.1}$$

Thus intensity is the flux per unit solid angle; it is a measure of flux concentration. The unit in which it is measured is called the CANDLE because in early days it was in fact a candle satisfying certain conditions. This was later replaced by a standardised pentane lamp and now (1948) the standard is an enclosed black body radiator operating at the freezing point (2046° K) of platinum, this having a brightness of exactly 60 candles per square cm.

> The unit of luminous flux is the LUMEN, which is the luminous flux emitted in unit solid angle by a uniform source of one candle.

The luminosity curve of Fig. 18.1 tells us that the radiant power needed to produce a given quantity of light varies with the wavelength. It is found that to produce one lumen at wavelength 555 $m\mu$ where the luminosity factor is a maximum, requires 0·00154 watt; or, at this wavelength and assuming the conversion of energy occurs

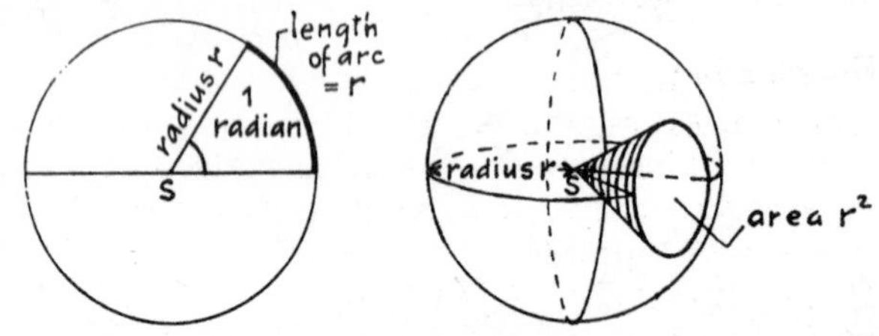

FIG. 18.4—UNIT ANGLE (RADIAN) AND UNIT SOLID ANGLE (STERADIAN).

without loss, the amount of light produced is 650 lumens per watt (650 = 1 ÷ 0·00154).* At λ 610, where the luminosity factor is 0·5, the power-light equivalent is 325 lumens per watt. An ordinary gas-filled tungsten filament lamp gives 10 to 18 lumens per watt, according to size, which shows how inefficient temperature radiation is in providing light. Most of the energy is infra-red and is lost. A high efficiency electronic flash lamp will give 40 lumens per watt which is a little more efficient.

A circle of radius r drawn with S as centre has a circumference of $2\pi r$ (Fig. 18.4). The unit of angle called the *radian* is the angle subtended at the centre by an arc equal in length to the radius and so there are 2π radians in the complete circle. A sphere of radius r has surface area $4\pi r^2$. The unit of solid angle, called the *steradian*, is the solid angle subtended at the centre by an area equal to the square on the radius, i.e. r^2. Thus the total solid angle

* Actually this power-light equivalent has not been finally agreed, but 650 is close to the mean of the most likely results.

around the centre S is 4π steradians; and the total flux radiated by a uniform point source of one candle is, therefore, 4π lumens.

On the surface of a sphere of twice the radius ($2r$) one steradian would mark out an area $A = (2r)^2 = 4r^2$. If the cone of solid angle ω (Fig. 18.3) has a cross-sectional area A at the point B distant l from S, then $\omega = \frac{A}{l^2}$; A and l^2 are to be expressed in the same unit. Strictly we should take the *spherical* area at B but the plane area will usually differ from the spherical by a negligible amount. Thus a circular area of 3 mm. radius distant 20 cm. from the source S subtends at the latter a solid angle $\omega = \frac{\pi \times 9}{(20 \times 10)^2} = 7{\cdot}068 \times 10^{-4}$ steradian.

18.5. Illumination.

Any surface, or aperture, on which luminous flux falls is said to be illuminated; the illumination is measured by the quantity of flux in lumens received by unit area of the surface or aperture.

> If luminous flux F falls on a small area A surrounding a point on a surface, the ILLUMINATION at that point is given by E where

$$E = \frac{F}{A} \qquad (18.2)$$

If the surface is distant l from the luminous source of intensity I (in that direction) then

$$E = \frac{F}{A} = \frac{\omega I}{\omega l^2} = \frac{I}{l^2}$$

Thus illumination is somewhat analagous to intensity in that it expresses the flux density at a certain place. It is concerned with the flux *received* and is quite independent of the nature of the surface, which may indeed be an aperture or the entrance pupil of an instrument or the eye. Illumination is measured in lumens per unit area, the actual unit depending upon the unit of length employed. Thus we have units such as

1 lumen per square metre or 1 lux or 1 metre-candle.

1 lumen per square cm. or 1 phot.

1 lumen per square foot or 1 foot-candle.

The illumination on this page, if being read in artificial light, is probably between two and ten lumens per sq. foot.

Referring to Fig. 18.3, if the point A is half-way between S and B, the cone has area A at B and area $\frac{1}{4}A$ at A. Each of these areas receives the same amount of flux and so the illumination at A is four times the illumination at B; that is, the illumination from a point source is inversely proportional to the square of the distance from the source; which is the *inverse square law.*

If a surface receiving the flux at B were tilted through an angle i as shown in diagram (a), the area of the surface intercepted by the cone of solid angle ω would be increased from A to $A/\cos i$. The same flux falls on these two areas and so the illumination is decreased to

$$E = \frac{F}{A} \cos i = \frac{I}{l^2} \cos i \quad (18.3)$$

which is sometimes called the cosine law of illumination.

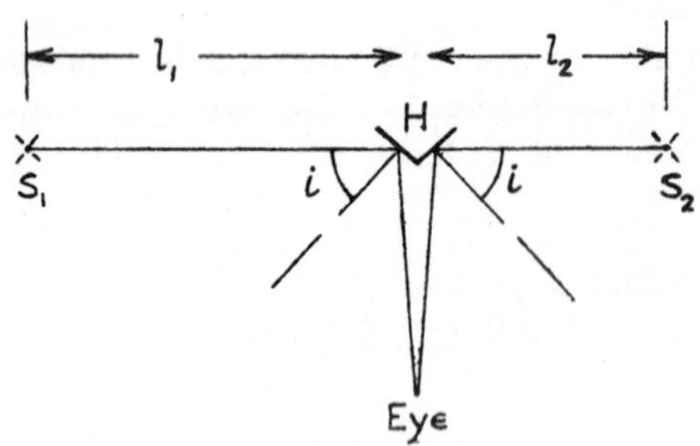

Fig. 18.5—The Principle of the Photometer.

In photometers intended for measuring luminous intensity it is arranged that the source to be measured and the standard source with which it is to be compared illuminate adjacent areas of a diffusely reflecting surface which is mounted in some kind of photometer head H. The form of the head varies in different types of photometer, but the principle of them all is illustrated in Fig. 18.5. If S_1 is the standard source of intensity I_1 in the direction S_1H and S_2 is the unknown source of intensity I_2 in the direction S_2H, then the illumination they produce on the two areas of the head are

$$E_1 = \frac{I_1}{l_1^2} \cos i \qquad \text{and} \qquad E_2 = \frac{I_2}{l_2^2} \cos i$$

When the distances are adjusted by moving the head or one of the sources along the line S_1S_2 until the two areas appear to have the same brightness, the illuminations are equal, assuming the reflection factor is the same over the two areas; then we have

$$\frac{I_1}{l_1^2} = \frac{I_2}{l_2^2} \tag{18.4}$$

The method is based on the assumption that the sources are point sources; provided the greatest dimension of the source is not greater than one twentieth of its distance from the photometer head, this is justified. Certain precautions and careful observation are necessary to attain an accuracy of one to two per cent. It is also assumed that the sources are of approximately the same colour; special procedure, one of which is the flicker method, are needed when the colours are different; the procedure is then called *heterochromatic* photometry.

In *spectro*-photometry the light from the sources is dispersed into two spectra and these are compared wavelength by wavelength. In *physical* photometry the eye is replaced by a photoelectric cell or a photographic plate.

18.6. Brightness or Luminance.

The conception of a point source is useful in that it simplifies calculations, but it is important to realise that in practice all sources* and illuminated objects have finite and measurable size; and it is with such finite objects that we are now dealing. If, to a normal observer, one of two adjacent similar objects appears brighter than the other, this means that the retinal image of the one is receiving more flux per unit area than that of the other. Thus the apparent brightness or luminosity of an object, be it a self-luminous surface or one that is reflecting or transmitting light (the term brightness or luminance is used in relation to any of these) depends upon the illumination of its retinal image. And since to each elementary area of the image there corresponds a certain area of the source or object, the brightness of the latter depends upon the flux emitted by it per unit area.

Suppose the small radiating surface of area S at S (Fig. 18.3) is observed normally by an eye at B. The luminous intensity in the normal direction SB is I candles. If the pupil of the eye, of area a, subtends a solid angle ω at S, then within this cone

---

* **Except stars.**

flux emitted by surface $= F = I\omega$ lumens; equ. (18.1)

flux emitted per unit area of surface $= \frac{F}{S} = \frac{I}{S}\omega$ lumens.

Suppose the radiating surface is viewed, at the same distance l, from a position K and that along this direction, inclined at angle α to the normal SB, the intensity of the surface is I_α candles, which will be smaller than I. Since the surface is viewed obliquely its apparent area, i.e. its area projected on a plane perpendicular to the direction of observation (or its orthogonally projected area) will be reduced from S to $S \cos \alpha$. The eye's pupil subtends the same solid angle as before so within the cone of solid angle ω

flux emitted by surface along SK $= F_\alpha = I_\alpha\, \omega$

$$\left.\begin{array}{l}\text{flux emitted per unit apparent} \\ \quad\text{area of surface}\end{array}\right\} = \frac{F_\alpha}{S \cos \alpha} = \frac{I_\alpha}{S \cos \alpha} \cdot \omega.$$

The quantity $\frac{I}{S}$ in the one case and $\frac{I_\alpha}{S \cos \alpha}$ in the other, appertaining to the radiating surface, is called the brightness or luminance of the surface in the particular direction.

Thus the brightness (luminance) B of a surface element in a given direction is the luminous intensity of the element in that direction per unit of apparent (orthogonally projected) area, i.e.

$$B = \frac{I_\alpha}{S \cos \alpha} \tag{18.5}$$

$$= \frac{I}{S} \quad \text{in the normal direction.}$$

It is measured in candles per unit area, the actual unit depending upon the unit of length employed. Thus we have units such as

1 candle per sq. metre	1 candle per sq. cm. = 1 stilb.
1 candle per sq. foot	1 candle per sq. inch.

Tables of conversion factors of units, brightnesses of various sources and illuminations for various purposes are given in the Appendix.

18.7. The Perfect Diffuser. Lambert's Cosine Law.

It is an experimental fact that most self-luminous surfaces and many reflecting and diffusing surfaces (except those with a high polish) appear almost equally bright in all directions. A heated metal sphere or the sun appear equally bright over their entire surface, for example. A surface that has the same brightness in all directions is called a perfect diffuser. A block of magnesium carbonate is the nearest approach to this in practice. - It follows from equ. (18.5) that for such a surface

$$\frac{I_a}{S \cos a} = \frac{I}{S} \quad \text{or} \quad I_a = I \cos a \tag{18.6}$$

or the luminous intensity in any direction varies as the cosine of the angle between that direction and the normal to the surface; which is known as LAMBERT'S *cosine law of emission* (1760).

If a surface element of area S had the same luminous intensity in all directions, like the ideal uniform point source, it would radiate $2\pi I$ or $2\pi BS$ lumens over a complete hemisphere, i.e. $2\pi B$ lumens per unit area of the surface. It can easily be shown* that for a surface obeying Lambert's law, i.e. a perfect diffuser, which has the same *brightness* in all directions, the total flux radiated over the hemisphere is equal to πB lumens per unit area of the surface, where B is its brightness in candles per unit area.

No surface reflects all the light incident upon it; white blotting paper reflects up to 80 per cent, which is called its REFLECTION FACTOR. If the illumination on a *perfectly diffusing surface* of reflection factor ρ is E, the surface receives E lumens per unit area and it reflects ρE lumens per unit area; hence its brightness is $\rho E/\pi$ candles per unit area; or E lumens per unit area. Thus B (ft.L) $= E$ (lum./ft.^{2}) x l.

There are advantages, especially when dealing with such non self-luminous surfaces, in expressing brightness in another unit, namely in *lumens* per unit area rather than candles per unit area. The actual unit depends upon the unit of length employed; thus for a perfectly diffusing surface (emitting or reflecting)

1 lambert ≡ 1 lumen per sq. cm.
1 foot-lambert ≡ 1 lumen per sq. foot

and from the above discussion we have

1 candle per sq. cm. = π lamberts
1 candle per sq. foot = π foot-lamberts.

18.8. Illumination of Image in Instrument or Eye.

Within wide limits and neglecting atmospheric absorption, the illumination of the retinal image of a surface is the same at whatever distance it is viewed. The truth of this may appear to be evident but we will establish it with the

* See Example, §18.11.

aid of Fig. 18.6, which will be useful in other connections. The diffusely radiating surface of area S and luminance B candles per unit area is at a distance l from a lens which forms an image of area S' on a screen placed at the conjugate distance l'. The aperture of the lens, of area a, subtends the solid angles ω and ω' at the object and image respectively. The linear magnification of the image is given by $m = \frac{l'}{l}$ so that the *areas* of image and object are in the ratio $\frac{l'^2}{l^2}$.

i.e. $\frac{S'}{S} = \frac{l'^2}{l^2}$; also $\omega = \frac{a}{l^2}$ and $\omega' = \frac{a}{l'^2}$

so that $$\frac{S'}{S} = \frac{\omega}{\omega'} \qquad (18.7)$$

flux reaching lens aperture $= I\omega = BS\omega$ lumens.

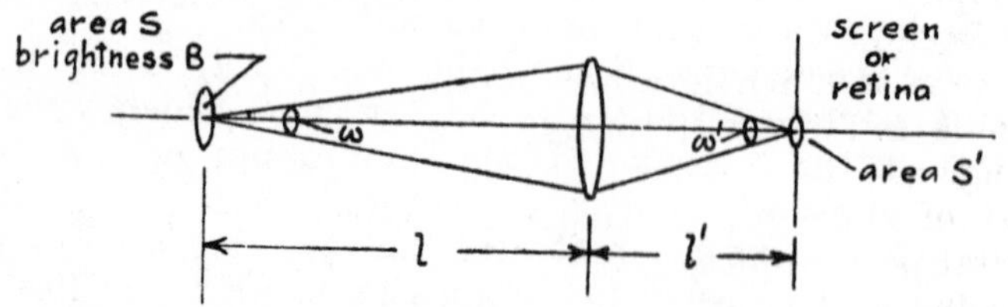

Fig. 18.6—Apparent Brightness or Luminosity. Illumination of image is independent of distance of object.

Neglecting the losses that occur in traversing the lens, this flux reaches and is spread over the image, so that

$$\text{illumination of image } E' = \frac{BS\omega}{S'}$$
$$= B\,\omega' \text{ lumens per unit area.} \qquad (18.8)$$

The lens and screen may serve to represent the optical system and retina of an observing eye which is focusing on the object.* Thus the illumination of the retinal image is independent of the distance and depends only on two factors, namely the " physical " brightness or luminance, B, of the object and the solid angle of the image cone. It is true that if the object distance were increased the

* In this case the only difference is that the image space, within the eye, has refractive index n', so that

$$m = \frac{l'}{n'l};\ \frac{S'}{S} = \frac{l'^2}{n'^2 l^2} = \frac{1}{n'^2}\cdot\frac{\omega}{\omega'} \text{ and } E' = n'^2 \,.\, B\omega'$$

which does not affect the argument.

solid angle ω would be decreased and less flux would enter the lens (or eye); but the area of the image would be decreased in the same proportion and so its illumination would be unchanged. The flux would be spread over fewer retinal elements.

If, with the object at a given distance, the aperture of the lens (or eye) is reduced, or if for some reason the aperture is not filled with light, then the image cone angle ω' is reduced and the illumination of the image and, therefore, in the case of the eye, the apparent brightness of the object, will be decreased. This question of filling the aperture of the lens or optical system is of importance in the design of projection systems.

We have been dealing above with sources and objects of finite area the images of which are spread over, and stimulate, a number of retinal elements. When the source or object is very small or so far removed from the eye as to subtend a small angle of the order of a few minutes at the eye (e.g. a star), it approximates to a point. Its image then is a diffraction pattern the size of which does not change as the "point" is moved further from the eye; most of the light in this image is concentrated over the central portion of the central disc of the diffraction pattern so that the stimulation is largely confined to a single retinal cone or rod. As such a "point" object moves further away, the solid cone of light entering the eye diminishes, the single element is less stimulated and the visibility *does* decrease with distance; the object finally becomes invisible because the stimulation falls below the threshold of vision.

Note that the term brightness or luminance refers to the stimulus and the term apparent brightness or luminosity to the sensation.

18.9. Heterochromatic Photometry. Flicker Method.

Reference has been made more than once in this chapter to the difficulty experienced in determining the equality of luminosity of two lights when they differ appreciably in colour; and though it does not fall within the scope of this book to describe methods of photometry, a brief mention of the photometry of differently coloured lights, i.e. heterochromatic photometry, will be useful. We shall see later that the physiological basis of flicker phenomena is not clearly understood, but it is found experimentally that considerable precision is obtained by the method if certain precautions are observed.

The flicker photometer is so designed that the two coloured lights to be compared are presented alternately to the eye in the same field of view ; the principle of the instrument is shown in Fig. 18.7. Light from one of the sources to be compared, S_1, is directed to illuminate a screen H which is coated with magnesium oxide. B is a sector disc, which may be of the form shown at (a), also coated with magnesium oxide and illuminated by light from the second source S_2 ; it can be rotated at varying speeds which are under sensitive control. The eye at E observes B and H through a clear-cut bevelled aperture at D which subtends an angle of 2° at E. The interior of

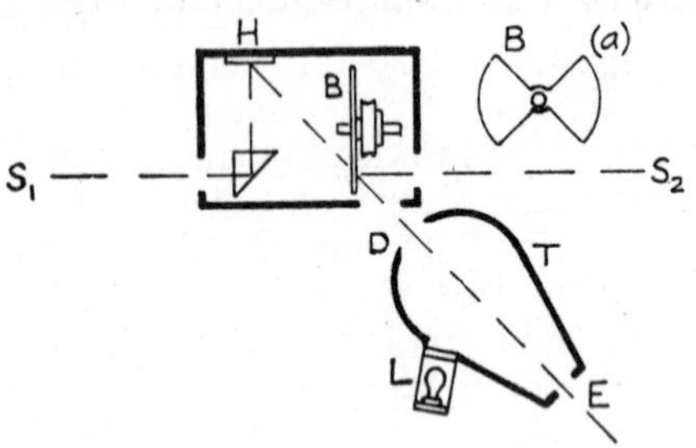

FIG. 18.7—FLICKER PHOTOMETER (GUILD).

the observing tube T is coated like B and H and maintained at an even brightness of about 2·5 foot-lamberts by means of a lamp L provided with an opal glass. The two sources are positioned so that the aperture D appears of about the same brightness as the interior. When the disc B is revolved slowly, the eye sees H and B alternately and the field flickers whether the two lights are equally bright or not. As the speed of rotation is raised the flicker becomes less pronounced ; it can be made to disappear by adjusting the speed and the distances of the sources from the photometer head. The test source S_2 is fixed and the comparison source S_1 moved towards or away from the head, the speed of rotation being reduced until the flicker is just on the point of disappearing. The brightnesses of H and B are then equal and the relative intensities of S_1 and S_2 can be calculated from their recorded distances from the head.

The basis of this flicker method is that when two lights differing both in luminosity and colour are alternated, the flicker due to the colour difference disappears at a lower speed than the flicker due to luminosity difference. Thus the equality of brightness can be judged without hindrance from the colour difference. The results are reliable only: when the field of view does not exceed 2°, so that a limited area of the retina is concerned in the observation; when the brightness of the test patch is not less than about 2·5 foot-lamberts so that we are working above the so-called Purkinje range; and when the surrounding field is of about the same brightness, since this conduces to comfort in observation.

18.10. Concerning Units and Sources of Brief Duration.

Units of Luminance (Brightness) and Illumination.

For the sake of uniformity and to help the student to make comparisons more readily, in most of the graphs and examples quoted in later chapters the luminance of a surface or an object will be expressed in millilamberts or foot-lamberts; these two units are nearly equal. The illumination of a surface or aperture will usually be stated in lumens per sq. foot (foot-candles). The connection between these and other units is given in Table II or can be calculated from the data given in 18.5 to 18.7.

For example:

$$1 \text{ millilambert} = \frac{1}{1000} \text{ lambert}$$

$$= \frac{1}{1000\,\pi} \text{ candles per sq. cm. (§18.7).}$$

$$= \frac{100 \times 100}{1000\,\pi} = \frac{10}{\pi} \text{ candles per sq. metre.}$$

Retinal Illumination: the photon.

In §18.8 we found that, neglecting losses in the eye, the illumination (E') of the retinal image depends upon the luminance (B) of the source or object and the size of the solid angle (ω') of the cone of light travelling to each point of the retinal image; and that since this solid angle is directly proportional to the area (a) of the pupil, the retinal illumination varies with the pupil size. Thus, when stating the effect at the retina oι a stimulus of given luminance it is necessary also to specify the pupil size. This has been done in defining a unit of retinal illumination called the PHOTON,* which is the illumination of the retina when a surface of luminance one candle per sq. metre is viewed by an eye through a pupil having an area of one sq mm.

Thus, in the case of a surface of luminance B millilamberts (1 m.l. $= \frac{10}{\pi}$ can./metre²) observed through a pupil of diameter d mm., we have

$$\text{retinal illumination } E' = \left(B \times \frac{10}{\pi}\right) \times \frac{\pi}{4} d^2 \text{ photons}$$

$$= B \times \frac{5}{2} d^2 \text{ photons.}$$

A surface of luminance one millilambert observed through a 4 mm. diameter pupil gives a retinal illumination of $2{\cdot}5 \times 4^2 = 40$ photons.

Steady Sources and Flash Sources.

It has already been explained (§18.2) that the lumen is a certain standard rate of flow of light; a certain quantity of light radiated per second in a flow which is continuous and steady for at least a few seconds. There are sources which emit light in very short flashes lasting, maybe, less than a thousandth of a second; in modern flash discharge tubes the total discharge per flash, during which the rate of radiation rises to a maximum and falls to zero, is completed in $\frac{1}{5000}$th of a second, or less. If the flashing source is a distant one, such as a navigation signal, it may appear very faint, just above the lower limit or "threshold" of visibility; whether a sensation will result, so that the source is seen, will depend ultimately upon whether a sufficient number of light-quanta reach and are absorbed by the receptors in the retina. This is discussed in more detail in §21.2.

In the case of a steady source the retina is receiving a flow of light at a more or less steady rate; the flash source delivers a packet of light, as it were, in one burst. But in both cases the physiological result is the discharge of a train of impulses along the optic nerve fibres to the brain and it seems that it is the rate at which the brain receives these impulses that determines the resulting visual sensation. Even in the case of the flash source the sensation takes time to grow to its maximum and it lasts for a longer period than the period of the flash. And so it is that the sensation we experience is of exactly the same kind in the case of both types of source. Hence we may legitimately compare a flash source with a continuous source, such as a star or a candle; an example will be found in §18.11.

*** Because of the risk of confusion with the light-quant, which was earlier, and still is, called the photon (see §17.8), it has been proposed in America to give the name *Troland* to the unit of retinal illumination; the desirability of the unit was first suggested by L. T. Troland.**

Luminosity of Radiations on Quantum Basis.

The luminosity curve of Fig. 18.1 shows the relative magnitudes of the visual effect produced by light of various wavelengths when the amount of *energy* (e.g. in ergs) radiated by the source is kept constant at all wavelengths; i.e. when the radiating source is an equal energy source. We have seen (equ. 17.2) that the quantum of energy is greater for short than for long wavelengths; for example, for wavelengths 545, 550 and 555 $m\mu$ respectively it has the values $3 \cdot 632 \times 10^{-12}$, $3 \cdot 598 \times 10^{-12}$ and $3 \cdot 566 \times 10^{-12}$ erg. The luminosity factors for these wavelengths as given by Fig. 18.1 or Table V are 0·980, 0·995 and 1·000 respectively; that is, these are the relative visual effectivities of these three wavelengths when the energy is kept constant. But if we take into consideration the relative values of the quantum at each of these wavelengths, their relative visual effectivities for each quantum delivered to the retina, i.e. "on a quantum basis", are:

$\lambda 545 : 0 \cdot 980 \times 3 \cdot 632 = 3 \cdot 560$ on quantum basis
$\lambda 550 : 0 \cdot 995 \times 3 \cdot 598 = 3 \cdot 580$,,
$\lambda 555 : 1 \cdot 000 \times 3 \cdot 566 = 3 \cdot 566$,,

The smallest amount of energy that a molecule of any substance can emit or absorb is one quantum. It has been shown that in numerous chemical reactions each molecule absorbs just one quantum of energy. If, as experiments show to be probable, this is true for visual purple, it follows from the above figures that the most visually effective radiation is not $\lambda 555$ but a wavelength very close to $\lambda 550$.

Similarly in relation to the scotopic luminosity curve to be discussed in Chapter XX, the wavelength of greatest luminosity under dark conditions is about $\lambda 510$ on an equal energy basis and little more than $\lambda 500$ on a quantum basis.

18.11. Examples.

1 (*a*) Two small lamps are separated by 2 metres. Along the direction joining them their intensities are 40 and 90 candles respectively. Find the position between them of a photometer head when the illuminations on it due to the two lamps are equal; i.e. the photometer is in "balance".

(*b*) When the 90 candle lamp is covered with a sheet of neutral glass it has to be moved 20 cm. nearer to the photometer head to restore balance. Find the percentage light transmission of the glass.

Answer: (*a*) With photometer in balance

$$\frac{I_1}{l_1^2} = \frac{I_2}{l_2^2} \quad \text{and} \quad l_2 = 2 - l_1 \text{ metres.}$$

$$\frac{40}{l_1^2} = \frac{90}{(2 - l_1)^2} \quad \text{or} \quad 5l_1^2 + 16l_1 - 16 = 0$$

$$\therefore\ l_1 = \frac{4}{5} \text{ metre} = 80 \text{ cm.} \qquad l_2 = \frac{6}{5} \text{ metre} = 120 \text{ cm.}$$

(*b*) Let x = fraction of light transmitted by neutral glass; then

$$\frac{I_1}{l_1^2} = \frac{x\, I_2}{(l_2 - 20)^2} \qquad l_1 \text{ and } l_2 \text{ in cm.}$$

$$\frac{40}{80^2} = \frac{x \, . \, 90}{100^2} \qquad \therefore\ x = \frac{4}{9} \cdot \frac{100}{64} = \frac{25}{36} = 69 \cdot 4 \text{ per cent}$$

2. (a) A source of light, small enough to be treated as a point, emits light uniformly in all directions. If its luminous intensity is 50 candles, what is the total luminous flux radiated by it in lumens and what illumination will it produce on a screen distant $66\frac{2}{3}$ cm.?

(b) If a $+1$ D spherical lens of 2 cm. aperture is set up at this distance and the screen moved to a position 50 cm. beyond the lens and perpendicular to the optical axis, find the illumination on the screen. Neglect lens aberration.

Answer : (a) Area of sphere $= 4\pi r^2$.
Total solid angle around point $= 4\pi$.
Total flux radiated $= 4\pi I = 4\pi \,.\, 50 = 628\cdot 3$ lumens.

This is spread uniformly over surface of any sphere with source as centre, so

$$\text{Illumination} = E = \frac{4\pi I}{4\pi r^2} = \frac{I}{r^2}$$

If $r = 66\frac{2}{3}$ cm. $\quad E = \dfrac{50}{(66\frac{2}{3})^2} = 0\cdot 01125$ lumens/cm.^{2} or phots.

(b) Area of lens $= \pi$ cm.^{2}
Flux incident on lens $= \cdot 01125 \times \pi = 0\cdot 0353$ lumens.

Light leaves lens with vergence $-1\cdot 5 + 1 = -0\cdot 5$ D, diverging from a virtual image point 200 cm. back from lens.

$$\left.\begin{array}{l}\text{area of pencil of}\\ \text{light on screen}\end{array}\right\} = \text{area of lens} \times \left(\frac{250}{200}\right)^2 = \pi \,.\, 1\cdot 5625 \text{ cm.}^2$$

$$\text{illumination on screen} = \frac{\text{flux}}{\text{area}} = \frac{\cdot 01125 \,.\, \pi}{1\cdot 5625 \,.\, \pi} = 0\cdot 0072 \text{ lumens/cm.}^2$$

3. (a) Calculate the illumination in lumens per sq. metre at the earth's equator at noon, given that the sun is 93 million miles from the earth, its radius is 433,000 miles, its brightness is 165,000 candles per sq. cm. and ten per cent of the light is absorbed by the atmosphere.

(b) If a strip of perfectly diffusing white material of reflection factor $0\cdot 8$ is laid on the ground, what will be its brightness ?

Answer : Assume 1 metre $=$ 40 inches.

(a) Area of sun's surface $= 4\pi r^2$
$= 4\pi(433 \times 10^3 \times 1760 \times 36 \times 2\cdot 5)^2$ cm.^{2}

Assuming radiation according to Lambert's cosine law:
Flux from each sq. cm. $= 165{,}000\pi$ lumens.
Area of sphere of radius 93×10^6 miles

$$= 4\pi\left(93 \times 10^6 \times 1760 \times \frac{36}{40}\right)^2 \text{ metre}^2$$

$$\text{Flux on one sq. metre} = \frac{9}{10} \cdot \frac{\pi \,.\, 165 \,.\, 433^2 \,.\, 2\cdot 5^2 \,.\, 16 \,.\, 10^{11}}{93 \,.\, 93 \,.\, 10^{12}}$$

$= 101{,}100$ lumens.

(b) Flux radiated by strip $= 0\cdot 8(101100)$ lumens per metre^2

$$\text{brightness} = \frac{80880}{\pi} = 25{,}750 \text{ candles per metre}^2$$

$= 2\cdot 575$ candles per cm.^{2}

4. Show that the total luminous flux radiated over the hemisphere by a perfect diffuser of brightness B candles per cm.^{2} is πB lumens per cm.^{2}; i.e. πB lamberts.

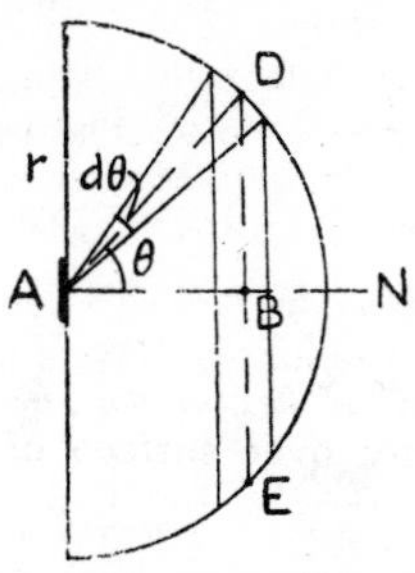

FIG. 18.8—ILLUSTRATING EXAMPLE 18.4.

Answer : In Fig. 18.8 the surface of area S is at A and is radiating over the hemisphere to the right. The luminous intensity of the surface along direction AD, inclined at θ to the normal AN is I_θ candles. If radius of hemisphere is r cm., illumination at D is

$$E = \frac{I_\theta}{r^2} = \frac{B \,.\, S \,.\cos\theta}{r^2} \text{ lumens per cm.}^2$$

Illumination is uniform all over the zone DE which has radius DB $= r\sin\theta$.

Area of zone $= r\,d\theta \,.\, 2\pi r\sin\theta$ cm.^{2}

Flux over zone $= E \times$ area $= 2\pi\, B \,.\, S \,.\, \sin\theta \,.\, \cos\theta \,.\, d\theta$ lumens.

$$\left.\begin{array}{r}\text{Total flux within cone}\\ \text{of semi-angle } \theta\end{array}\right\} = \pi BS\int_0^\theta 2\sin\theta \,.\, \cos\theta \,.\, d\theta$$

$$= \pi BS \sin^2\theta \text{ lumens.}$$

Total flux over hemisphere $(\theta = 90) = \pi BS$ lumens

$$\text{or}\quad \left.\begin{array}{l}\text{Flux radiated per unit}\\ \text{area of surface}\end{array}\right\} = \pi B \text{ lumens per cm.}^2$$

$$= \pi B \text{ lamberts.}$$

5. (*a*) A sight testing chart is observed by an eye the pupil diameter of which is 4 mm. On a certain area of the chart the illumination is 100 lumens per sq. metre ; its reflection factor is 0·7. Find the amount of luminous flux entering the eye, the illumination of the retinal image, the flux and the energy in watts falling on each foveal cone. Assume 7500 cones in the foveal area.

(*b*) If the illumination out of doors due to the sun and sky is 40000 lumens per sq. metre, find the flux entering the eye and the illumination of the retinal image when the eye is observing an object the reflection factor of which is 0·4, the pupil diameter now being 2·5 mm.

Answer : (*a*) Assume diffuse reflection.

Brightness of chart $= B = \cdot 7 \times 100 = 70$ lumens/metre^2

$$= \frac{7}{10^3} \text{ lamberts}$$

Area of pupil $= a = 4\pi$ mm.^{2}

If l = distance from eye to chart
l' = length of eye, of refractive index $n' = 4/3$
ω = solid angle subtended at chart by eye's pupil
ω' = solid angle subtended at retina by eye's pupil
S' = area of fovea = $0\cdot06$ mm.^{2} say
S = area of region of chart conjugate to fovea

we have $\omega = \dfrac{a}{l^2}$; $\omega' = \dfrac{a}{l'^2}$; $\dfrac{S'}{S} = \dfrac{l'^2}{n'^2 l^2} = \dfrac{1}{n'^2} \cdot \dfrac{\omega}{\omega'}$

Assuming eye is emmetropic and of power $F_e = 60$ D, its axial length $l' = f'_e = \dfrac{n'}{F_e} = \dfrac{n'}{60}$ metre $= n' \times \dfrac{100}{6}$ mm.

$$\omega' = \frac{a}{l'^2} = \frac{4\pi}{10^6} \cdot \frac{3600}{n'^2} = \frac{0\cdot04525}{n'^2} \text{ steradian.}$$

Flux reaching pupil $= BS\omega = BS'\omega' n'^2$ lumens

$$= \frac{70}{10^6} \times \cdot06 \times \cdot04525 = \frac{1\cdot90}{10^7} \text{ lumens}$$

Assuming that 5 per cent of incident light is lost by reflections at the cornea and crystalline lens and by absorption in the ocular media

$$E' \text{ on fovea} = \frac{95}{100} \cdot \frac{1\cdot9}{10^7} \cdot \frac{1}{06} \text{ lumens per mm.}^2$$

$$= 3\cdot01 \text{ lumens per metre}^2$$

$$\text{Flux on one cone} = \frac{95}{100} \cdot \frac{1\cdot9}{10^7} \cdot \frac{1}{7500} = \frac{2\cdot41}{10^{11}} \text{ lumen}$$

Assuming that for all wavelengths present in the white light illuminating the chart 1 watt = 250 lumens (see §18.4).

$$\text{Energy on one cone} = \frac{1}{250} \cdot \frac{2\cdot41}{10^{11}} = \frac{9\cdot64}{10^{14}} \text{ watt.}$$

(*b*) Brightness of object $= B = 0\cdot4 \times 40{,}000 = 16{,}000$ lumens per metre^2

Area of pupil $= a = \pi \times 1\cdot25^2 = \pi \times 1\cdot5625$ mm.^{2}

$$\omega' = \frac{a}{l'^2} = \frac{\pi \times 1\cdot5625}{10^6} \cdot \frac{3600}{n'^2} = \frac{0\cdot0177}{n'^2} \text{ steradian.}$$

Flux reaching pupil $= B\,S'\omega' n'^2$

$$= \frac{16{,}000}{10^6} \times \cdot06 \times \cdot0177 = \frac{1\cdot7}{10^5} \text{ lumen}$$

$$E' \text{ on fovea} = \frac{95}{100} \cdot \frac{1\cdot7}{10^5} \cdot \frac{1}{\cdot06} \text{ lumens per mm.}^2$$

$$= 269 \text{ lumens per metre.}^2$$

6. Assuming that under favourable conditions the normal eye can detect a small source of whitish light when this sends 500 quanta of radiant energy into the eye, calculate the distance at which a standard candle would just be detected. Neglect atmospheric absorption; assume a pupil diameter of 6 mm. and one watt equivalent to 250 lumens for white light.

Answer : Assuming under these conditions a mean wavelength of 510 $m\mu$, we have from equations (17.1) and (17.2):

$$1 \text{ quantum} = \frac{h \cdot c}{\lambda} = \frac{1979 \times 10^{-12}}{510} \text{ erg} = 3 \cdot 881 \times 10^{-12} \text{ erg}$$
$$= 3 \cdot 881 \times 10^{-19} \text{ watt-sec.}$$

Eye has to receive 500 quanta

$$\equiv 500 \times 3 \cdot 881 \times 10^{-19} = 1 \cdot 940 \times 10^{-16} \text{ watt-sec.}$$

Thus (§18.10) the candle must radiate to the eye

$$1 \cdot 940 \times 10^{-16} \times 250 = 4 \cdot 85 \times 10^{-14} \text{ lumen}$$

If candle is l mm. from eye, $\omega = \dfrac{\text{pupil area}}{l^2}$

$$= \frac{9\pi}{l^2}$$

Flux from small source of intensity I candles within solid angle ω is $F = I\omega$ lumens,

$$\text{i.e. } 4 \cdot 85 \times 10^{-14} = 1 \times \frac{9\pi}{l^2}$$

$$l^2 = \frac{9\pi \times 10^{14}}{4 \cdot 85} \text{ mm}^2.$$

$$l = 2 \cdot 415 \times 10^7 \text{ mm.}$$

$$= \frac{2 \cdot 415 \times 10^7 \times 39 \cdot 37}{10^3 \times 36 \times 1760} = 15 \cdot 0 \text{ miles.}$$

[Prentice Reeves (1918) found the distance to be about 13 miles. Astronomical observations give about 20 miles under optimum conditions.]

EXERCISES. CHAPTER XVIII.

1. Show on a diagram the form of the luminosity curve for the normal eye and explain its meaning. Use it to explain the relationship between radiant energy and luminous flux.

2. State Lambert's cosine law of emission. Explain what is meant by a perfectly diffusing surface.

The brightness of a flat perfectly diffusing surface of area 2 sq. mm. is 25 candles per sq. mm. What is its luminous intensity along (*a*) the normal direction ; (*b*) a direction inclined at 60° to the normal ?

If the light leaving the surface normally falls normally on a circular screen 2 cm. in diameter and 50 cm. from the surface, what amount of luminous flux, expressed in lumens, will fall on the screen ?

(S.M.C.)

3. Give clear definitions of : illumination of a surface ; brightness of a surface.

A table four feet square is illuminated by a single lamp placed six feet vertically above its middle point. What must be the candle-power of this lamp in order that the illumination on the table shall not fall below two lumens per square foot at any point ? (S.M.C.)

4. If a luminous plane surface is observed first from a distance of one metre and then from twice that distance, its brightness appears unchanged. Explain this statement.

Two lamps of 50 candle-power and 9 candle-power are placed at distances of 50 and 30 cm. respectively from a photometer head and on the same side of it. At what distance on the other side of the head must a third lamp of 27 candle-power be placed in order that both sides be equally illuminated ? (S.M.C.)

5. Two equal small sources of light of 30 candles intensity are placed on a photometer bench, each one metre from the photometer head and on opposite sides of it. One source is brought a little nearer to the head; approximately how far could it be moved before the eye could detect the difference in illumination on the two halves of the head ?

6. A source of light is suspended over a desk which slopes at 30° to the horizontal, the source being 2 metres above the point of the desk vertically below it. The illumination at this point is 32 metre-candles. Find the total light flux emitted by the source in lumens, if it emits uniformally in all directions. (S.M.C.)

7. The illumination on a surface is 10 lumens per sq. metre; express this in foot-candles.

Two small lamps A and B give equal illuminations on the two sides of a photometer when their distances from the photometer are in the ratio 4 : 5. A sheet of glass is then placed in front of B and it is found that equality of illumination is obtained when the distances of A and B are in the ratio 16 : 19. Find the percentage of light transmitted by the glass. (S.M.C.)

8. A source of light is suspended 5 feet vertically above the middle point of the back edge of a writing desk which is 20 in. wide from back to front and slopes at 30 degrees to the horizontal. The intensity of illumination at the middle point of the front edge of the desk is not to fall below 2 foot-candles. By taking measurements from a scale diagram, find the maximum candle-power of the source, which is assumed to be equally bright in all directions. (S.M.C.)

9. A lighting unit is mounted on a standard 25 feet above the roadway. Suppose that such a source were required to yield a uniform horizontal illumination on the surface of the roadway up to a distance of 75 feet from the foot of the standard. Calculate the candle-power that the lighting unit must have in various directions inclined at intervals of 10° to the vertical, if the horizontal illumination required is 0·2 foot-candles. Draw the polar curve of candle-power.

10. The illumination of the earth at noon is 9000 lumens per sq. foot. Calculate the brightness of a strip of ground covered with white paint which is a perfect diffuse reflector.

If you were given a 5000 candle-power floodlight, how high from the ground would you place it to produce the same illumination as the sun produces at noon ?

11. Explain why you would expect the illumination on a screen, illuminated by a small source, to vary inversely with the square of its distance from the source.

If a photographic print can be made with 4 seconds exposure at a distance of 4 feet from a 32 c.p. lamp, what exposure will be required if the negative is held at 2 feet from a 16 c.p. lamp ?

12. Establish the following conversion factors:

Illumination :

1 lux	=	0·0929 lumens per foot^2
1 milliphot	=	10 lumens per metre^2
1 lumen per foot^2	=	10·764 lumens per metre^2

Brightness

1 millilambert	=	3·183 candles per metre^2
1 candle per foot^2	=	3·382 millilamberts
1 stilb	=	3142 millilamberts
1 foot-lambert	=	3·427 candles per metre^2
	=	1·076 millilambert

13. A test chart is hung vertically on a wall. A lamp of candle-power I is fixed at the same height as the top edge of the chart and at a perpendicular distance of x feet from the middle point of this top edge. Show that the illumination at a point on the middle vertical line of the chart and h feet below the top edge is given by

$$E = \frac{Ix}{(x^2 + h^2)^{3/2}} \qquad \text{(S.M.C.)}$$

14. Explain in what main respect the eye differs from other selective detectors of radiation. Can you describe another important difference ?

15. On what characteristics of the stimulating radiant energy does (*a*) the magnitude and (*b*) the quality of visual sensation depend ?

Quote figures which give a measure of the sensitivity of the eye to radiation. Draw a curve which illustrates how the quality of the sensation is related to the radiation.

16. What do you understand by the term heterochromatic photometry ? Describe briefly various methods of subjective comparison that have been employed. (S.M.C.)

17. A " point " source of light is found to produce an illumination of 100 ft. can. at a distance of x feet from the source, and 1 ft. can. at a distance of $(x + 36)$ feet from the source. Determine the two distances and evaluate the candle-power of the source. If the source has the same candle-power in all directions, determine its total luminous output in lumens.

18. Explain the terms : brightness or luminance ; apparent brightness or luminosity ; luminosity factor ; reflection factor.

19. What is the relationship between radiant flux in general and luminous flux ; and between the watt and the lumen ?

It is desired to improve the illumination of the image produced by a certain lens system. What are the two basic steps that can be taken ?

20. Of the various possible methods for comparing the intensities of sources of different colour, describe the flicker method and the apparatus used in carrying out the method. What is the principle of the method ?

STIMULUS AND SENSATION

CHAPTER XIX

COLOUR

19.1. Colour, the Quality of Sensation.

WHEREAS variations in the magnitude of visual sensations depend upon the quantity of luminous flux reaching the retina, their *quality*, which we appreciate as differences in colour or hue, is determined by the wavelength* of the stimulating light or, if the light is composite, by the combination of wavelengths in it, i.e. its spectral distribution. All ordinary everyday objects are secondary sources,† rendered visible by the light which they reflect or transmit to our eyes ; this light forms the stimulus. The sensation depends upon the magnitude and spectral composition of this stimulus and upon the properties of the visual apparatus.

From well-known experiments on dispersion and interference we know that light of high frequency and short wavelength gives rise to blue and violet sensations and that light of lower frequency and longer wavelength evokes a yellow or a red sensation. If light from the sun or an electric lamp is spread out into a continuous spectrum by passing it through a spectrometer, when this is observed in direct, foveal, vision by a visually normal individual, the colour sensations aroused by the different wavelength ranges are as set out in the accompanying table, in which are given the hues that stand out prominently.

Approx. λ limits, $m\mu$	390–440	440–500	500–560	560–600	630–750
Colour sensation or hue	Violet	Blue	Green	Yellow	Red
Fraunhofer line contained . .	G	F	E	D	C

* Strictly by the frequency, to which the wavelength in vacuo is inversely proportional.

† §18.3.

Any visual sensation is completely described, apart from its duration, by specifying (a) its luminosity; (b) its hue; and (c) the saturation of the hue.

LUMINOSITY: the intensity or magnitude of luminous sensation.

HUE: that attribute of certain visual sensations by which we distinguish red, green, blue, yellow, purple, etc. from one another and by which the eye distinguishes different parts of the spectrum.

SATURATION: the vividness or fullness of a hue—as opposed to paleness when it is mixed with white.

If we use a sodium flame or lamp to illuminate the slit of a spectrometer we see a line (or double line) of pure

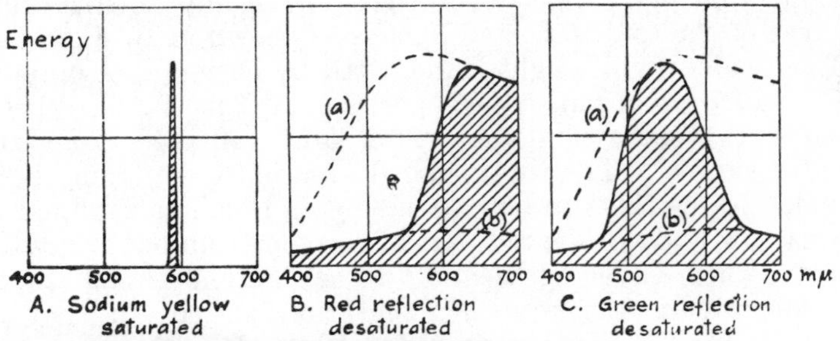

FIG. 19.1—PURE LIGHT GIVING SATURATED LINE (A) AND IMPURE LIGHT REFLECTED FROM SECONDARY SOURCES GIVING DESATURATED LIGHT (B AND C).

yellow, uncontaminated with any other hue. A hue of such purity or fullness is said to be saturated. The light emitted by the source is in this instance confined to a narrow band of sodium D light lying at the mean position $\lambda\, 589 \cdot 3$, as depicted by A in Fig. 19.1; it is described as pure or homogeneous or monochromatic light.

The hues of the spectrum are the most saturated that we encounter in ordinary vision, though more saturated sensations can be evoked in special ways (e.g. after-images*).

By comparison, the light sent into our eyes by secondary sources, be they natural or artificial objects, is much less pure. Whatever the object may be, the retinal image of it depends upon the composition of the light that it reflects

* §20.6.

into our eyes; and this in turn depends upon the light by which it is illuminated and how much of this it respectively absorbs and reflects. Suppose a "red" rose is seen in ordinary daylight; some of the incident light from the sun, sky and clouds, which we describe as white light, is reflected as white light from the outer surface of the rose. The remaining incident light penetrates its outer layers before being reflected and emerges robbed of some of its constituent wavelengths, namely "violet", "blue", "green" and much of the "yellow" light. Which wavelengths are absorbed depends upon the chemical constitution of the object. The total reflected light is thus a mixture of white light containing all wavelengths and the restricted range of wavelengths, namely "yellow" and "red" light, that were not absorbed. The energy distribution curve of the total reflected light is as shown in B, Fig. 19.1. The incident white light is indicated by curve (a)—compare Fig. 17.7; the unshaded portion of this is absorbed; curve (b) represents the white light reflected from the outer surface. The total shaded area is the emerging light which forms the stimulus to the eye. It is not confined to a narrow band in the red part of the spectrum but is diluted with other wavelengths and to that extent is said to be desaturated; the resulting sensation is red but not so vividly red as spectrum red; it tends either towards pink or a dull dark red.

If this same red rose were illuminated by "green-blue" light, apart from the small proportion reflected from the outer surface, it would all be absorbed; only the small proportion of surface-reflected light would enter the eye and the rose would appear nearly black, or at least a dull gray.

Curve (C) shows the energy distribution of the reflected light in the case of a "green" object, such as a leaf, illuminated by white light. Whereas in both cases (B) and (C) all wavelengths are present in the reflected light, there is a predominance of red in one case and green in the other, with corresponding peaks in their distribution curves. If we are supplied with the energy distribution curve of a sample of light, we can in most cases predict reasonably well the colour sensation that will be aroused by it. If the curve shows a peak, the colour will tend to correspond to that part of the spectrum where the peak occurs, though this is not always the case. If the curve is smooth and not appreciably higher at one end than the other, the sensation will tend towards white.

It will be clear from the above why a coloured fabric does not present the same appearance under the artificial illumination of a shop as it does when examined in daylight, because the light by which it is illuminated differs in the two cases (Fig. 17.7). For this reason artificial daylight lamps are employed for such purposes. In these the light from the electric lamp is made to pass through a specially prepared bulb or filter, or is reflected from a shade treated with specially prepared pigments. Compared with daylight the light emitted by the lamp filament is too rich in the longer (red) wavelengths and the filter or pigment absorbs some of these so that the spectral distribution of the finally emerging light approximates to that of daylight. It is to be noted that the correction is carried out by absorption and so the original brightness is reduced by these devices.

This raises the question as to what we mean by white light and why white holds its unique position amongst the sensations of colour. In the broadest sense the term colour is used not only to include those sensations like red, green, etc. which possess the attribute of hue and which are called *chromatic colours* or sensations; but also the white, gray and black sensations which are devoid of the attribute of hue and are called *achromatic colours* or sensations. White is unique presumably because it is the sensation aroused by the light from the sun, in the presence of which we have evolved and which provides the background and is responsible for all the colours of nature. It would usually be described as the sensation evoked by daylight. The colour of daylight, however, is most variable; it varies with place, with time of year, time of day, distribution of cloud, etc. For accurate colorimetric work it has therefore become essential to settle upon standard white. This was done in 1931 by the Commission Internationale de l'Eclairage (C.I.E.). This committee specified three illuminants called sources S_A, S_B and S_C. S_A is to represent an average artificial illuminant and is a gas-filled tungsten lamp run at a colour temperature of 2854° K. S_B and S_C are intended to correspond to two grades of daylight of colour temperatures respectively 4800° K and 6500° K; they are obtained by using certain specified liquid filters in conjunction with source S_A. A third filter has since (1934) been proposed which when used with S_A provides an illuminant giving the same colour as the equal energy source.*

It will be observed that colour terms such as red, green, etc., have been used above to describe the stimulating light and the object from which it comes. It is well to be aware that strictly this is wrong though it is almost universally done to avoid circumlocution. In the case of the leaf, for example, neither the leaf nor the light coming from it is green; the quality of greenness arises only in the brain of the observer and even then only when the conditions are suitable. We *should* say " when radiation lying somewhere between the approximate limits λ 500 and λ 560, or predominantly of this range, enters a normal light-adapted eye, a sensation of green is aroused ". That colour is a purely subjective phenomenon is well illustrated by BENHAM'S top; this has nothing on it but black and white markings, yet when rapidly rotated it appears in vivid hues.†

Except in special circumstances, the human visual apparatus responds only to radiations within the λ 390 to λ 750 range of the visual spectrum. It follows that

ALL COLOUR SENSATIONS ARE DUE TO MIXTURES, IN VARYING PROPORTIONS, OF THE CONSTITUENT RADIATIONS LYING WITHIN THE VISUAL SPECTRUM.

The eye can detect so many different spectral hues, and each hue may be degraded with so many detectable degrees of desaturation, that a vast number of different colours result, as everyone knows from experience with the objects around us.

19.2. Spectral Composition and Visual Sensation.

When all the constituent wavelengths present in the sun's radiation are mixed together, as they are in ordinary sunlight, we experience a simple single sensation of white. Although this is such a common experience it is nevertheless a remarkable phenomenon. The stimulating radiation contains components which, separately, arouse the sensations of violet, blue, green, yellow and red and many other intermediate hues of the blue-green, green-yellow and orange variety lying between these prominent hues; but

* For particulars of these sources and for an excellent and authoritative account of colour measurement see *The Measurement of Colour* by W. D. WRIGHT, Adam Hilger Ltd., 1944.

† §20.3.

when they all stimulate the eye together there is no trace of this complexity in the resultant sensation ; it is simply white ; just as simple as, say, the green sensation due to monochromatic λ 546 light. Somewhere in the retinal receptors or in the path from them to the brain or in the brain, the effects of this tremendous range of radiations undergo some kind of integrating process which finally arouses in consciousness a single sensation quality, which we call white.

Further ; simple experiments show that exactly the same white sensation is aroused when the stimulus contains only two wavelengths such as λ 472 (blue) and λ 574

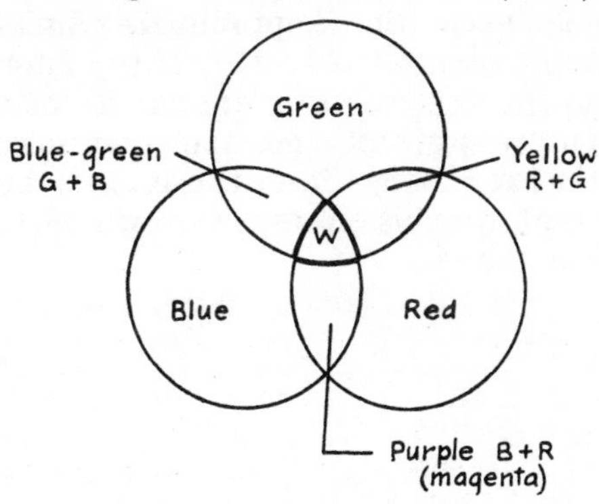

FIG. 19.2—SIMPLE SENSATIONS FROM COMPOSITE STIMULI. W APPEARS WHITE WHEN R, G AND B ARE IN SUITABLE PROPORTIONS.

(yellow), providing the proper proportions of these two lights are used ; and there are many other pairs of wavelengths which will produce the same result.

Again : if we stimulate the eye with " green " light and " red " light in suitable proportions the sensation is yellow, exactly the same as the sensation aroused by monochromatic sodium light of λ 589·3.

The sensations resulting from the addition of separate stimuli or from the " mixing of colours " as it is usually described, can be qualitatively demonstrated to an audience in the following way. Suppose we arrange that by using three lanterns we throw three over-lapping circular patches of light on to a white screen,* the lanterns being provided with colour filters so that they throw respectively " red " light, " green " light and " blue " light. As indicated in

* By a suitable arrangement of prisms the three patches may be obtained from one lantern.

Fig. 19.2, the circles will appear red, green and blue. The part of the screen where the red and green discs overlap is sending "red" light plus "green" light to our eyes, yet the sensation aroused is a simple yellow colour practically identical with the sensation produced by homogeneous D light of the spectrum. Similarly, "green" light plus "blue" light evokes a sensation described as blue-green, which again may be aroused by a simple homogeneous radiation of wavelength lying between the λ 560 and λ 390 lines of the spectrum. The sector where the "red" and "blue" lights overlap appears purple or magenta. In the centre of the screen where all three discs overlap the appearance approximates to white. If the filters have been chosen to transmit the appropriate ranges of wavelengths and the correct quantity of each, the sensation can be made to agree with whatever has been chosen as standard white.

The important conclusion to be drawn from the above observations is that

THE SAME VISUAL SENSATION MAY BE EVOKED BY ENTIRELY DIFFERENT PHYSICAL STIMULI.*

In this respect the eye behaves quite differently from the ear. Whereas the eye cannot distinguish the difference if we substitute yellow for a compound of green and red, the impression aroused in the brain by the piano note D is quite different from the double impression created by the notes C and E sounded together. The ear differentiates and analyses; the eye cannot analyse a complex stimulus; the two senses are fundamentally different.

Complementary Colours.

The separate colour sensations due to two lights which when mixed result in a third colour are said to be complementary with respect to the third colour. Ordinarily the term complementary is applied to those colours which together produce white.

Suppose that by some arrangement we can illuminate the left-hand half of a photometer head or colorimeter, Fig. 19.3, by the white light we have agreed to adopt as standard white and the right-hand half with successive pairs of spectrum colours, the wavelengths and luminosities

* It is also true that exactly the same stimulus may evoke entirely different sensations in different parts of the retina of a given eye or even on the same part of the retina according to the state of adaptation at the moment; these phenomena are studied in Chapters XX and XXI.

of which we can vary at will. If then we vary the two wavelengths on the right, and their relative luminosities, until the right field matches the white on the left, the lights of these two wavelengths are complementary. Observations of this kind made by HELMHOLTZ, KÖNIG

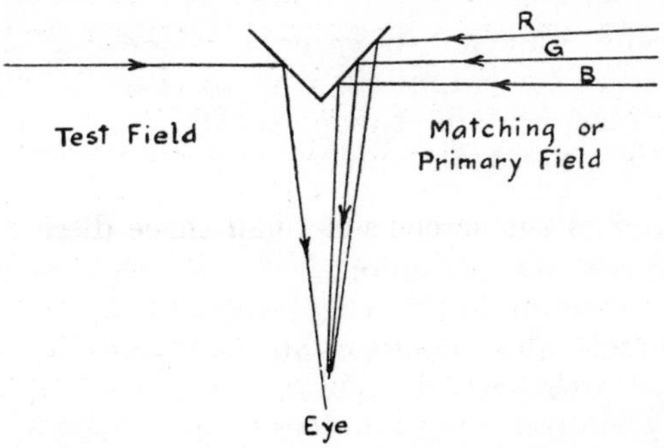

FIG. 19.3—COLORIMETER—DIAGRAMMATIC.

and others differ among themselves probably because of variations in the " white " they used and differences in the observers. Later results by SINDEN (1923) are given in the following table.

COMPLEMENTARY SPECTRAL COLOURS: SINDEN (1923)

Complementaries

λ_1	650	609	591	586	580	578·5	576·5	575·5	574	573	572	570·5
λ_2	496	493·5	490	487·5	482·5	480·5	477·5	474·5	472	466·5	459	443

Relative Luminosities

L_1	42·1	52·4	67·1	73·8	82·7	85·5	87·7	90·3	92·0	94·2	96·1	97·5
L_2	57·9	47·6	32·9	26·2	17·3	14·5	12·3	9·7	8·0	5·8	3·9	2·5

From the figures in the table it will be observed that:

(i) there are no spectral hues complementary to the greenish hues between λ 570 and λ 496; as will be clearer when the colour chart is discussed, this range must be mixed with purple hues in order to produce white. Purple results from mixtures of red and blue, or violet.

(ii) the relative luminosities differ greatly for different complementary pairs. Whereas two lights of λ 609 and λ 493·5 must be of approximately equal luminosities, the yellow of λ 570·5 must have a luminosity about forty times greater than its complementary violet of λ 443. That is, although as is shown by the luminosity curve, Fig. 18.1, the luminosity factor of violet is very small, its contribution to the *colour* quality of a sensation is very strong.

In carrying out the above experiment the field of view in the photometer is limited to 2° so that only a restricted retinal region containing the fovea takes part in the observations; this restriction applied also in §18.9.

19.3. The Tristimulus Basis of Colour Sensation.

Experiment reveals another remarkable fact and this is the most striking in the whole range of colour phenomena. Whatever light we introduce into the left (test) field of our colorimeter, whether it be a monochromatic radiation taken from the spectrum or a compound light with any spectral distribution whatsoever, it can be matched in hue and luminosity by introducing into the right (matching) field not more than three appropriate lights in suitable proportions. For practical reasons the three lights that we choose for the matching side of our colorimeter are red, green and blue. Within these limits we have a wide choice. In the actual instrument, as in the Donaldson colorimeter for example, they may be compound lights obtained by the use of coloured filters. We may suppose they are the monochromatic radiations 650 $m\mu$, 530 $m\mu$ and 460 $m\mu$ which are used by W. D. Wright in his colorimeter.* All three are thus physically precisely defined. We will call them the MATCHING STIMULI† and represent them by the symbols R, G and B.

The colour sensations resulting from mixing these three matching stimuli are broadly as explained in the lantern experiment, but depend upon the relative proportions of each. If we use only R and G we obtain a hue lying somewhere between them in the spectrum, i.e. orange or yellow or yellow-green according to the relative amounts of R and G in the mixture. Using G and B we obtain one of the green-blue hues of the spectrum lying between the green and blue. If, however, we mix together the R and B stimuli, which are further apart in the spectrum, we obtain

* See §19.8.

† It has been customary to call them primary colours or lights, but it is now suggested that this term be discontinued.

one of the purple hues which are not to be found in the spectrum at all, a circumstance to be referred to again. If we use all three matching stimuli in certain proportions, we obtain white; if then we were slowly to increase the proportion of R in the mixture the white would take on a pale pink tint (a much desaturated red) which would gradually increase in redness, but which would never become a full saturated red unless the green and blue matching lights were reduced to zero.

If we introduce into the test field a monochromatic blue-green spectrum radiation of wavelength, say, $\lambda\,500$ lying between the $\lambda\,460$ and $\lambda\,530$ of B and G, we should find that whereas we could match it in hue with these two matching stimuli, we could not quite match it in saturation. The mixture in the matching field would have the same hue as the test colour but would be paler, as if white had been added to it. In order to secure a complete match in hue *and* saturation it would be necessary to desaturate the test colour, which we can do by adding white to it, or as we shall see more clearly presently,* by adding a quantity of R. In other words, we can still match it completely with our three matching stimuli, but one of them, in this case the red, would have to be introduced into the *test* field; which is equivalent to saying that a negative amount of R is needed in the matching field. The significance of this will be better appreciated when the trichromatic equation and colour chart are discussed below.*

If we match one test light C_1 by mixing R, G and B in our matching field in quantities represented by r_1, g_1 and b_1; and a second test light C_2 with quantities r_2 of R, g_2 of G and b_2 of B; then the two test colours C_1 and C_2 introduced together will be matched by $(r_1 + r_2)$ of R, $(g_1 + g_2)$ of G and $(b_1 + b_2)$ of B. This additive law of colour mixture was stated by ABNEY and is sometimes called ABNEY'S law.

Such colour mixing experiments, with whatever apparatus carried out, lead to the following two fundamental laws of colour mixture:

A. Over an extensive range of luminosities (excluding very low and very high luminosities†) and with the reservation that highly saturated

---

* §§19.4 and 19.6.

† I.e. the luminosity level must not be so low that the Purkinje phenomenon operates, nor so high that glare results; see §20.6.

colours must be desaturated to some extent, any colour sensation can be matched by using a suitable mixture of three selected radiations.

B. If C_1 and C_2 are two lights which have been separately matched by mixtures of three selected radiations, then the two lights C_1 and C_2 together will be matched by the sum of the two previous mixtures.

The three chosen radiations or matching stimuli must be such that no one of them can be matched by a mixture of the other two; this is equivalent to stating that white can be matched by a mixture of the three in suitable proportions.

Prominent among the pioneer investigators in the field of colour were YOUNG, MAXWELL, HELMHOLTZ, KÖNIG and ABNEY, using colour tops and discs and the spectrometer in their experimental work. More refined apparatus and a better appreciation of the calculations involved have enabled modern physicists such as H. E. IVES, J. GUILD, T. SMITH and W. D. WRIGHT to put colorimetry on an exact scientific basis.

We see from the above that SO FAR AS STIMULI ARE CONCERNED, NORMAL COLOUR VISION IS TRICHROMATIC.

The physiological processes in or behind the retina must therefore, it is argued, possess some kind of triple mechanism, as suggested by YOUNG and supported by HELMHOLTZ. What is the nature of this mechanism? There are such possibilities as: (a) the existence of three different photo-chemical substances in or around the retinal cones, with absorption maxima located at different points in the visible spectrum; (b) three types of bipolar cell in the retina; (c) three types of nerve fibre in the pathway from retina to brain; (d) three types of cone. The experimental evidence is as yet inconclusive, but we have to assume that associated with the cones there are ultimately three light-sensitive systems of some kind,* each of which responds to a wide range of spectral radiations; one with maximum sensitivity in or towards the red, one in the green and the third in or near the blue. The relative extents to which these three systems respond

* It has also been suggested (HARTRIDGE) that there may be more than three, perhaps seven, types of receptor and three types of nerve fibre; and that the types of receptor are distributed differently as between the fovea and the peripheral zones of the retina.

when light strikes the retina depends upon the distribution of energy in the stimulus. If the stimulus is, for example, the light from a leaf with the spectral distribution shown in Fig. 19.1 (C), the green system of the eye will be greatly stimulated and the red and blue systems only slightly affected. These three responses converge towards the brain, where a sensation compounded of the three is aroused ; it is found to be a somewhat desaturated green sensation.

As the physiologists provide more detailed information about the processes that occur in the retina when it is stimulated by light, or about the nerve impulses that travel along the fibres of the optic nerve to the brain, it may be possible to obtain a clearer picture of the nature of this triple response system in the visual apparatus.*

19.4. The Measurement of Colour. Trichromatic System.

Enquiry into the nature of the triple physiological mechanism and its mode of action belongs to another part of the subject. Here, although the very existence of colour is due to the properties of the visual mechanism, our direct concern is with the stimulus. We want to devise a scheme whereby each of the enormous number of colours can be accurately measured and specified, preferably on a basis of numbers, so that a given colour sample may be assigned its proper place in the adopted classification and be capable of exact reproduction at any time and place by technical men. This opens up an important branch of Applied Optics called COLORIMETRY. It is a complex subject, of great importance in industry. At least an outline of its principles is required by the optical practitioner since it is fundamental to a clear understanding of colour vision and its anomalies.

The observations in the previous sections supply an adequate basis for setting up such a trichromatic system of colour measurement. It will be understood that if we were to determine, in terms of three universally agreed matching stimuli, the trichromatic specification of radiation of each wavelength throughout the visible spectrum, making allowance for the luminosity of each radiation (Fig. 18.1), we could *calculate* the trichromatic specification of any light in terms of the three agreed stimuli when we know its spectral energy distribution. There is, however,

* §21.10 and Chapter XXII.

a more direct and less laborious method of measuring and specifying colour experimentally with the colorimeter.

Our problem is to measure, i.e. to determine the trichromatic specification of, an unknown light, the test light, which we will call C. The observer is supposed to be a normal observer. We first introduce into the test field of the colorimeter a certain quantity, say one lumen, of the agreed standard white light, W. This can be provided by a tungsten lamp and special filter as already explained (§19.1). The R, G and B matching lights are admitted into the matching field and their quantities manipulated, by means of the slits, sectors or other means provided in the instrument, until there is a complete match, in hue and in luminosity, between the two fields and they appear exactly alike. Suppose the number of lumens of R, G and B are respectively $l_R = 0\cdot36$ lumen, $l_G = 0\cdot63$ lumen and $l_B = 0\cdot01$ lumen ; we can write the " colour equation " for standard white in terms of light flux as

$$1\cdot0\ \text{W} \equiv 0\cdot36\ \text{R} + 0\cdot63\ \text{G} + 0\cdot01\ \text{B}.$$

The amount of light is the same on both sides of the equation ; this is the case in all colour equations.*

Although the quantities of *light* contributed by the three matching stimuli are decidedly unequal, their mixture has produced a resultant (white) which is neutral, devoid of hue. It is therefore logical, and it leads to simplification in calculations, to assess their contributions as *equal* quantities of *colour* quality. The scale readings of the colorimeter to give this white match are then considered equal.

We now introduce the unknown light C into the test field. It may be monochromatic or compound ; it may come direct from a luminous source or it may have been transmitted through a coloured filter or reflected from some surface ; in any case it arouses a sensation of some definite colour quality. Suppose that it needs 0·44 lumens of R, 1·54 lumens of G and 0·1667 lumens of B to match it completely. The number of lumens in each field is 2·147 and so the equation for C in terms of light flux is

$$2\cdot147\ \text{C} \equiv 0\cdot44\ \text{R} + 1\cdot54\ \text{G} + 0\cdot1667\ \text{B}.$$

To express the colour equation in terms, not of luminosity units, but of the new units, called TRICHROMATIC UNITS,

* There is disagreement amongst colour authorities as to the sign that should be used in these colour " equations " ; meanwhile I have used the equivalence sign $\equiv$.

obtained from the white match, we must divide the flux quantities of R, G and B by 0·36, 0·63 and 0·01 respectively, giving the quantities of R, G and B in trichromatic units as $\frac{11}{9}$ of R, $\frac{22}{9}$ of G and $16\frac{2}{3}$ of B; that is $20\frac{1}{3}$ trichromatic units of colour altogether. We can therefore write

$$20\tfrac{1}{3}\,\mathrm{C} \equiv \tfrac{11}{9}\,\mathrm{R} + \tfrac{22}{9}\,\mathrm{G} + 16\tfrac{2}{3}\,\mathrm{B}$$

or $$1{\cdot}0\,\mathrm{C} \equiv 0{\cdot}06\,\mathrm{R} + 0{\cdot}12\,\mathrm{G} + 0{\cdot}82\,\mathrm{B}$$

which is called the UNIT TRICHROMATIC EQUATION; and the coefficients of R, G and B are the TRICHROMATIC COEFFICIENTS, which always add up to unity. The trichromatic unit is a colour unit as distinct from a unit of light.

The equation states that one trichromatic unit, or one T unit, of the test colour C is equivalent in colour and luminosity to the colour resulting from the mixture of 0·06 T unit of R, 0·12 T unit of G and 0·82 T unit of B —on the arbitrary but agreed basis that the quantities in T units of the matching stimuli required to match the agreed standard white are accepted as equal.

Expressing the above in symbols: if l_R, l_G, and l_B are the quantities in lumens of R, G and B to give a complete match of the test colour C, the equation for C in terms of light flux is

$$l_C\,\mathrm{C} \equiv l_R\,.\,\mathrm{R} + l_G\,.\,\mathrm{G} + l_B\,.\,\mathrm{B} \qquad (19.1)$$

in which $$l_C = l_R + l_G + l_B \qquad (19.2)$$

If the amounts of R, G and B expressed in trichromatic units are u, v and w ($\frac{11}{9}$, $\frac{22}{9}$, $16\frac{2}{3}$ in the above example), then the trichromatic coefficients may be expressed by r, g and b (0·06, 0·12, 0·82 in the example) which are such that

$$r = \frac{u}{u+v+w} \qquad g = \frac{v}{u+v+w} \qquad b = \frac{w}{u+v+w} \qquad (19.3)$$

and

$$r + g + b = 1 \qquad (19.4)$$

The unit trichromatic equation is*

$$\mathrm{C} \equiv r\,.\,\mathrm{R} + g\,.\,\mathrm{G} + b\,.\,\mathrm{B} \qquad (19.5$$

Also, the equation for standard white in trichromatic units is clearly*

$$W \equiv \tfrac{1}{3}\,\mathrm{R} + \tfrac{1}{3}\,\mathrm{G} + \tfrac{1}{3}\,\mathrm{B} \qquad (19.6)$$

---

* It is usual to omit the coefficient 1·0 for the test colour in unit trichromatic equations.

In a unit trichromatic equation the three coefficients add up to unity; thus if we know two of them, say r and g, the third, b, can be found by subtracting their sum from unity; i.e. $b = 1-(r + g)$.

19.5. Trichromatic Coefficients of the Spectrum Hues.

The procedure just described has been used to determine the trichromatic specification of each wavelength of the visible spectrum from one end, λ 390, to the other, λ 750. Very narrow bands of wavelengths from a carefully produced pure spectrum are allowed, in succession, to illuminate the test field. For each band the instrument is manipulated to introduce the necessary quantities of R, G and B to provide an exact match. It is found, since the spectrum hues are highly saturated hues, that no combination of R, G and B introduced into the matching field will provide an exact match; it will be possible to match each spectrum radiation in hue, but not in saturation. Thus it is necessary to desaturate the spectrum radiation in the test field. This could be done by adding our standard white to it; it is usual, however, in practical colorimeters, to achieve the desaturation by providing an arrangement for in. troducing any of the matching stimuli into the test field- That this secures the same result as desaturating with white will be understood if we consider a numerical example.

Using the monochromatic matching stimuli of wavelengths 650, 530 and 460 $m\mu$ and adopting the S_B source (4800° K) as standard white, WRIGHT found (see Table V) that the spectrum radiation λ 500, for example, was matched by using 0·772 T unit of G and 0·461 T unit of B in the matching field and by adding 0·233 T unit of R to the test light (λ 500) in the test field. That is, representing λ 500 by the symbol C, he found its unit trichromatic equation to be

$$1\cdot00\,C + 0\cdot233\,R \equiv 0\cdot772\,G + 0\cdot461\,B \qquad (a)$$

or

$$1\cdot00\,C \equiv -0\cdot233\,R + 0\cdot772\,G + 0\cdot461\,B$$

Now we know that for standard white

$$1\cdot00\,W \equiv 0\cdot333\,R + 0\cdot333\,G + 0\cdot333\,B$$

so

$$0\cdot333\,R \equiv 1\cdot00\,W - 0\cdot333\,G - 0\cdot333\,B$$

$$0\cdot233\,R \equiv 0\cdot699\,W - 0\cdot233\,G - 0\cdot233\,B$$

$$\therefore\ 1\cdot00\,C + 0\cdot699\,W \equiv 1\cdot005\,G + 0\cdot694\,B \qquad (b)$$

Equations (a) and (b) are equivalent to one another and tell us that we can match radiation of λ 500 by desaturating it either with white light or with R light, in suitable quantity in each case.

The results obtained by WRIGHT in this manner for wavelengths 390, 400, 410 . . . 700 $m\mu$ are given in Table V. They are also plotted in Fig. 19.4 giving curves described as the *trichromatic coefficient curves.* Radiations other than

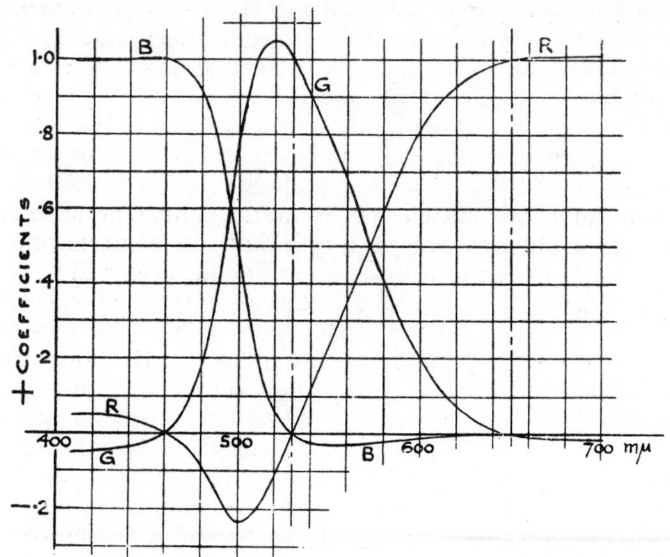

FIG. 19.4—TRICHROMATIC COEFFICIENTS. R : 650, G : 530, B : 460 $m\mu$. EQUAL QUANTITIES GIVE WHITE (4800° K)—W. D. WRIGHT.

λ 650, λ 530 and λ 460 could have been used. In that case a different set of coefficients and curves of different shapes would have been obtained ; but in all cases where real physical radiations are used as matching stimuli, one of the coefficients, for each spectral light, is negative.

19.6. The Colour Chart or Chromaticity Diagram.

The information given by the unit trichromatic equation concerning any colour C may be presented graphically in another manner as in Fig. 19.5. Only two coefficients, say red and green, need be plotted ; the red coefficient is represented by the horizontal axis and the green vertically. Diagrams of this kind, sometimes called colour triangles, are very useful. The white adopted as standard white is represented by the point W, the co-ordinates of which are

(0·333, 0·333). The point C represents a colour with co-ordinates (0·2, 0·3); it will be a considerably desaturated blue-violet hue.

Neither the trichromatic equation nor the colour chart gives any information regarding the luminosity of the sensations. In terms of trichromatic units, based upon the convention that equal quantities give white, they give the *proportions* in which the selected matching stimuli have to be mixed in order to match the test light in hue and saturation.

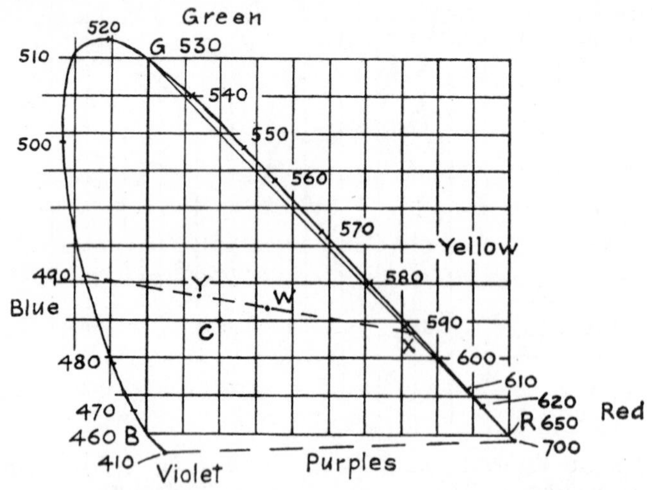

FIG. 19.5—COLOUR CHART. WRIGHT'S DATA. EQUAL QUANTITIES OF MATCHING STIMULI MAKE WHITE (W). COMPARE FIG. 19.7.

W. D. WRIGHT'S coefficients of the spectrum colours, given in the Table, are plotted on the chart. The red matching stimulus, R, of λ 650, for which $r = 1 \cdot 0$, $g = 0$, $b = 0$, has co-ordinates (1·0, 0·0). G similarly has co-ordinates (0·0, 1·0) and B (0·0, 0·0). Every other spectrum hue lies outside the triangle RGB since, as the table shows, one of the three coefficients is negative in every case. The point λ 500, for example, is 0·772 upwards from the zero, which is the positive direction for green; and 0·233 to the left of the zero, which is the negative direction for red. The curved line joining all these points is called the SPECTRUM LOCUS, which is extremely useful in helping to visualise the relative positions of the various colours; and in other ways.

The bulge outside the GB side of the triangle tells us that negative quantities of R are required to match spectral lights lying between λ 460 and λ 530; and the less pronounced bulge outside the RG side that small negative quantities of B are needed to match spectral lights between λ 530 and λ 650.

When the colour chart, with the spectrum locus and white point, has once been obtained from reliable and specified data, it provides a mathematically accurate specification of colour just as equation (19.5) does, if it is drawn to a sufficiently large scale; and it helps to visualise the results of colour mixing.

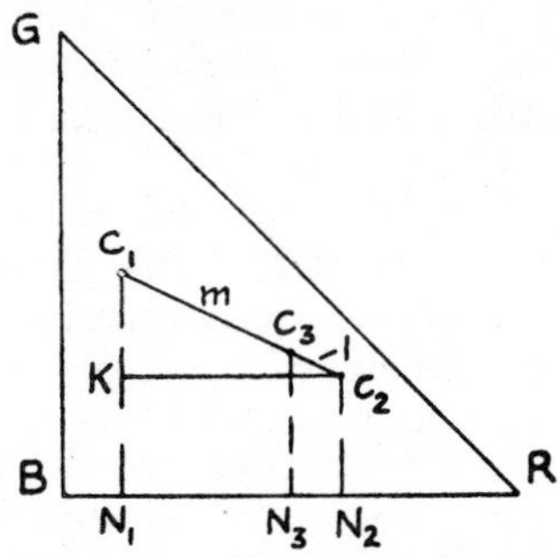

Fig. 19.6—Mixture of one T unit of colour C_1 and m T units of colour C_2 gives $(m + 1)$ T units of colour C_3.

It is an interesting fact that the purple colours of many natural objects are not present in the spectrum. The chart shows that these colours result from the mixture of red and blue, or red and violet. The actual hue of the purple, whether crimson, rose-pink, magenta, etc., depends upon the relative proportions of the two constituents.

Consideration of this physiological gap, as it were, in the spectrum and the facts of complementary colours led in the past to the construction of colour charts in which the spectrum hues were arranged around the circumference of a closed figure, frequently a circle (e.g. Newton); white was placed at the centre and green opposite the purple gap between red and violet. Such charts were the forerunners of the colour charts of the present.

Suppose we have two colours C_1 and C_2, the unit trichromatic equations of which are

$$1\cdot0\, C_1 = r_1 . R + g_1 . G + b_1 . B$$

and

$$1\cdot0\, C_2 = r_2 . R + g_2 . G + b_2 . B$$

and we mix 1 T unit of C_1 with m T units of C_2. The resultant colour, C_3, will be represented by

$$(1 + m)\,C_3 = (r_1 + mr_2)\,R + (g_1 + mg_2)\,G + (b_1 + mb_2)\,B$$

and the unit equation for C_3 will be

$$1 \cdot 0\,C_3 = r_3 \,.\, R + g_3 \,.\, G + b_3 \,.\, B$$

where

$$r_3 = \frac{r_1 + mr_2}{1 + m}; \quad g_3 = \frac{g_1 + mg_2}{1 + m}; \quad b_3 = \frac{b_1 + mb_2}{1 + m}$$

This result can be obtained very simply from the colour chart. Let the points C_1 and C_2 (Fig. 19.6) represent the given colours. If we mark a point C_3 on the line C_1C_2 such that it divides C_1C_2 in the proportion $C_1C_3 : C_2C_3 :: m : 1$, then the point C_3 represents the resultant colour given by the mixture. The point C_3 is the centre of gravity of particles of masses 1 and m placed at C_1 and C_2 respectively.

To prove this, consider the green coefficients. The perpendiculars C_1N_1, C_2N_2 and C_3N_3 dropped on the BR line represent g_1, g_2 and g_3 respectively. Draw the line C_2K parallel to BR. Then

$$\begin{aligned} C_3N_3 &= C_2N_2 + C_1K\,\frac{1}{1 + m} \\ &= C_2N_2 + \frac{C_1N_1 - C_2N_2}{1 + m} \\ &= \frac{m \,.\, C_2N_2 + C_1N_1}{1 + m} \end{aligned}$$

or

$$g_3 = \frac{g_1 + m \,.\, g_2}{1 + m}$$

The same method of proof can be used for the red coefficients.

It follows that a straight line drawn on the colour chart (Fig. 19.5) and passing through the white point W intersects the spectrum locus in two points which represent complementary hues; and that any point on such a line lying between W and the spectrum locus represents a colour of the same hue as the spectral colour, but desaturated with white to an extent proportional to the distance of the point from the spectrum locus. Thus the broken line through W in Fig. 19.5 shows that wavelengths 490 $m\mu$ and 591 $m\mu$ are complementary—compare with SINDEN'S table of complementaries, §19.2. Mixtures of R and G lie along the line RG and mixtures of G and B along the line GB. The colour represented by the point X where the broken line intersects the RG side of the triangle will be of the same orange hue as that evoked by light of λ 591, but very slightly desaturated. And the colour represented by the point Y will have the blue hue corresponding to λ 490, but it will be very considerably desaturated, i.e. very pale, since it contains more white than saturated blue.

The fact that combinations of lights from the RG range are so nearly saturated explains why it is so easy to obtain materials and fabrics with bright, highly saturated colours in the red, orange, yellow and yellow-green group. In the GB range we cannot obtain a resultant colour lying near to the spectrum locus unless the two component stimuli are spectral lights lying close together. Hence for a coloured material to have a highly saturated colour in the green-blue range, it must absorb all except a short region of the spectrum. Since it absorbs so much of the light incident on it, it will be a dark material; moreover, some of the incident light will always be reflected from the outer surface layer of the material and so will desaturate the emerging light. Thus we rarely find highly saturated blue-greens amongst natural objects.

Since all colour sensations are due to positive mixtures of the spectrum hues in varying proportions, it follows that they are represented by points on the colour chart lying within the area bounded by the spectrum locus and the straight line joining its two red and violet extremities. This area may be called the *colour field*; within it every possible colour has a definite location—saturated hues along the boundaries, white at the centre and desaturated colours in the intermediate regions between W and the boundaries.

When deciding on the three lights to be used as matching stimuli in a colorimeter, two of them, the red and blue, are chosen near the ends of the spectrum and the third near the sharp bend in the spectrum locus, which is in the green region (Fig. 19.5). The area enclosed by the RGB triangle is then large and practically all colours found in commerce lie within it and so can be matched by direct mixtures of the matching lights. A point not too far round the bend of the spectrum locus is selected for G so that the straight line RG lies close to the spectrum locus and the important colours in this range are provided by the colorimeter in a highly saturated state.

Even with the above limitation there is a fairly wide choice of matching stimuli to be used in a given colorimeter. For example, whereas W. D. WRIGHT used the spectrum radiations λ 650, λ 530 and λ 460, in the colorimeters designed by J. GUILD and by R. DONALDSON, different sets of red, green and blue filters were used.

19.7. Standard Reference Stimuli. The C.I.E. System.

If a given test colour C were matched in two colorimeters, one with matching stimuli described as R, G, B and the other with a different set of matching stimuli called, say, X, Y and Z, there would result the two unit trichromatic equations

$$C \equiv r \,.\, R + g \,.\, G + b \,.\, B$$

and

$$C \equiv x \,.\, X + y \,.\, Y + z \,.\, Z$$

The coefficients r, g, b would differ from the coefficients x, y, z because of the difference between the spectral compositions of the two sets of matching stimuli; and if the two instruments were used by two different observers whose colour vision characteristics are not identical, there would be a further variation.

If we can assume a normal observer and if the physical composition of the two sets of matching stimuli are precisely known, or the composition of one set known in terms of the other set, the second trichromatic equation can be obtained from the first by purely mathematical methods. In order that the results obtained with different colorimeters throughout the world may be compared, it is necessary to agree upon the definition of the normal observer and on the accurate specification of one standard set of matching stimuli, which are then conveniently called the *reference stimuli*, in terms of which all colour matches can be expressed. (Such standardisation is needed in all measurement; and so we have units like the metre, the dioptre, the ampere, and so on.) It was carried out in the case of colour by the Commission Internationale de l'Eclairage in 1931. These hypothetical reference stimuli called X, Y, Z, and known as the C.I.E. reference stimuli, as well as a standard observer, were defined. The stimuli were chosen so that the coefficients in the unit trichromatic equation all have positive values for the spectrum hues.

On the C.I.E. colour chart, therefore, (Fig. 19.7), in which X is plotted horizontally and Y vertically, the spectrum locus lies entirely *within* the triangle XYZ. Figs. 19.5 and 19.7 provide the same information. It will be observed, for example, that a sharp bend occurs in both curves at λ 520 and wavelengths situated at opposite ends of straight lines drawn through W (complementaries) are the same. The reference stimuli X, Y, Z are not realisable in practice, but that does not invalidate their usefulness as standards. If trichromatic coefficient curves were plotted for them, there would be no negative portions below the axis as there are in Fig. 19.4. No actual physical radiation can stimulate one of the receptor systems in the eye without also activating the other systems.

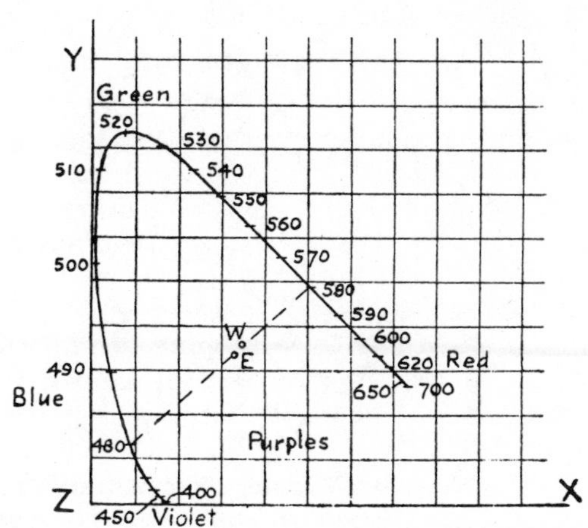

FIG. 19.7—COLOUR CHART. C.I.E. DATA. EQUAL QUANTITIES OF MATCHING STIMULI MAKE E. COMPARE FIG. 19.5.

The centre of the X, Y, Z triangle, with co-ordinates (0·33, 0·33), is marked E because the white used as standard on this system is that given by the hypothetical equal energy source. The white adopted as standard in Fig. 19.5 is indicated on the C.I.E. chart by the point W.

The choice of matching or reference stimuli for colorimetric purposes must not be confused with the spectral sensitivities of the three physiological response systems assumed to be present in the visual apparatus. We can choose the former as we please, to suit practical convenience; the latter are a property of the human visual mechanism and are not certainly known.*

19.8. The Wright Colorimeter.

It will be of interest to give a brief description of the apparatus designed by W. D. WRIGHT in 1926 and improved by him in 1938.† He has used it not only for measuring the trichromatic coefficients of the colours throughout the spectrum (§19.5) but for many other investigations concerned with colour discrimination, defective colour vision, adaptation, etc.

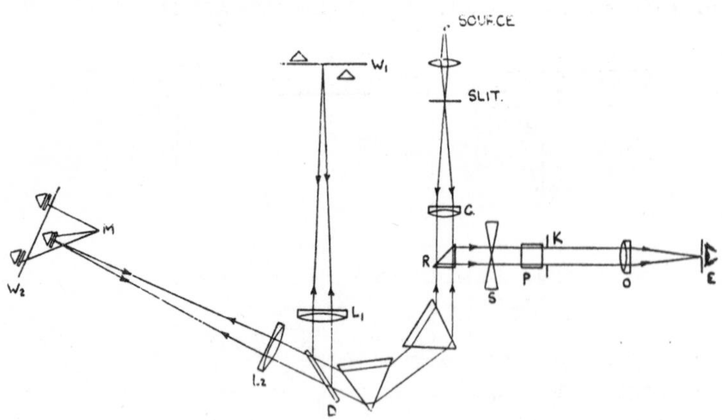

FIG. 19.8—THE WRIGHT COLORIMETER.

The optical system of the later model is shown in Fig. 19.8. A ribbon filament lamp is used as the source and an image of the lamp is formed by a condenser lens on the slit of a collimator. The parallel beam from the collimator objective C is refracted through the top half of two 60° dispersing prisms and is then incident on a dividing mirror D. This mirror, shown in Fig. 19.8A (a), divides the beam into two halves, one half being reflected by the strip of mirror p_1 into the lens L_1, to be focused in the spectrum

* §21.10.

† W. D. WRIGHT, *Trans. Opt. Soc.*, 29, 225, 1927; and *Journ. Scient. Insts.*, 16, Jan. 1939.

W_1, while the other half is allowed to pass through the hole p_2 into the lens L_2 to be focused in the spectrum W_2. The dispersing prisms are of extra dense flint glass. Each of the lenses L_1 and L_2 has a focal length of 47 inches and forms a spectrum 9·5 in. long between the wavelengths 400 $m\mu$ and 750 $m\mu$. In W_1 two roof reflecting prisms are mounted, by means of which two strips of spectrum can be reflected back and the light made to retrace its path through the dispersing system. In W_2 three reflecting prisms are mounted, the light reflected from these also returning through the dispersing system. The reflected beams, however, return at a lower level from the incident beam so that the beam from W_1, which was originally reflected from the strip p_1 of the dividing mirror, now

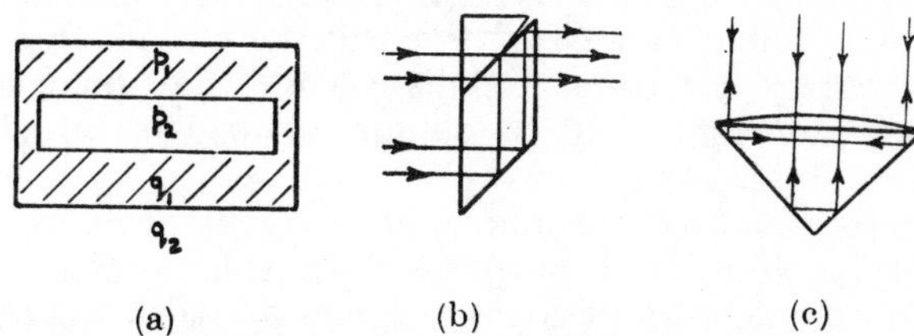

FIG. 19.8A.—WRIGHT COLORIMETER. DETAILS OF MIRROR AND REFLECTING PRISMS.

strikes strip q_1 while the beam from W_2, which initially passed through the space p_2, now returns through the space q_2 below the strip q_1. After the returning beams have re-traversed the dispersing prisms they are received by a prism R and reflected into a photometer prism P, shown in Fig. 19.8A (b). A rectangular diaphragm K limits the aperture of the beam which is subsequently focused by an objective O to form, at E, an image of the roof prisms in W_1 and W_2. An enlarged view of the roof reflecting prisms is shown in Fig. 19.8A (c).

The intensities of the three matching stimuli can be controlled by the observer through the operation of three photometer wedges M suspended in front of the reflecting prisms in the W_2 spectrum. The heights of these wedges can be manipulated by the observer by means of strings which pass over pulleys and are wound on drums mounted conveniently to the observer's hand; each wedge mounting has a scale and pointer and each wedge is previously carefully calibrated.

The two reflecting prisms in the W_1 spectrum provide the test colour (T.C.) and the desaturating primary (D.P.) —see §19.5. These reflectors can be moved to different parts of the W_1 spectrum as required. The intensities can be controlled also by neutral filters placed in front of the two reflecting prisms and, in addition, a rotating sector can be used at S to intercept the light from the W_1 spectrum and reduce its intensity by a factor given by the angular opening of the sector.

The two beams (matching and test) arriving at the photometer prism P from the spectra W_1 and W_2 are seen by the eye at E as two half-fields separated by a sharp dividing line; one half-field is filled by a mixture of the three matching stimuli and the other half-field by a spectral colour of any desired wavelength mixed with the desaturating colour, which can be of the wavelength of any one of the matching radiations. This second half-field can be filled by any light, e.g. a coloured surface, which it is desired to test.

The DONALDSON colorimeter, however, is probably better adapted for industrial purposes. In this instrument the three matching stimuli are obtained by the use of three colour filters carefully selected to give highly saturated colours and to be stable in quality. The intensities are controlled by slides which expose varying areas of these filters and the mixing of the three lights is carried out by admitting them into an integrating sphere the inner surface of which is silver-plated and then covered with a coating of magnesium oxide.

19.9. Subtractive Colour Mixture.

To those who have been accustomed to mixing water-colours it may come as a surprise at first to learn that the adding of, say, blue light to yellow light gives rise to a sensation of white, whereas the mixing of blue and yellow water-colours gives green. These facts are not contradictory, however, and follow quite simply from the principles already described. It is necessary only to bear in mind that the colours which water-colours and other pigments appear to have result from the wavelengths that they *absorb*; this has already been described in §19.1 in connection with natural objects seen by reflected light. The light finally emerging from all these objects is the residue after the absorbed wavelengths have been *subtracted* from the original incident light.

If a red filter is placed in one lantern and a green filter in another and the two beams of light are made to overlap on a white screen, the light reaching the eye is that which has been transmitted by the red filter, which is predominantly red but probably also contains orange, *plus* that transmitted by the green filter, which is predominantly green but probably includes a little blue (see Fig. 19.1). This additive mixture arouses a sensation of yellow, though it will be desaturated to a greater or less extent. (The colour chart shows that if the blue is small in amount, the desaturation will not be very marked.) If the two filters are now placed together (say red first) in one lantern, the light reaching the screen and hence the eye is the red and orange transmitted by the red filter minus the red and orange absorbed by the green filter; the result is practically zero. Little or no light passes through the combination.

By choosing three pigments or dyes very carefully, a wide range of colours can be obtained from their mixture. The three usually chosen are blue-green (or minus red), magenta (or minus green) and yellow (or minus blue), which are sometimes described as the SUBTRACTIVE PRIMARIES. The blue-green absorbs red and yellow; the magenta absorbs yellow and green; the yellow absorbs blue and violet. These subtractive primaries are used in three-colour printing, photography and television.

19.10. Filters. Density.

Reference has frequently been made in this chapter to the absorption of light by filters, pigments, etc. For certain purposes—industrial, medical, photographic, colorimetric, eye protection—it is necessary to obstruct some part or parts of the optical range of electromagnetic radiation emitted by the sun or artificial sources. A device for effecting such obstruction may be called a FILTER; it prevents the unwanted radiations from passing, either by absorbing them or reflecting them, or both. Most filters are of the absorbing type. They are made of glass containing various metallic compounds, or of plastics or gelatine containing dyes; they may be thin films deposited on glass or plastic material; or they may consist of various materials such as quartz, rocksalt, sylvine, paraffin, etc.

The accompanying table gives a convenient grouping of filters according to their effects on radiation with brief references to their applications.

TABLE. FILTERS

Symbol	*Description*	*Usual Constitution*	*Applications*
U.V.A.	Ultra-violet absorbing	Glass	Eye protection against scattered or reflected sunlight; mercury lamps; welding arcs.
V.A.G.	General absorption of visible	Glass	Eye protection against glare, scattered or reflected sunlight, especially if eyes used for close work.
V.A.S.	Selective absorption of visible	Glass; plastic; gelatine	Colours for photography, microscopy, signals, theatres, perimetry.
I.R.A.	Infra-red absorbing	Glass	Eye protection against direct sunlight, furnaces, glass blowing and other industrial techniques; roof lights.
U.V.T.	Ultra-violet transmitting	Glass	Bulbs for U.V. lamps; windows for clinics; optics for U.V. photography.
I.R.T.	Infra-red transmitting	Glass; quartz; rocksalt; sylvine	Optics for I.R. apparatus; windows for radiometric apparatus; I.R. signalling and safety devices.
NEUT.	Neutral	Glass; plastic; gelatine	Photometry; colorimetry; special and experimental purposes.
MONO.	Monochromatic	Glass; plastic; gelatine	Photography; spectroscopy; special and experimental purposes.
REFL.	To increase reflection	Thin films	Surface reflection mirrors.
ANTI-REFL.	To decrease reflection	Thin films	Coatings for prisms and lenses to increase transmission.

The colour of a filter is not a sound criterion of the radiation it is transmitting; thus a red glass may be transmitting all the visible (e.g. §19.1) as well as U.V. and I.R. radiations, its red colour being due to the fact that it transmits red more copiously than other wavelengths. It is difficult to make "pure" or monochromatic filters which will transmit just one narrow band of the spectrum to the exclusion of other wavelengths.

The filters classed as neutral are more scientifically constructed than the ordinary commercial " smoke " glasses sometimes used for eye protection.

It is sometimes convenient, especially in the case of deep neutral or coloured filters, such as are used in photometry and colorimetry, to specify the transmission and absorption in terms of a quantity called DENSITY which is defined as

the logarithm, to base 10, *of the opacity.*

If a quantity I_0 of luminous flux of a given wavelength is incident on a filter, a certain proportion of it is reflected; if r = the reflection factor, the reflected flux is rI_0 and an amount $I_E = (1 - r)I_0$ enters the material of the filter. Of this, some is transmitted, the remainder being absorbed or scattered. If unit thickness transmit a fraction p, twice this thickness transmits p^2 and thickness t units transmits the fraction p^t. The luminous flux transmitted is given by $I_T = I_E \cdot p^t$.

$$\text{Transmission factor (or Transparency)} = \frac{\text{lum. flux transmitted}}{\text{lum. flux entering}}$$

$$= \frac{I_T}{I_E} = p^t$$

$$\text{Opacity*} = \text{reciprocal of transmission factor} = \frac{I_E}{I_T}$$

$$\text{Density} = d = \log_{10}\frac{I_E}{I_T} = \log_{10}\frac{1}{p^t}$$

Thus if a certain filter transmit 10 per cent of the luminous flux entering it, i.e. $\frac{I_T}{I_E} = 0{\cdot}1$, then its density $d = \log_{10}10 = 1{\cdot}0$. If a filter transmit 1 per cent, $\frac{I_T}{I_E} = 0{\cdot}01$ and density $d = \log_{10}100 = 2{\cdot}0$. If this latter filter has unit thickness, then a filter of the same material but twice the thickness, or two filters of unit thickness in contact, will have density given by

$$d = \log_{10}\frac{1}{{\cdot}01^2} = \log_{10} 10{,}000 = 4{\cdot}0.$$

The density increases directly with the thickness; the combined density of a number of absorbing media in series is equal to the sum of their individual densities.

* The transmission factor is always less than unity and the opacity greater than unity.

The above remarks deal with the transmission and density for a certain wavelength. If the transmission factor and density were the same for all wavelengths the material would be a neutral material. If the material is coloured it has different transmission factors for different wavelengths and increasing the thickness will narrow down the transmission curve (such as Fig. 19.1 C, for example) so that its colour will become more saturated as the thickness increases.

EXERCISES. CHAPTER XIX.

1. (*a*) Explain why a disc marked with yellow and blue sectors appears almost white when it is rapidly rotated.

(*b*) Explain the meaning of the terms: complementary colours; saturation.

2. (*a*) A buttercup and a sodium flame both appear yellow. Explain the difference between the two yellows and how the difference arises.

(*b*) Objects normally described as (i) white, (ii) blue, (iii) red, are observed through a piece of red glass. Explain how they will appear.

3. (*a*) Explain why a piece of glass which appears coloured when in one piece appears practically white when crushed to a powder.

(*b*) Why is it preferred to match coloured fabrics out-of-doors or with the help of an artificial daylight lamp?

(*c*) Why do purple fabrics appear redder in artificial light than in daylight?

4. Explain each of the following:

(*a*) Yellow and blue paints mixed together produce green paint, but yellow and blue lights projected on to a screen produce white light.

(*b*) Materials with bright saturated colours can be obtained in the red-orange-yellow range, but in the green-blue range the colours may be saturated but not bright. (S.M.C.—part question.)

5. What is light and what is colour?

Discuss the significance and limitations of the statement: "Any colour sensation can be matched by mixing not more than three suitable spectral lights in varying proportions".

How would you proceed to prove the statement experimentally? (S.M.C.)

6. When radiation within the wavelength range 200 to 2000 millimicrons is incident on a body, the radiation and the body are affected in ways dependent upon the direction and intensity of the radiation and upon the nature of the body and the condition of its surface. Describe concisely what these effects are in the case of (*a*) optical glass; (*b*) uranium glass; (*c*) a metal such as zinc; (*d*) a "black body". (S.M.C.)

7. Give an account of the radiation emitted by the filament of an electric lamp as its temperature is gradually raised to the practical limit.

Explain (*a*) the term white light; (*b*) why the colours of natural objects are generally unsaturated; (*c*) what will be the colour of a paint produced by mixing yellow paint and blue paint. (S.M.C.)

8. Define the term white light. Is the light emitted by a carbon filament lamp the same as that emitted by a modern tungsten filament lamp? If not, describe the difference and state the cause of it.

Yellow light from a pure spectrum is admitted to one part of the field of a colour matching apparatus and a mixture of red and green spectrum lights to the other part of the field of the instrument. Explain whether it is possible to adjust the red and green lights to match the yellow light completely in hue, saturation and luminosity. (S.M.C.)

9. Explain what is meant by the energy distribution curve of the light emitted or reflected by a body and how the appearance of the body depends upon the shape of the curve. Draw curves showing the energy distribution of the light in the following cases:

(*a*) the light emitted by a sodium flame;
(*b*) the light emitted by the sun;
(*c*) the light emitted by an incandescent lamp;
(*d*) the light transmitted by a cheap green glass and by a good green glass with a sharp "cut-off" when white light is incident.
(*e*) the light reflected by a purple fabric in daylight.

10. Explain the difference between matching stimuli as used in a colorimeter and the spectral sensitivities of the three physiological response systems assumed to exist in the human visual apparatus.

With the aid of the colour chart explain the considerations that govern the choice of red, green and blue for colorimetric matching stimuli.

11. With the aid of the colour chart, showing the spectrum locus, explain the meaning of the term complementary colours. State the approximate wavelengths of the hues that are complementary to hues of wavelengths (*a*) 450, (*b*) 490, (*c*) 600 $m\mu$ respectively.

Comment on the luminosities of the two complementary lights in cases (*a*) and (*b*).

12. State and explain the two fundamental laws on which trichromatic colorimetry or "colour mixing" depends.

13. Operations with a trichromatic colorimeter enable the unit trichromatic equation of an unknown colour to be obtained in terms of three matching stimuli on the basis that the quantities, expressed in trichromatic units, of these stimuli required to match the agreed standard white are equal.

Explain this statement, making clear the meaning of the terms trichromatic unit, unit trichromatic equation and standard white.

14. Explain the meaning of the following colour equations:

$$160\,\mathrm{R} + 120\,\mathrm{G} + 180\,\mathrm{B} = 100\,\mathrm{W}$$
$$90\,\mathrm{Y} + 10\,\mathrm{G} + 200\,\mathrm{B} = 100\,\mathrm{W}$$

Deduce the equation for yellow in terms of the three primaries. (B.O.A.)

15. A certain green radiation C was matched in a colorimeter with matching stimuli R, G and B and the resulting unit trichromatic equation was

$$\mathrm{C} = 0{\cdot}232\,\mathrm{R} + 0{\cdot}797\,\mathrm{G} - 0{\cdot}029\,\mathrm{B}$$

Discuss the significance of the negative quantity of the blue matching stimulus and find the U.T. equation for C in terms of W (white), R and G.

16. (*a*) Construct a colour chart and on it plot the spectrum locus.

(*b*) Mark on it the position of the colour C_1 which results from mixing 0·6 T unit of the green matching stimulus and 0·4 T unit of the blue matching stimulus. What will be the hue and state of saturation of this colour ? What wavelength of the spectrum will have the same hue ?

(*c*) Mark the position of the colour C_2 formed by mixing 0·7 T unit of the red matching stimulus and 0·3 T unit of the green matching stimulus. Describe this colour similarly.

(*d*) Mark the position of the colour C_3 formed by mixing equal quantities, in T units, of C_1 and C_2. Describe this colour and state its co-ordinates on the chart.

(*e*) If 0·74 T unit of C_3 are mixed with 0·26 T unit of the colour which has co-ordinates (0·285, 0), what will be the resultant colour ?

17. (*a*) Find the densities of filters with percentage transmission factors of 100, 50, 10, 5, 1, and 0·001.

(*b*) The transparency of a 2 mm. thick filter is 30 per cent ; what is the density of a filter of the same material and 10 mm. thick ?

18. Explain the meaning of the term optical density as applied to an absorbing medium. Illustrate by finding the density of a filter which transmits 20 per cent of the light flux incident on it.

What will be the transparency (i.e. percentage of light transmitted) and optical density of a filter of the same material and twice the thickness ? (S.M.C.)

19. (*a*) In the case of vision the same sensation may be evoked by entirely different physical stimuli ; in the case of hearing this is not so. Discuss this statement.

(*b*) A person with a red glass before the right eye and a glass of "complementary" green before the left observes a white card ruled with red lines. What does he see with each eye ?

20. What connection is there between the wavelength of light and its colour ? What do you call (*a*) light of greater wavelength, (*b*) light of shorter wavelength than that of visible light ? How can these lights be obtained ? Is there any connection between the colour of a hot body and its temperature ? (B.O.A.)

21. Write an essay on the apparatus and laws of colour mixing. (S.M.C.)

22. Describe apparatus suitable for matching the colour and obtaining the colour equation of a given piece of material. Explain clearly how the equation is obtained. (B.O.A.)

23. What are (*a*) the colour triangle ; (*b*) a colour equation ? How are these related ? the colour triangle what colours are indicated (*a*) by points on the sides of the triangle ; (*b*) by a point near the centre of the triangle ? Explain your answers. (B.O.A.)

24. Explain on the three-colour theory of vision the meaning of complementary colours. Name pairs of such colours. (B.O.A.)

25. What is the colour triangle ? Plot on a colour triangle the following colours and say in general terms what each colour is :

(*a*) $+ 0 \cdot 3\,R + 0 \cdot 6\,Gr + 0 \cdot 1\,B$; (*b*) $- 0 \cdot 05\,R + 0 \cdot 6\,Gr + 0 \cdot 45\,B$; (*c*) $+ 0 \cdot 35\,R + 0 \cdot 35\,Gr + 0 \cdot 3\,B$.

Draw a diagram of, and describe briefly, the apparatus by which these equations are obtained. (B.O.A.)

26. Explain on the three-colour theory of colour vision the reason for the difficulty of matching colours by artificial light. What conditions must be fulfilled by the artificial light to enable such matches to be made with accuracy? (B.O.A.)

27. In what various ways can a colour be specified in actual numbers? Explain the underlying principles of such specifications. (B.O.A.)

STIMULUS AND SENSATION

CHAPTER XX

THE DEVELOPMENT OF SENSATION

20.1. Stimulus, Eye, Sensation.

THE student should first revise Chapter I which describes the visual mechanism in outline and contains some necessary definitions.

In everyday life the human visual mechanism is presented with rapidly varying scenes which are built up of numerous elements varying in brightness, colour and position. Each element emits light which is refracted by the eye's optical system into an image on the retina which forms the stimulus; in response to this stimulation there arises a simple visual sensation. It is the integration of such elementary visual sensations with information reaching the brain simultaneously from other senses and from the organs of the body which results in the general appraisement of the scene called a percept.*

Each simple sensation has three attributes: (1) duration; (2) magnitude (luminosity); (3) quality (colour—hue, saturation). It arises in consciousness through the mediation of three main agencies, namely: (A) the stimulus, light; (B) the visual mechanism; (C) the mind. These three agencies have characteristics, as below, *all of which play their part in determining the nature of each sensation.*† In any visual act a number of these characteristics will be in operation simultaneously in combination, affecting the sensation in its three attributes. Bearing in mind also that the visual mechanism is a delicate living organism, continually varying as it "adapts" itself to the changing external and internal conditions, it can be appreciated what a bewildering variety of sensations is possible; and how complicated may be the process by which the sensation is built up in the brain even when the stimulus is simple, such as a single flash of light.

---

* §§ 1.2 and 1.4.

† To save continual repetition in this and subsequent chapters the student should keep this constantly in mind.

The characteristics are:

A. THE STIMULUS.

(1) its duration; single and intermittent stimuli
(2) its intensity and distribution of light over it
(3) its size
(4) its spectral composition

} these are not independent of one another

(5) its form or contour
(6) the condition of the optical system and pupil.

B. THE VISUAL MECHANISM.

(a) the sensitivity varies regionally over the retina: foveal, para-foveal and peripheral.
(b) time is needed for sensation to grow and decay; persistence of vision.
(c) the condition of the stimulated region is influenced by
  (i) previous stimulation (temporal induction) and by
  (ii) simultaneous stimulation of other regions of the retina (spatial induction) or of the other eye.
(d) the acuteness of the light sense, form sense and colour sense.
(e) the eye is in continual motion when fixating.
(f) the sensation is influenced by the general physiological condition of the body.

C. THE MIND.

Experience; memory; interest; other senses.

When investigating the accurate quantitative relationships between stimulus and sensation, the conditions of each experiment must be carefully controlled; attention must be confined to a defined region of the retina and that region must be maintained in a prescribed condition. Experimenters are restricted at the outset by the fact that we cannot measure sensations; we cannot measure a taste, a smell or a light sensation. Of two objects it is possible to distinguish that one appears to be brighter than the other, but we are unable to decide by how much one is the brighter. The eye* is merely a comparator;

* See footnote, §18.1.

it can decide, to a certain degree of precision, when two visual sensations are equal with respect to some attribute such as hue or luminosity, but this does not measure the sensation in any physical unit. The only kinds of experiment we can perform consist in simple tasks such as comparing stimuli which evoke a just perceptible sensation, i.e. the liminal or THRESHOLD value of the stimulus ; or measuring the change of stimulus which evokes a just perceptible change in the sensation, i.e. the DIFFERENTIAL THRESHOLD value of the stimulus.

Such experiments, be it noted, tell us nothing about the *nature* of the sensations ; nothing about how they arise in consciousness in response to the impulses transmitted from the retina.

In studying this subject the student should keep in mind the intimacy of the retina and brain ; the former is a projection outwards of the latter, the nerve fibres being the axons of the second neurones (ganglia) of the nervous chain; the brain and retina operate together as a unit.

20.2. Rod Vision and Cone Vision. The Duplicity Theory.

The existence of the two types of receptor, rods and cones, in the human retina and the anatomical investigation of MAX SCHULTZE (1868) on the rods and cones in vertebrate retinæ generally ; the discovery of visual purple by H. MÜLLER in 1851 and of the bleaching effect on it of light (BOLL, 1876) ; together with numerous visual phenomena such as those mentioned in §§ 1.7 to 1.11 led KRIES to propose in 1896 that there are two distinct mechanisms in the retina : the ROD OR SCOTOPIC MECHANISM which, in conjunction with the visual purple, is responsible for vision at low levels of illumination ; and the CONE OR PHOTOPIC MECHANISM which comes into operation at ordinary and high levels of illumination. So much evidence has since accumulated in support of this so-called duplicity theory that its broad acceptance is practically universal. A selection of such evidence may be summarised as follows.

The rods and cones are distributed over the human retina in the manner shown by Fig. 20.1 from which it is seen that within the rod-free area of about 45 minutes radius surrounding the central fovea the cones are densely packed : their population is about 150,000 per sq. mm. The cone density falls very rapidly in the para-foveal region. The rods begin to make their appearance at the edge of the rod-free area and their density rises to a maximum, stated to be also about 150,000 per mm.[2] at about 20° from the fovea.*

We know from common observation that in daylight and under bright conditions generally the fovea is easily the most sensitive part of the retina. Whenever an object engages our attention, it is not until we have rotated the eyes until that object is imaged on the fovea that we can distinguish its fine detail and recognise its variations of colour. Under these bright conditions all three senses—light, form and colour—are much more acute at the fovea than elsewhere and it seems to be essential to employ the cones in our visual tasks.

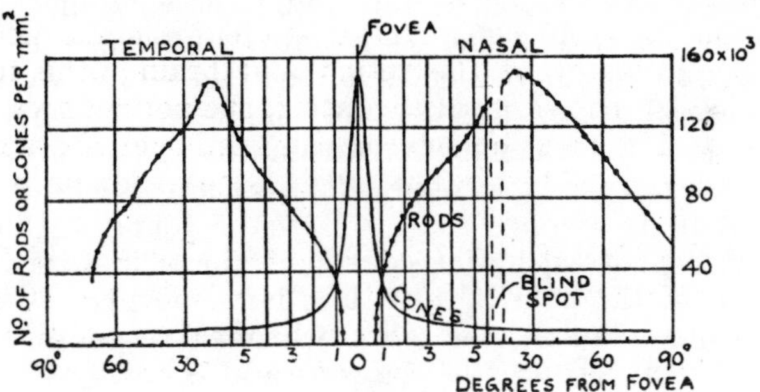

Fig. 20.1—Approximate Distribution of Rods and Cones across Human Retina. (Note enlarged scale of abscissæ up to 5°).

In dim illumination it is quite otherwise; we cannot read or distinguish fine detail; colour vision is absent, all objects appearing grey and varying only in apparent brightness. Such vision as is possible under these conditions, such as the detection of faint lights and the movements of things about us, is not achieved by the fovea but by the para-foveal and peripheral regions of the retina where the rods predominate. The cones seem to have gone out of action.

The evidence seems irresistible that under photopic conditions vision is mediated primarily by the cones, which are responsible for form vision and colour vision; and that in scotopic conditions it is the rods that are active, as detectors of light and movement. It is to be

* This figure and the graph of Fig. 20.1 would give a total number of rods over the whole retina, however, far exceeding the 120 millions or so usually quoted.

expected, therefore, that the nature of a sensation will depend on the location of the retinal region that is stimulated [B (a) of §20.1], since this determines the relative numbers of rods and cones concerned in the response.

It may be the case, nevertheless, that the distinction between the two mechanisms is not absolute; that they exert reciprocal actions one on the other. The evidence is not sufficiently conclusive to rule out the possibility, for example, that the rods *may* play some part in colour vision. Certain photochemical substances with properties akin to those of visual purple have been found in the cones of certain species,* and until more is known about their character and distribution, the finer points of the relationship between the rod mechanism and the cone mechanism cannot be settled. The structural differences between the rods and the more slender of the cones that are found in the foveal region are not very definite. Neither is it very clear as to whereabouts within the rod or around it the visual purple is located. The Stiles-Crawford effect would seem to require that it is to be found within the rod, and the corresponding cone substances likewise within the body of the cone; there is other evidence, however, which suggests that the photo-chemical substances are located on the surfaces of the rods and cones.

When the variation of sensitivity as between the cone-populated fovea and the periphery of the retina is under discussion, the presence of the yellow " pigment " which covers an area extending somewhat beyond the fovea must be taken into consideration. This substance seems to absorb in that part of the spectrum extending from the violet to the yellow-green region. Since its amount varies between individuals, CLERK MAXWELL suggested long ago that this would cause variations in colour matching between different individuals. This is one of the reasons for limiting the field of view in colorimeters to 2 degrees.† We will use the generally accepted term pigment when referring to this substance though it is on the whole too transparent to be called pigment.

20.3. Effect of a Single Stimulus. The Primary Image.

We will suppose that the eye has remained in the dark for an appreciable period so that the activity aroused in the retina by previous stimulations has subsided. The eye is

* §22.2. † §19.2.

then said to be dark-adapted.* When a brief stimulus falls on a certain area of the retina of such an eye the equilibrium of this area (which we will call the test region) is disturbed; there arises almost immediately a sensation called the PRIMARY IMAGE: this is the only image that is noticed in ordinary vision and is the one by which we recognise the object from which the stimulating light comes. The disturbance continues and with the passage of time the region undergoes a sequence of rhythmical changes which give rise to corresponding sensations called *after-images* and which also modify the manner in which this region will respond to any succeeding stimulus which may fall on it [B (c) i of §20.1]. The process by which this temporal series of events is induced in the test region by the original stimulus is called TEMPORAL INDUCTION.

The effects of the stimulus, however, are not confined to the test region on which it falls; in consequence of the nervous inter-connections within the retina the stimulus induces changes also in other regions of the retina, perhaps over the whole retina, and maybe even in the retina of the other eye. The process by which these effects are induced between one region and another is called SPATIAL INDUCTION [B (c) ii].

Thus a single stimulus, even a very brief one such as a flash of light, is responsible for a complex series of events in the retina.

We limit ourselves at present to temporal induction, to the test region; and consider first the primary image. In order that a stimulus shall evoke a sensation at all and be perceived it must exceed the liminal value: i.e. it must be of sufficient size and intensity and must act for a sufficient period of time. From the moment when such a stimulus strikes the retina of a dark-adapted eye, the above mentioned sequence commences. First there is a LATENT PERIOD before any sensation is appreciated; the sensation then rises, more or less rapidly according to the stimulus intensity, to a certain maximum value, from which it immediately begins to fall and, with a brief stimulus such as we are considering, it gradually decays to zero. This rise and fall of the initial sensation constitutes the primary image; it persists for some time after stimulation has ceased.

* Adaptation is discussed in §20.7.

The rise and fall of the primary image are illustrated in Fig. 20.2 by two curves connecting sensation with time for a weak and a strong stimulus respectively. Referring first to the weak stimulus, it is supposed to commence at the instant marked O and to cease after a period Ot_1. No sensation is experienced until after the latent period Oa_1; the sensation then rises and will reach a maximum value at M_1 after a period Om_1 provided the stimulus acts for at least this length of time. The period Om_1, the least period during which a stimulus must act in order to evoke the maximum sensation of which it is capable, is the ACTION TIME

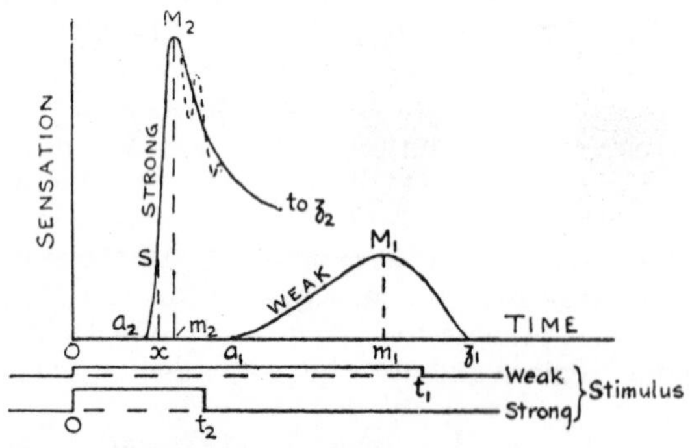

FIG. 20.2—THE PRIMARY IMAGE WITH WEAK AND STRONG STIMULUS RESPECTIVELY. Oa_1 AND Oa_2 ARE THE LATENT PERIODS: Om_1 AND Om_2 ARE THE ACTION TIMES OF THE STIMULI.

of the stimulus. The maximum value having been reached the sensation falls; and if the stimulus ceases soon after the expiration of the action time, it falls to zero at z_1. The stimulus being a weak one, nothing further happens.

The second curve shows the sequence for the case of a stronger stimulus, acting over a period Ot_2. The latent period Oa_2 and the action time Om_2 are shorter and the maximum value or peak of the primary image at M_2 is greater. If the stimulus ceases at or just after its action time at m_2 the decay of the sensation may be accompanied by rapid fluctuations of darkness and brightness; these are suggested by the broken line superimposed on the graph. During the building up of the primary image throughout the period Om_2 the effect of the light is cumulative; were the stimulus to cease after a shorter period Ox, the sensation would only reach the value xS, even though the stimulus is at full strength.

If the stimulus lasts for some time the curve will proceed parallel to the x axis for a while before dropping to zero at z_2.

The latent period varies from 0·05 to 0·2 second for ordinary intensities of stimulus. It is shorter: in extra-foveal regions of the retina, in the dark-adapted eye, for stronger stimuli and for light of longer wavelength. The primary image lasts for about the same length of time as the latent period, i.e. 0·05 to 0·2 second. It is shorter for strong stimuli than weak ones. This is surprising, but has received partial explanation as the result of electro-physiological investigations, to be described later.

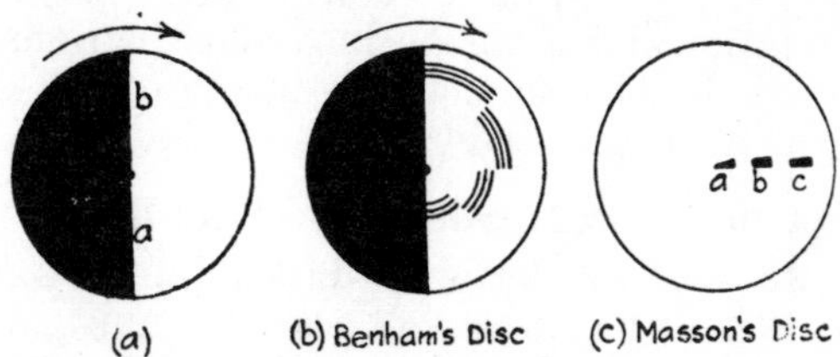

FIG. 20.3—BLACK-AND-WHITE DISCS WHICH, WHEN REVOLVED, ILLUSTRATE VARIOUS VISUAL PHENOMENA—SEE TEXT.

These properties of the primary image and its latent period may be responsible for some unexpected colour effects which can be observed even though the stimulus is achromatic—a white light or a white and black rotating disc. The effects can be obtained by gazing steadily at one point of a rotating black and white disc under adequate illumination, such as those depicted at (a), (b) and (c) in Fig. 20.3. Referring to the first of these, if the disc is rotated in the direction of the arrow, then at a certain speed of rotation which depends upon the illumination, the forward edge a of the white sector appears reddish and the following edge, b, bluish. This may be accounted for by the fact, stated above, that the latent period is shorter for red light than for blue. The same kind of effect is observed with BENHAM'S disc* in which, when rotated at a certain speed, the central portion appears red and the outer portion blue or blue-green.

Discs of this kind, fixed to a wheel capable of being revolved at various speeds, were used extensively by early

* Described by C. E. BENHAM (1894).

experimenters on visual phenomena and are most useful for student's laboratory work. In more precise experiments great care has to be exercised in controlling the variables associated with the stimulus and the eye. For example, to ensure that conditions B (a) and B (c) of §20.1 can be put under control as needed, the individual under test may be put in a closed compartment or a box provided with a small aperture through which he observes the test object or light. Matters are so arranged that the interior white walls of the box may be illuminated to known extents and the observer's eye, therefore, conditioned (i.e. light- or dark-adapted) as required before and during the experiment. A fixation light can be moved to various positions on the wall of the box so that the image of the test object may be formed on selected regions of the retina.

20.4. Effect of a Single Stimulus. After-Images (Positive).

The eye we are considering is dark-adapted and remains in the dark after the impact of the stimulus. Unless the stimulus is very weak the primary image already described is followed by an after-image, which passes through a sequence of phases. When special methods of investigation are employed it is found that the earlier phases occur very rapidly, occupying less than one second of time ; but that these are followed by later phases which may last for several seconds or even minutes* and may pass through a sequence of colour changes. The sequence may vary considerably according to the individual and to the intensity, spectral composition and duration of the stimulus.

After-images are so interesting and sometimes, when the conditions are suitable, so startlingly vivid, that they have received a great deal of attention ; moreover, they are of considerable theoretical significance. Unfortunately, however, attempts made to explain them have led to the introduction of confusing terminology, which will as far as possible be omitted here. The kind of after-images we are discussing are usually described as positive after-images. They are similar in kind to the primary image ; if the original stimulus is white—a flash of white light, or a piece of well-illuminated white paper on a dark ground, or a window, etc.—the after-image is white on a dark ground. If the original stimulus is coloured, the after-image has the same hue.

* The after-image may last for hours if the stimulus has been *very* intense.

The sequence is illustrated graphically in Fig. 20.4. The primary-image decays to zero at z (compare Fig. 20.2), to be succeeded by the series numbered 1 to 5, the ordinates giving a rough idea of the brightnesses in relation to that of the primary image. Nos. 1 and 5 are of the same hue as the primary image. No. 3, sometimes called the Purkinje after-image or Bidwell's ghost, is usually of the same hue also but (an example of the vagaries of these phenomena) may be of complementary hue, especially if the stimulus were of high intensity.

Suppose the dark-adapted eyes are completely shielded from a small source (spot) of white light by the hand, which is rapidly removed and replaced and the eyes closed. The first sensation, the primary image, will be white and will be succeeded after a short interval by a white after-image, i.e. No. 5 in Fig. 20.4. This will sometimes be so

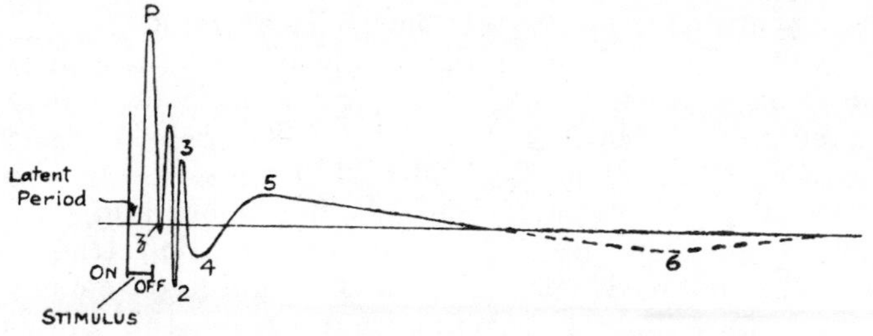

FIG. 20.4—PRIMARY AND AFTER-IMAGES FOLLOWING A SHORT STIMULUS.

bright and vivid that it appears as if the source were still being observed, and the hand transparent. As it fades away it may pass through a sequence of colours, frequently in this order: blue or greenish-blue, violet, orange. The rapid early phases 1 to 4, lasting less than a second, will not be noticed in a simple experiment of this kind.

20.5. Spatial Induction.

Because the visual mechanism possesses the property that the impact of a stimulus falling on one area of the retina influences the sensitivity of other regions (§20.3), it follows that if two adjacent areas of the retina are stimulated by two separate lights, the sensation arising from each area is different, in hue or luminosity, from what it would have been had the other light been absent. It is found that the sensations from the two areas induce effects in each other which tend generally to accentuate the contrast between them, though this depends upon the nature of the boundary which separates the two areas.

The phenomenon is called *spatial induction* or *simultaneous contrast* and has been well appreciated for centuries. Painters especially are familiar with the reciprocal action between juxtaposed colours and use it to good effect in their pictures. The following are a few of the numerous simple ways in which the phenomenon can be exhibited; if a little care is exercised in choosing the papers and arranging the conditions of illumination, the effects are sometimes most striking.

1. A strip of grey paper laid partly on a white and partly on a black background appears darker against the white than against the black.

A coloured strip of paper, say red, appears brighter and more saturated against the black background.

A grey strip on a blue ground appears to be tinged with yellow, on a green ground it appears purple or pink and on a red ground, bluish-green. The effects are best observed by covering the whole field with thin white tissue paper. If we call the background the inducing colour and that to which it gives rise in the object of attention (the grey strip) the induced colour, then the induced colour is always approximately complementary to the inducing colour.

If a sheet of black paper containing a small hole is held between the eye and a bright sky, the hole appears brighter than the sky as seen round about the paper.

2. The shadow method: with an arrangement similar to the Rumford shadow photometer, the two sources are ordinary electric lights, one bulb being white and the other coloured (say yellow); the lights are adjusted for distance until the two shadows cast on the white screen are about equally dark. Except where the two shadows fall the white screen is illuminated by both sources and will appear yellowish. The shadow cast by the yellow source is illuminated only by the white source; it does not appear grey (dull white), however, but bluish because of the inductive effect of the yellowish surround. If this shadow is observed through a tube, thus eliminating the inducing surround from the field of view, it appears grey instead of blue.

3. The method of after-images: if, after the eyes have been closed and rested for a while, a pencil dot on a small square of white paper on a large green background be steadily fixated for two minutes or so and the gaze then transferred to a white surface, an after-image will presently appear which is purple or pink except over the small area corresponding to the white square; here the appearance will be green, complementary to the purple of the surrounding after-image. If the experiment is repeated with a red instead of green surround, the after-image will have a blue-green surround with a red square corresponding to the white square of the original stimulus.

The reasons for these appearances will be better understood after the discussion of the so-called negative after-image in the following section (20.6).

The student should also observe that as the two minutes' fixation of the white square progresses, its apparent brightness decreases; it becomes grey tinged somewhat with the hue of the background. This grey image will be seen to move relatively to the actual white square, due to the involuntary movements of the eyes round about the point of fixation.

The simultaneous contrast effects above described, whether of luminosity or of hue, are most marked near to the border between the two adjacent fields. A row of grey strips, the strips being of successively darker grey, appears like a succession of flutings because of the accentuation at each border.

No adequate explanation of these spatial induction effects has yet been advanced. HELMHOLTZ maintained that they are errors of judgment and are therefore brought about by a central, cortical, process. All normal people experience the phenomena in the same way, however; and colour contrast has been obtained under the illumination of a flash lasting no more than 10^{-6} second, a time too short for any kind of judgment, true or false. Hence the consensus of modern opinion is in favour of a physiological explanation. It is anticipated that current electrophysiological researches will throw light on the interaction between different regions of the retina, which is believed to be the basic cause of the phenomena.

Whatever may be the explanation of the effects, they are always present and are of great importance in everyday vision and in the use of optical instruments. The fact that the visual acuity of the visual mechanism is as good as it is in spite of the imperfections (aberrations and diffraction) of the eye's optical system must be due in part to the accentuation of contrast at the boundary between one part of an image and another ; and there is ample evidence of the effect that the brightness of the surround has on visual acuity* and on the efficiency and comfort of the individual in all kinds of visual tasks. Glare, which will be discussed later, is an obvious illustration of this last remark. The influence of spatial induction is of importance in connection with the general and local illumination and the colours of machines and workbenches in factories, especially when work involving fine detail is concerned ; in camouflage ; in the use of test charts, etc. ; and in the design and use of telescopic instruments, particularly night glasses.

With regard to telescopes, L. C. MARTIN and T. C. RICHARDS found (1928) that for picking up objects in dim illumination the field of view of the instrument should be as large as possible ; a small object not discernible against the background in a small field may become easily visible when the size of the stimulated retinal area is increased by enlarging the field of view of the instrument. It is suggested (indeed has been put into practice) that in night glasses it would be desirable to stimulate the extra-foveal regions of the retina artificially by introducing a ring of illumination, such as phosphorescent paint, around the circumference of the field stop of the instrument.

On the other hand, if the object is a dark one on a brighter background, then the speed and accuracy of observation is improved by reducing the size of field. This occurs in the case of glasses for marine use, where a ship may be under observation in a bright field of sky and water.

The inductive effect of two adjacent areas on one another seems to be affected by the nature of the boundary between them ; in the experiment with a grey strip on a coloured ground, for example, the appearance of the induced complementary colour is to a large extent prohibited if the outline of the strip is marked on the coloured background with pen or pencil. This boundary effect arises whenever a comparison is being made between two areas differing in hue or luminosity. In those cases where there is a *gradual*

* §2.10.

variation across the field the eye has the property of endeavouring to ignore the variation. In the field of view of a telescope the brightness is greatest over a limited central area and falls gradually to half this value or less at the edge of the field* : yet to most people the field appears to be uniformly bright all over.

20.6. Modified (Negative) After-Images.

It was stated in §20.3 that the original stimulus induces effects in neighbouring regions of the retina (spatial induction) and temporal effects within the test region. In consequence of the latter, if the eye is subjected to a second stimulus, which we will call the secondary stimulus, the response of the retina will not be the same as it would have been in the absence of the original stimulus. In general the temporal induction effect of the original stimulus is to inhibit further sensations of the same kind as the primary image and encourage those of opposite kind.

The sensation that will be evoked by the secondary stimulus will clearly depend upon a variety of factors associated with the two stimuli and with the location of the retinal region(s) stimulated by them. Very little precise quantitative research has been done on this problem. Most of the published work, practically all of which is qualitative, is concerned with the special type of case where the original stimulus acts on the fovea and parafoveal region and the secondary stimulus, following immediately and continuing for some time, acts upon a considerable area of the retina, including the fovea, and is of a lower brightness than the original stimulus. In these circumstances the primary image evoked by the original stimulus is followed by an after-image, usually called a negative after-image, which passes through a sequence of phases differing from the sequence of the positive after-image already described.

For example, if the spot of white light in the simple experiment of §20.4 is steadily fixated for a minute or so and the eyes are then directed to a white sheet of paper, the after-image consists of a black spot seen against the white surround ; it fades and returns, sometimes appearing violet in colour. If, after the original steady fixation, the eyes are closed and shielded from further stimulation, the

---

* §7.1.

after-image is black with a yellowish border seen against a dark ground which, however, is not so black as the small central after-image; the after-image fades and returns, becoming violet as in the previous case.

If a small square of red paper on a black background is fixated for a minute or so and the gaze then directed to a white sheet, the after-image is blue-green, approximately complementary to the original red stimulus. If, after the fixation, the gaze is transferred to a sheet of green paper, the after-image will appear of a distinctly more saturated green than the green background.

The general nature of these negative after-images can be studied by exposing small pieces of paper of various colours and sizes on backgrounds of various colours and then transferring the gaze to a second paper background which is also varied in colour and size. It will be readily appreciated that according to such variations, and remembering that differently coloured lights evoke sensations with different latent periods and rates of growth and decay, these after-images can be very complex. Before their cause and significance can be properly understood, however, much work will be needed under controlled scientific conditions.

Suitable arrangement of the simple experiments will reveal that the after-image may be unexpectedly vivid and pure, more saturated than the spectrum hues or any hues we experience in nature. If, for example, we produce a pure spectrum of good extent and provide means such as a slit in the plane of the spectrum for isolating different restricted regions of it, we can expose the eye to a small area of, say, the blue-green region. If we then expose the red part of the spectrum and transfer the gaze to it, the after-image is seen to stand out as a red patch (complementary to the blue-green original stimulus) which is purer than the surrounding spectrum red; the latter is somewhat whitish by comparison. On the assumption of a triple response system in the retina (§19.3),* a partial explanation of this high saturation of the after-image might be suggested. Monochromatic blue-green light of wavelength, say, 500 $m\mu$ will stimulate the blue and green response systems to a much greater extent than the red system. The two former will consequently become

* See also §21.10.

"fatigued" more than the latter, in the sense that the photo-chemical substances* through which they operate will be broken down or bleached more than the "red" substance. The contributions of the blue and green response systems to subsequent stimulation by the secondary stimulus will consequently be reduced below the normal amounts and the preponderance of the red response system will evoke a purer red than is normally experienced.

Because these after-images are opposite in kind to the primary image evoked by the original stimulus, black if the latter were white and of more or less complementary hue if it were coloured, the phenomenon is sometimes described as *successive induction* or *successive contrast.* It is to be noted, however, that when the secondary stimulus covers an extensive retinal area including the test region, the activity of the latter is due to three causes: the contemporary stimulation of it by the secondary stimulus; the spatial induction effect of the secondary stimulus falling on the surrounding area; and the temporal inductive effect of the original stimulus. It is not surprising, therefore, that the sequence of sensations varies widely with the conditions as to intensity, colour and extent of the two stimuli and according to the individual.

After-images as vivid as those experienced in specially arranged experiments would be most annoying if they occurred in daily life. But the effect of temporal induction in enhancing the sensitivity of the retina to a second stimulus of different kind from the original stimulus, the effect of spatial induction in accentuating the boundaries between adjacent retinal areas, the continual movement of the eyes from one part of the scene to another and the concentration of the individual's attention on that which he is observing at the moment, all conspire to submerge the after-images and prepare the eye for each new scene as it is presented. If this were not so, many visual acts, such as reading which we perform with such facility, would be impossible; the eye would be unable to distinguish the succeeding impressions one from another.

20.7. Adaptation.

In the interests of their self-preservation all surviving living organisms have, over the ages, become structurally

---

* Chapter XXII.

and physiologically adapted to deal more or less successfully with the environment in which they find themselves. Our eyes have developed to function mainly in out-of-door conditions where, on a bright day, the illumination may rise to 10,000 ft. candles; and yet they must function as well as may be in relative darkness when the illumination may be as low as 10^{-3} ft. candles, or less. This is a range of ten millions to one. The processes by which the visual mechanism is enabled to function effectively and sufficiently quickly over this enormous range of brightnesses are of considerable importance. Everyone is familiar with the dazzle and discomfort experienced when we move from a moderately-lighted room into bright sunlight and with the temporary loss of vision on entering a dark room (e.g. a cinema) from brighter surroundings. Though the eyes are at first unequal to the new conditions, they do adapt themselves in time; so much so that, except in extreme cases, the individual is scarcely aware after a while that any change in the level of brightness has taken place. This point was mentioned in §1.4 (B) and will arise again in §21.4.

During a period spent in surroundings of a certain general level of brightness, adjustments take place in a normal eye which enable it to control its response and so put it into a condition of balance with the prevailing conditions, enabling it, after a while, to deal effectively with stimuli at this level. These adjustments, the nature of which are described below, constitute the process called ADAPTATION.* Suppose a person is sitting well in the interior of an average room on a fine day: the illumination on objects round about him will be, say, 15 ft. candles; their reflection factors will vary but we may take their average brightness as, say, 10 ft. lamb. At this brightness level vision is photopic, the cones only are active and the fovea is in every way the most sensitive part of the retina; visual acuity and colour vision are good; as for the light sense, sources of brightness as low as 10^{-2} ft. lamb. or so will be discernible at the fovea. In other words, the light threshold at the fovea will be about 10^{-2} ft. lamb. If the person now moves near to the window or outside, the prevailing brightness level will be raised, maybe to 1,000 ft. lamb.; objects of this brightness will at first appear abnormally bright

* There is adaptation, and induction, in all the senses; see §21.2.

(glaring) because the retina is not adapted to them. Adjustments of the pupil and in the retina, described below, will at once commence to re-adapt the eye to the higher brightness level ; this process is usually called LIGHT ADAPTATION. Gradually, bright objects will assume a normal appearance ; visual acuity will probably improve. Vision is still photopic, but at a higher level.

Suppose now the person moves into a comparatively dark room where the general brightness level is only 10^{-4} ft. lamb. The eye, pre-adapted to 1,000 ft. lamb., will at first be unable to see the faintly illuminated objects in the dark room. Adjustments are again made, however, and the light threshold gradually falls until such objects become visible. This process is usually called DARK ADAPTATION. At and below this level vision is scotopic ; the rods only are active and foveal vision (cones) is suspended. There will be no colour vision and visual acuity will be very poor. Incidentally, we see how, according to the state of the eye, very different levels of brightness may cause equal sensations.

Between the approximate limits 10^{-1} to 10^{-4} ft. lamb. both rods and cones are in operation, to relative extents depending upon the particular circumstances.* At all times the sensitivity of a given area of the retina to light is conditioned by, amongst other factors, the stimulus or stimuli to which it has been previously subjected and by other regions of the retina.

The process of adaptation to higher levels—light adaptation—is relatively rapid ; only 2 or 3 minutes are required for the eye to become adapted to the highest levels ordinarily met with. Dark adaptation is a slower process ; 30 minutes or more are needed to become adapted to the conditions encountered on a dark night or in a cinema, for example. Indeed the sensitivity of the eye will continue to improve slightly over a period of hours.

To enable it to execute the process of adaptation, and so to prevent rapidly varying stimuli from proving too disconcerting, the visual mechanism is provided with at least two and probably three means of control : the two are the iris and the photo-chemical mechanism in the retina.

Immediately the eye is exposed to bright conditions the pupil begins to contract ; from the maximum diameter

---

* §20.2.

of 8 mm. to the minimum of 2 mm. or so the area is reduced to 16 times in a few seconds; but because of the smaller effectiveness of the rays refracted by the peripheral portions of the optical system and arriving at the retina obliquely (Stiles-Crawford effect*), the intensity of the light is reduced by less than 16 times. The protection thus provided by the pupil is probably useful because it operates so quickly but it is a very small fraction of the ten thousand to one change of intensity that may occur. The pupil size is probably more concerned with visual acuity than with assisting in the control of retinal response.

The second and more important means of control occurs in the retina. It is a complex photo-chemical process which is not yet fully understood but in broad outline is somewhat as follows. After a period spent in darkness the visual purple, and presumably such photo-chemical substances as may be associated with the cones, are present in maximal concentration. Their response to a given stimulus and hence the subjective sensation arising therefrom will also be a maximum; faint sources of light will initiate sufficient response to be appreciated. If now the external field be illuminated and light reaches the dark-adapted retina, there commences a decomposition or bleaching of these substances and the retina begins to be less sensitive to faint sources. As we are dealing with a normal eye so that the retina is intact and in contact with the pigment epithelium and choroid, the decomposition will be followed by the normal regenerative process to restore the substances back to maximum concentration. As the light stimulus continues the decomposition prevails over the regeneration for a while and the concentration is progressively diminished; the sensation arising from the stimulus is consequently reduced and the field no longer appears abnormally bright as it did at first. Gradually, as the concentration falls, the rate of decomposition slows down; eventually a balance is reached between the rates of decomposition and regeneration and the mechanism has become adapted to the new level of brightness; the light threshold has been raised. The difference between this new level and the old, and the area of retina chiefly concerned, depend upon the brightness and the extent of the stimulus that entered the field.

---

* §2.15.

If now the stimulus is removed or the individual enters a dark room, he is at first able to see very little. In the comparative absence of light, however, the rate of decomposition falls and regeneration is relatively accelerated so that presently the concentration of light sensitive material is sufficient for a small quantity of light to produce a noticeable response and the person is again able to see faint sources. The light threshold has been lowered again.

Research during the last twenty years or so on electrical changes in the retina and on nerve impulses* indicates that there is probably a third method of control, of an electrical nature, which is more rapid than the above photo-chemical control.

When the eye passes through the process of adaptation to a higher or lower level of brightness, all its functions are affected to a greater or less extent. References have been made to the effects on visual acuity and on colour vision; the influence on the eye's sensitivity to flicker will be mentioned later. At present we are concerned mainly with the effect on the light sense; and this varies in different regions of the retina. During dark adaptation, for instance, the sensitivity of the fovea to light increases less than a hundredfold whereas the peripheral regions, particularly an annulus round about 20° from the fovea, acquire a ten-thousandfold increase in light sensitivity. It is usual to study the progress of the adaptation process in terms of its effects on the light sense, for which purpose a test patch of simple shape is employed.

Though the terms light adaptation and dark adaptation are firmly established, they are rather vague and unsatisfactory. In any work laying claim to precision it is necessary to specify the brightness levels from and to which adaptation takes place, the spectral composition of the adapting stimulus and the period of time during which the eye has been exposed to each level; also to specify which region of the retina it is the functioning of which is under investigation (the test region) and which region has been subjected to the adapting stimulus. It is usually the whole retina, including the test region, which is concerned when we use the term adaptation; when the adapting stimulation is restricted in extent, as when a single glare source enters

---

* §22.3; this quicker electrical process of adaptation has been called α-adaptation and the slower photo-chemical process β-adaptation.

the field of view,* the effect is discussed as spatial induction. The border line between what may be called induction on the one hand and adaptation on the other is ill defined.

20.8. Dark Adaptation. Measurement.

To obtain reliable results in measuring the course of adaptation the conditions under which the experiment is carried out must be standardised. This can be done by placing the person to be tested in the closed box described in §20.3.† He first spends a stated period (say 30 minutes) in dim illumination, is then light-adapted for 5 minutes

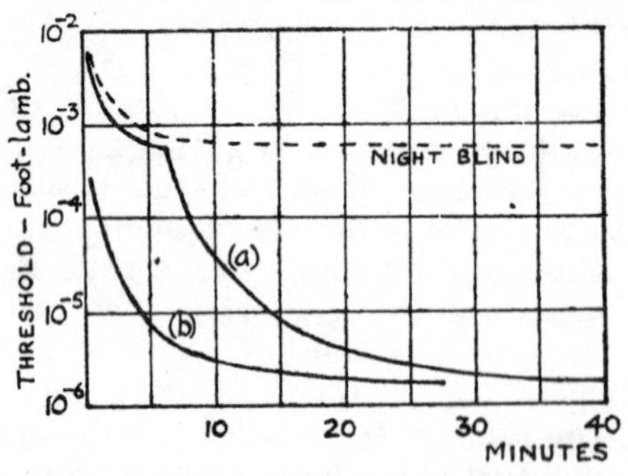

FIG. 20.5—DARK ADAPTATION (WHITE LIGHT). LEAST PERCEPTIBLE BRIGHTNESS, TO LOG SCALE, AGAINST TIME IN MINUTES. APPROX. PRE-ADAPTATION LEVELS: (*a*) 1000 FT. LAMB. (*b*) 10-20 FT. LAMB. BROKEN CURVE APPLIES TO NIGHT-BLIND PERSON.

by raising the brightness of the interior walls of the box to a given level (maybe up to 1,000 ft. lamb.) and then, in complete darkness, is presented for a brief interval with the test stimulus, adjusted to known brightness, through the small aperture. The time is recorded when this test patch becomes perceptible. It is presented at successive intervals, its brightness being reduced by definite steps at each exposure. Thus we measure the threshold at successive intervals. The commencing brightness of the test patch might be, say, 10^{-2} ft. lamb. and the final brightness in the region of 10^{-5} or 10^{-6} ft. lamb., which is about the normal lower limit, or threshold, of vision—the final rod threshold.

* §§ 20.5 and 21.3.

† Special instruments called adaptometers (e.g. the Crookes adaptometer) are available for the purpose also.

In this way curves of the type shown in Fig. 20.5, for a white test patch, are obtained: (a) when the 5 minutes pre-adaptation brightness is 1,000 ft. lamb.; (b) when it is only in the region of 10 ft. lamb. The former curve is seen to consist of two distinct parts; for the first six or seven minutes both rods and cones, mainly the latter, are regenerating; the second part of the curve is due to the continued adaptation of the rods only. In the case of curve (b) only the rod recovery is evident; the test has commenced at a brightness level too low for the small amount of cone action that would take place to be recorded.

These curves apply to normal individuals. There are people whose gain in light sensitivity is much smaller or whose recovery is slower. People suffering from night-blindness* are an extreme case; their dark-adaptation curve is of the form shown by the broken line in Fig. 20.5. It has been found that there is often a deterioration of dark adaptation with age. Whether the course of dark adaptation in one eye is retarded if the other eye continues to be illuminated has not been conclusively settled. There are certain ocular and general diseases and nutritional and metabolic defects, which cause deficiency in light sensitivity in dim illuminations; the testing of dark adaptation, therefore, has many practical applications. An adaptometer can be used for carrying out perimetry at low brightness levels; by exploring a number of meridians a sensitivity contour for the whole retina may be plotted if desired.

The course of dark-adaptation and the value of the final threshold reached is affected by the presence or absence of ultra-violet in the pre-adapting radiation. If ultra-violet between the limits 285 to 400 $m\mu$ is filtered out of this radiation, the threshold becomes lower at every point of the dark-adaptation curve, in both cone and rod portions. Whereas the final threshold shown for curve (a) in Fig. 20.5 has log. $\bar{6}\cdot25$, corresponding to a threshold of about $1\cdot8$ millionths of a foot-lambert, this would become, say, $\bar{6}\cdot0$, corresponding to $1\cdot0$ millionth ft. lamb.

20.9. The Purkinje Effect.

During the course of dark-adaptation the colour sense is markedly affected, particularly with respect to the relative luminosity of the different colours. The student

---

* §21.12.

may have observed that a red flower which appears brighter than a blue flower in daylight becomes dark and appears definitely less bright than the blue flower during the onset of twilight; as the darkness deepens the red flower becomes black and the blue flower grey. This effect was first noticed by PURKINJE in 1825 and is known as the PURKINJE EFFECT. Again, in photopic conditions the spectrum appears brightest in the yellow-green region at wavelength 555 $m\mu$* ; this applies for brightness conditions exceeding about 10^{-1} ft. lambert. If the illumination is gradually decreased the brightest part shifts towards the blue end to wavelength

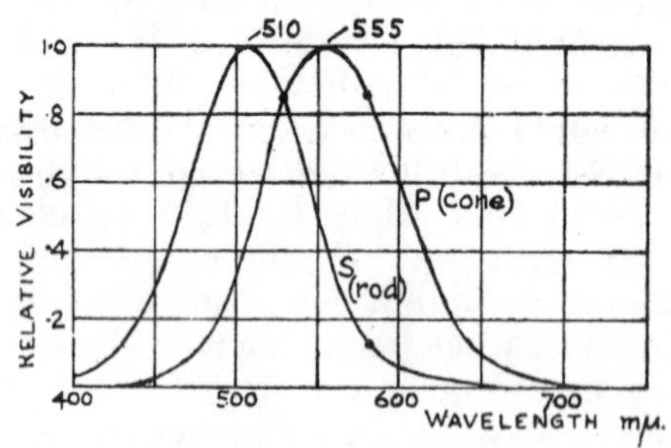

FIG. 20.6—PHOTOPIC (P) AND SCOTOPIC (S) LUMINOSITY CURVES, FOR EQUAL ENERGY SOURCE, ILLUSTRATING THE PURKINJE EFFECT; MAXIMUM ORDINATES MADE EQUAL FOR THE TWO CURVES; SEE TEXT.

510 $m\mu$ or lower and at brightnesses less than about 10^{-3} ft. lamberts all colour disappears from the spectrum; it appears of a uniform grey or slightly bluish-grey colour, varying only in apparent brightness—the scotopic spectrum.

Thus we see that the photopic luminosity curve, showing the relative visibilities of the different wavelengths under daylight conditions, does not apply at low illuminations. A curve can be plotted showing the relative visibility of different wavelengths under these dark, scotopic, conditions below 10^{-3} ft. lamb. or so; the threshold value of the stimulus is determined as already explained for a selection of wavelengths across the spectrum and the reciprocals of these values plotted against wavelength. The curve is called the SCOTOPIC LUMINOSITY CURVE and it takes somewhat the same shape as the photopic curve described in §18.1, but its maximum is shifted towards the blue end to a position rather below 510 $m\mu$. In the experiment

* §18.1.

the observations are made, not by the fovea, but by a parafoveal region removed some 2° to 3° from the fovea. The scotopic and photopic curves are shown together in Fig. 20.6; their ordinates have been adjusted so that the maximum in both cases equals unity, though the scotopic sensitivity of the eye is really much greater than the photopic.* If we take two wavelengths such as λ 530 and λ 580, which, having equal ordinates on the photopic curve, appear equally bright under daylight conditions, it is seen from their positions on the scotopic curve that the λ 580 light now appears far less bright. It follows that in darkness the threshold for red light does not fall so low as for the blue light; if dark adaptation curves were determined separately for lights of different wavelengths, those for blue would drop to a lower level than is shown in Fig. 20.5 whilst those for red would not drop so much. The curves of Fig. 20.5 apply to white light.

At brightness levels below 10^{-3} ft. lambert or so the cones are believed to be out of action; thus the scotopic curve describes the performance of the rod mechanism. The photopic curve, applying to brightness levels exceeding 10^{-1} ft. lambert, describes mainly the performance of the cone mechanism, though the rods may still be in operation to some extent. Between these brightness levels both rods and cones are active and colour is still perceived. The luminosity curve for this intermediate range of brightnesses would be somewhere between the two curves of Fig. 20.6.

The Purkinje phenomenon proper, i.e. the shift from cone vision to rod vision, cannot occur at the fovea since rods are absent, but recent work† indicates that when vision is restricted to the fovea there *is* a slight shift of the maximum towards the shorter wavelengths: this is a phenomenon of some theoretical significance.

Much useful information is summarised in these luminosity curves. They show at a glance, for example, the superior sensitivity of the rod mechanism to light of short wavelength and of the cone mechanism at long wavelengths. Because of this the dark-adapted eye may be exposed to long wavelength red light of appreciable intensity without materially upsetting the state of dark-adaptation, and yet the intensity is sufficient for the cone mechanism to function so that the person can read. Thus night-fighter pilots were

* See also §21.5.

† WALTERS and WRIGHT, *Proc. Roy. Soc.* (1943).

supplied with goggles with red filters, with a sharper cut-off in the red than indicated in Fig. 19.1 B; with these they could read in a reasonably illuminated room and yet were well dark-adapted when they emerged from the room to set off on a night flight.

The scotopic luminosity curve has been of great service in investigating the photo-chemical processes in the retina.* It exhibits the main characteristic of dark-adapted rod vision. The Purkinje effect has been observed by electrical methods (GRANIT) in the frog's eye.†

20.10. Foveal Adaptation. Binocular Matching.

Within the photopic range of vision the process of adaptation to high brightness levels and recovery of sensitivity upon lowering the brightness are comparatively rapid and it is difficult to measure the course of these processes by the threshold method described in §20.8. WRIGHT has introduced an interesting binocular matching method for investigating these photopic adaptations. In this method the observer uses both eyes; one, say the left, is maintained in a constant state‡ of dark adaptation and is used as a reference standard against which to compare the changes induced in the right eye by varying degrees of light-adaptation.

The procedure is somewhat as follows: both eyes are dark-adapted for 30 minutes; a test patch of a certain brightness is then presented to the right eye and the brightness of a second (comparison) patch seen only by the left eye is adjusted until the two appear equal. Call this apparent brightness a. The right eye is then subjected to the adapting radiation of some measured high brightness A for 3 minutes and again presented with the original test patch. This will now appear much fainter than before and the comparison patch in front of the still dark-adapted left eye will have to be reduced to some figure a_0 in order to obtain a match. The ratio a_0/a is the factor by which the light sensitivity of the right eye has been reduced. When a_0 has been satisfactorily measured (certain precautions are necessary) and the adapting radiation A removed, the course of the recovery of sensitivity in the right eye is recorded by making a series of rapid matches

* §22.2. † §22.3.

‡ The left (comparison) eye will remain constant in so far as it is unaffected by the varying stimulations of the right eye.

at successive intervals. Eventually the original value a is reached again.

Such tests can be carried out for various values and colours of the adapting radiation A and of the test patch. A typical result for a white adapting radiation of about 200 ft. lamb. (6000 photons*) is shown by curve A in Fig. 20.7. Giving to a the arbitrary value 10, a_0 (after light-adaptation) was reduced to 0·8, about $\frac{1}{12}$th of a. The curve is a dark-adaptation curve for the fovea ; it follows a straight line course at first and recovery of sensitivity is nearly complete after about 2 minutes.

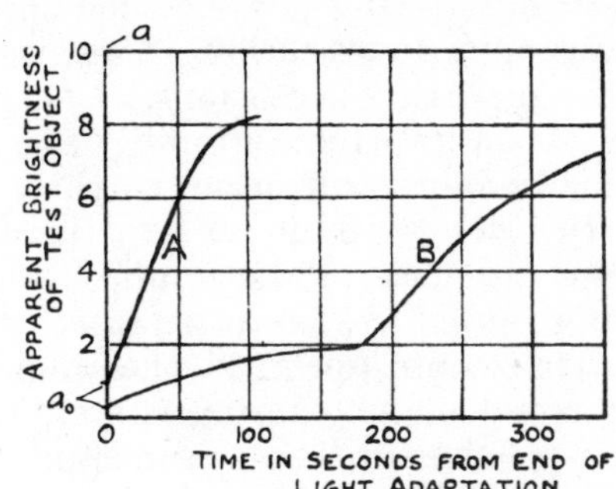

FIG. 20.7—DARK ADAPTATION OF PHOTOPIC MECHANISM. RECOVERY OF SENSITIVITY AFTER LIGHT-ADAPTATION TO WHITE RADIATION OF (A) 6000 QUANTA, (B) 23,000 QUANTA (WRIGHT).

When the adapting intensity A is higher, the sensitivity is reduced to a lower value a_0 ; moreover, the curve (B) is no longer linear but shows a break which is probably due " to some breakdown in the photo-chemical system in the cones " (WRIGHT). Fig. 20.7 gives the same kind of information as Fig. 20.5 ; in the former the ordinates express sensitivity whereas in the latter they express threshold, which is proportional to the reciprocal of sensitivity.

20.11. Periodic Stimuli. Flicker and Fusion.

The sensation that will arise when the eye is subjected to a succession of short stimuli of equal intensity repeated at regular intervals depends upon the usual stimulus and eye characteristics (§20.1) and also upon the rapidity with which the stimuli follow one another. If the time interval

* §18.10.

between successive stimuli is greater than the time taken for the peak response to develop (am, Fig. 20.2), the observer will experience a succession of separate sensations. If the successive stimuli follow one another more rapidly, the interval between them being less than this peak development time, then the impression due to the second stimulus will commence before the first primary image has appreciably decayed and the observer will experience a continuous but pulsating sensation of flicker. As the frequency of the stimuli is increased the coarse unpleasant flicker becomes finer and more tremulous until at a certain stage called the CRITICAL FREQUENCY the flicker ceases, the individual sensations having now become completely fused into a continuous uniform sensation. The visual mechanism is integrating the successive sensations. Everyday examples of this fusion of intermittent stimuli have already been quoted* and many more will occur to the student.

To provide the rapid stimuli in experiments on flicker, and to vary the intensity of a stimulus in other kinds of investigation, an episcotister is often used, i.e. a rotating opaque disc with sector openings the angular widths of which can be varied at will during the experiment.

These flicker phenomena have been studied by TALBOT (1834), PLATEAU (1835), FERRY (1892), PORTER (1898) and later by H. E. IVES (1912) and LYTHGOE (1929). Two laws have been experimentally established:

(a) The TALBOT-PLATEAU law, which states that the continuous impression resulting from the fusion of rapidly varying stimuli is the same as if the total light were uniformly distributed throughout the whole period; in other words, the resultant impression is the mean of the periodic impressions.

The law applies except at very low or very high intensities of the stimuli and provided the eye is exposed to light for at least 3 per cent of the cycle. Suppose for example, a sector disc with a 60° open sector is rotated sufficiently rapidly in front of a bright white patch of luminance† say 24 m.l. that the critical frequency has been passed and a continuous uniform sensation is experienced; then this sensation will be equal to that obtained when the eye observes a steady white patch of luminance $\frac{60}{360} \times 24 = 4$ m.l.

* §1.10. † i.e. brightness; see §§ 18.4 and 18.6.

(b) The Ferry-Porter law: the critical frequency of flicker increases directly with the logarithm of the luminance of the field.

Representing the critical frequency by f_c and the intensity (luminance) of the stimulating light by B, the law may be written

$$f_c = k \log B + p$$

and may be plotted as in Fig. 20.8, in which are shown two pairs of curves, one pair relating to the dark-adapted eye and the other to an eye which is light-adapted, the surrounding field being adjusted throughout to the same brightness as the test patch. The two curves of each pair apply respectively to the fovea (cones) and to a region removed 10° from the fovea (mainly rods). The constant

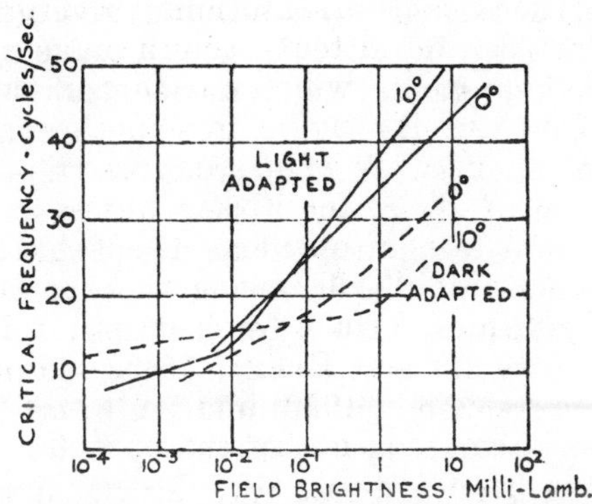

Fig. 20.8.—Variations of Critical Frequency of Flicker with Brightness of Field, at the Fovea (0°) and 10° from Fovea. Full lines: light-adapted eye, surround brightness equal to test patch brightness. Broken lines: dark-adapted eye.

k and hence the slope of the curve depends upon the location and the size of the stimulated retinal region; the constant p depends upon the state of adaptation of this region and on the brightness of the surrounding field—all of which factors have a bearing on the critical frequency.

The curves reveal a difference between the foveal and extra-foveal regions; whereas for the former the curves have a more or less constant slope, for the latter they show a rather abrupt change of slope, occurring at about 0·01 m.l. in the light-adapted eye. This suggests that at this low intensity of the stimulus, the rod mechanism has come into operation. In the light-adapted eye we see that the critical frequency is higher in the extra-foveal region; as a consequence of this, as the student may have noted on occasion, a rotating spoked wheel may show no flicker when observed directly by foveal vision, but when the eyes are turned to one side so that the wheel is seen in indirect vision, the flicker appears.

We see also from Fig. 20.8 that for a fairly bright stimulus the sensitivity of the eye to flicker is reduced in dark adaptation, especially in the extra-foveal region of the retina. If, after fusion has been obtained with a surround as bright as the test patch, the illumination of the surround is gradually reduced, the critical frequency is lowered. Thus keeping the interior relatively dark in a cinema reduces the number of separate projections of the film per second needed to give a continuous sensation free from flicker. For artistic and æsthetic reasons also the surroundings should be kept dark; the more the general illumination is reduced, however, the worse are the seeing conditions for detail and contrast on the screen itself. A surrounding illumination of about one fiftieth of the screen illumination is therefore recommended as a suitable compromise.

The phenomena of flicker are more complex than this brief survey indicates. It is, for instance, surprising that when the intensity of the stimulus is increased it is necessary to increase the frequency of stimulation in order to achieve fusion. This is a consequence of the fact that the primary image resulting from a strong stimulus has a shorter duration than is the case with a weaker stimulus (§20.3). But why should this be so? It would appear more natural to expect the sensation caused by a strong stimulus to last the longer; it has been suggested that the explanation lies in the complex structure of the electrical impulses discharged along the optic nerve fibres.*

The critical frequency of flicker increases with the area of the stimulus. If the latter is provided by four test patches at the corners of a square, the frequency is higher than for each test patch presented singly. This is evidence of inter-action between adjacent retinal areas.

The above discussion has been concerned with equal stimuli separated by equal intervals of total darkness. If the alternations are between two lights of different intensities the frequency at which flicker disappears will depend upon

* §22.3.

the brightness difference of the two lights. Under favourable conditions a brightness difference of 1·5 per cent can be detected by this flicker method. The manner in which the method is used for heterochromatic photometry has already been discussed.*

Flicker phenomena have a bearing on problems concerned with signalling, navigation lights, rotating beacons, etc., but these cannot be discussed here.

EXERCISES. CHAPTER XX.

1. Describe a form of selective detector other than the eye. Discuss the respects in which the eye differs from other selective detectors of radiation.

2. Write a short essay describing in general terms the dependence of the attributes of a visual sensation on the various characteristics of the stimulus and the visual mechanism.

3. Describe the Stiles-Crawford effect concerning the effect of a visual stimulus on the retina. What bearing might this be supposed to have on the location of visual purple in the retinal receptors ?

4. Give an account of the duplicity theory of vision and the evidence on which it is based.

5. Describe, with the aid of a graph, the characteristics of the primary image that is experienced in response to a flash of light and how these characteristics are affected by the intensity and wavelength of the stimulus.

6. Discs carrying black markings on a white background may exhibit colour effects when rotated. Explain how these colours are thought to arise.

7. Write an essay on spatial induction, including a description of ways in which its effects may be exhibited experimentally.

8. Describe how the effects of spatial induction are of importance in everyday vision and in the design and use of visual instruments.

9. Discuss the evidence that the cones of the retina are responsible for the high acuity of vision in daylight while the rods are chiefly efficient in dim light and in detecting the movements of objects. (B.O.A.)

10. What is meant by temporal induction ? What are the conditions under which a negative after-image is experienced ?

11. Give a short account of simple experiments for exhibiting negative after-images. These are said to be sometimes more saturated than the spectrum hues. Explain how this might happen.

12. Explain how our facility in such visual tasks as reading is dependent upon the effects of temporal and spatial induction and other factors.

13. Give an account, in broad outline, of the photo-chemical process by which the visual mechanism adapts itself to the varying levels of brightness of the external field. What is the function of the pupil in this connection ?

---

* §18.9.

14. Give an account of the effects of dark-adaptation on the light sense, the colour sense and the form sense.

15. Describe how the course of dark-adaptation may be experimentally determined. What precautions are observed to standardise the conditions of the experiment? Give graphs exhibiting the general course of adaptation with time when the eye was pre-adapted to (*a*) a high brightness level, say 1 lambert; (*b*) a brightness level of, say, 10 milli-lamberts.

16. A person who has spent some time in bright sunlight enters a dark room. Describe the sensations he experiences during the next half hour or so and the events taking place in his retina to account for these sensations.

17. The change in light-sensitivity of the eye during adaptation depends upon the region of the retina concerned. Discuss this, quoting numerical values of the light threshold at the fovea and at 20° from the fovea.

18. Draw the photopic luminosity curve and the scotopic luminosity curve for the normal human eye. How, and under what conditions, are these curves determined? What is their significance?

19. Describe the so-called Purkinje effect which arises as the eye is dark-adapted. Is this phenomenon in evidence at the fovea? What effect has it on the appearance of the spectrum?

20. Aeroplane pilots are supplied with goggles fitted with red filters during the period preceding a night flight. Explain clearly the reason for this.

21. Explain what is meant by the critical frequency of flicker With the aid of graphs describe the factors associated with the eye and with the stimulus and its surroundings, on which the critical frequency depends.

22. State and discuss the TALBOT-PLATEAU and the FERRY-PORTER laws concerning the phenomenon of flicker.

23. Discuss the dependence of the critical frequency of flicker on the following factors:
(*a*) The region of the retina stimulated.
(*b*) The size of the stimulus.
(*c*) The state of adaptation of the eye.
(*d*) The brightness of the surrounding field.

24. Explain the basis of the application of the flicker method to heterochromatic photometry. Describe the construction and the use of the flicker photometer.

25. Discuss the following:
(*a*) Under suitable conditions a rotating spoked wheel exhibits no flicker when observed foveally, but flicker appears when the eyes are turned aside.
(*b*) If the general illumination in a cinema were raised whilst a picture is being shown on the screen, the viewing conditions would be unfavourable.

26. Describe the after-image formed on looking at a white screen after gazing at a bright coloured object. How is this appearance explained on the three-colour theory of vision? (B.O.A.)

27. Give a concise account of the rate and range of adaptability of the eye to various levels of brightness together with a short description of the measuring apparatus used. (S.M.C.)

28. How is the rate of adaptation of the eye to darkness measured ? Describe any instrument which enables it to be measured accurately. Of what use is the information so obtained ? (S.M.C.)

29. Explain the terms: flicker, critical frequency of flicker, flicker photometer. Give a brief description of any experimental results dealing with the dependence of critical frequency on illumination and spectral quality. (S.M.C.)

30. Describe the Purkinje effect and the scotopic luminosity curve. If red and blue lights are balanced photometrically by the dark-adapted eye, how will they appear when the eye is adapted to higher illumination ?

31. What do you know concerning the luminosity of spectral colours ? Indicate how it varies according to the state of adaptation of the eyes. (S.M.C.)

32. Describe in detail the variations in the structure of the retina between the fovea and periphery. How are these variations related to the visual acuity across the retina ? (B.O.A.)

33. Explain what is meant by the luminosity curve of the spectrum and describe the differences that are found among different observers. How is the Purkinje effect accounted for by the alteration in the luminosity curve as the illumination is reduced ? (B.O.A.)

34. What is the critical frequency of flicker ? How does it vary (*a*) with the level of illumination, (*b*) with the region of the retina illuminated, (*c*) with the wavelength of the light ? (B.O.A.)

35. Give an account of the phenomena of dark adaptation and of the physiological changes that take place during adaptation. (B.O.A.)

36. A beam of light of intensity I is allowed to enter the eye and stimulate the retina for time t. Describe how the visual response rises and falls during and after stimulation and indicate how changes in the magnitude of I and t affect the course of the response. (B.O.A.)

37. State the PLATEAU-TALBOT law and describe an experimental method, dependent upon the truth of this law, of measuring the light-difference sense and the light and colour thresholds.

38. Give an account of the succession of visual sensations which are produced when the eye is stimulated by a light of short duration such as a bright spot or line upon a rotating black disc. Explain why the sensation of flicker caused by an intermittent stimulus may be eliminated by altering the brightness of the stimulus without changing its frequency.

39. What bearing has the phenomenon of "after-images" upon the theories of (*a*) ocular movements and (*b*) colour perception ? (B.O.A.)

40. Describe experiments to illustrate and examine the phenomena of simultaneous contrast and successive contrast. State the kind of results that are found by these experiments and their explanation on the Young-Helmholtz three-colour theory. (B.O.A.)

STIMULUS AND SENSATION

CHAPTER XXI

DISCRIMINATION OF SENSATION. THE SENSES OF LIGHT AND COLOUR.

In the last chapter were described those characteristics of the visual mechanism which determine the development and general nature of the sensation. Detailed appreciation of the fine gradations of brightness, contour and colour between the various elements of the scene presented to the eye is possible only if the light sense, form sense and colour sense have precision and acute discrimination [B (d) of §20.1]. The form sense was discussed in Chapter II. Here we will consider first the light sense and enquire into :

(a) the magnitude of the stimulus which evokes a just perceptible sensation—the light threshold ;

(b) the difference or ratio between two stimuli which evoke a difference of sensation which can just be perceived—the differential light threshold.

THE LIGHT SENSE.

21.1. Limits of Visibility. Wavelength Limits.

At ordinary intensities radiation between the approximate limits 300 to 1500 $m\mu$ is transmitted in varying proportions by the ocular media and reaches the retina. Much of the ultra-violet up to λ 380 is absorbed by the crystalline lens in which a certain amount of fluorescence takes place ; in old people the absorption below λ 380 is practically complete. The wavelength limits of transmission vary, however, with the intensity of the radiation and cannot be precisely specified.

In ordinary circumstances it is only over the range from λ 390 to λ 750 that there is visual response, as shown by the photopic luminosity curve ; but in special circumstances and when the intensity is high there is visibility well outside this range. Spectroscopists report that spectrum lines of wavelengths down to 309·1 $m\mu$ are visible under suitable conditions; they appear blue or violet or blue-violet. In the case of an aphakic eye the luminosity of these ultra-violet lines is considerably increased, especially in the region of λ 365, because of the absence of the crystalline lens.

Less information is available concerning the other end of the spectrum; HELMHOLTZ reported that λ 850 could be made visible to him.

21.2. Intensity Limits of Visibility. The Light Threshold.

For each sense (seeing, hearing, touch, etc.) there is an adequate stimulus* and this has a threshold value and a differential threshold value. In the case of the sense of touch, for example, a certain minimum pressure, expressed in dynes or as a fraction of a pound, can just be appreciated. The value of this threshold will depend upon the area and location of the region that is stimulated, upon the condition of this region as "induced" by previous treatment and upon the duration of the stimulus; it will differ as between a blunt and a sharp instrument of pressure and will not be the same as applied to, say, the tip of the finger or to the thigh. If two separate pressure stimuli are to be distinguished and a comparison made between their magnitudes, they must be sufficiently separated and differ from one another by at least the differential threshold value. In each sense these threshold values can be expressed ultimately in energy units.

In the sense of light it is of theoretical and practical interest to know the value of the faintest source that the eye is capable of perceiving. Such information is of importance in astronomy, in connection with distant signals, lighthouses, searchlights, etc. The scotopic luminosity curve, Fig. 20.6, tells us that the dark-adapted eye is most sensitive to light of wavelength about 510 $m\mu$, hence the threshold will be lowest for this wavelength. For the faintest sources to be perceived the eye must be fully dark-adapted; it will not be the fovea that is responsible for the perception but a region of the retina removed some 10° to 20° from the fovea, where the rods predominate and are most densely packed. Even if we arrange for these most favourable conditions, the determination of the value

---

* §1.4.

of the threshold is not an easy matter. Certain physiological characteristics must be taken into consideration: because of the lateral inter-connections of the neurones within the retina there is summation of the responses from many rods along one nerve fibre and so the threshold intensity of a stimulus is bound up with its area; thus it is necessary to differentiate between "point" sources and sources of finite extent. With the former it is the steady flow of light on unit area of the retina and hence the intensity of the source that matters. With the latter it is, within certain limits of area, the total flow of light on the whole stimulated area which determines the threshold; if the stimulated area is doubled the threshold intensity is halved. Further, the sensational response to a flash of short duration is of such a character (§20.3) that with sources of this kind the threshold intensity depends upon the period of the flash; the total quantity of light during the period is the criterion. (These statements are to be taken as approximate guides; actually the problem is more complicated.) We will therefore deal separately with steady sources, of duration exceeding 0·5 second, subdivided into point sources and those of finite extent; and then with flash sources of less than, say, 0·05 second duration.

In making a determination of the light threshold account must also be taken of the fact that, even when the utmost effort is made by the observer to fixate the test source or object as steadily as possible, the eye is nevertheless in continual motion and does not remain stationary in any position for more than a tenth of a second or less. Thus it may so happen that over a comparatively long period of time no one set of receptors covered by the image of the source remains long enough in one position for the stimulus, consisting of light quanta, to reach the threshold value.

STEADY POINT SOURCES.

A star may be considered as a point source and its visibility decreases with distance (§18.8). Astronomers express what they call the "magnitude" of stars by means of an arbitrary scale which is based upon their apparent brightness. The higher the magnitude the fainter the star, the ratio of successive magnitudes being equal to $\sqrt[5]{100} = 2\cdot5$ approximately. If E_1 represents the illumination at the earth's surface of a star of the first magnitude and E_m the corresponding illumination by a star of magnitude m, then

$$E_m = E_1/(\sqrt[5]{100})^{m-1}$$
$$\text{or } \log E_m = \log E_1 - 0\cdot4(m-1) \qquad (21.1)$$

FABRY determined (1925) that the illumination produced at the earth by a star of the first magnitude is $7\cdot7 \times 10^{-8}$ lumens per foot². Ordinarily, stars of the sixth magnitude are just visible to the naked eye; but under optimum conditions, including precautions to eliminate the spatial inductive effect of the surrounding skylight, the eye can detect stars of magnitude 8·5. Calculation using the above equation shows that such stars give an illumination of $7\cdot7 \times 10^{-11}$ lumens per foot²; neglecting atmospheric absorption this illumination would be produced by a standard candle at a distance of 21·6 miles* and is equivalent to an energy flux of about 5×10^{-10} erg per second or 5×10^{-17} watt entering the eye. Laboratory experiments on artificial stars give a slightly higher threshold which we may take, therefore, as rather less than 10^{-16} watt, or about 200 quanta per second. It is difficult to grasp the utter minuteness of this quantity; it is less than a thousand million millionth of the power concerned in operating an ophthalmoscope lamp. A bolometer will record a millionth of a degree,† yet the eye is thousands of times more sensitive.

STEADY SOURCES OF FINITE EXTENT.

For sources subtending less than 10° the threshold brightness B_T of the stimulus decreases as the stimulus area a increases, though the law connecting B_T and a is not a simple one. Approximately, however, experiment shows that:

for sources subtending $<2°$ the product $B_T a$ is constant.
for sources between 2° and 10° the product $B_T\sqrt{a}$ is constant.
for sources subtending $>10°$ the threshold is independent of area and depends solely on the brightness of the stimulus; the results obtained by many investigators put the threshold brightness of such sources at about 10^{-7} foot-lambert.

A just perceptible small patch subtending less than 10° becomes invisible if its size is reduced unless its brightness

* §18.11, Ex. 6. † §17.8.

is proportionately increased; the increase will be in proportion to the area of the patch if it subtends less than 2° and in proportion to its linear dimensions if it subtends between 2° and 10°.

The extreme range of brightnesses over which the eye can normally operate with steady sources may be stated as:

Range of rod mechanism	10^{-7} to 10^{-1}	foot lamberts
Range of cone mechanism	10^{-4} to 10^{4}	,, ,,
Total Range	10^{-7} to 10^{4}	,, ,,

Flash Sources.

For a single stimulus of brief duration, its effect in evoking a visual sensation is cumulative during its action time (§18.1 footnote and §20.3). Whether a sensation will result and what its magnitude will be if it is aroused, depends upon the total quantity of light that is rapidly delivered to the retina during the flash. Because of the complexity of the photochemical and electrical reactions that are set up in the retina, the relationship between the intensity and duration of the flash in order to produce the most favourable delivery of the energy needed to arouse a visual response is probably not simple; but we may say that, except for very short flashes, the total energy in the flash and the visual response are directly proportional to one another. That is, the product of threshold intensity I and the duration t of the flash is approximately constant; if a flash of intensity I and duration, say, ·05 second reaches the threshold, a flash of duration ·005 second would need to have an intensity $10I$. For flashes of less than ·005 second the intensity has to be greater than the value given by this constant.

Ultimately, the arousing of a sensation will depend upon the reception in a brief period of time of a certain minimum (threshold) number of light quanta, each one striking a separate rod in the retina, so that the reaction is sufficient to initiate an adequate discharge of impulses along the nerve fibre (or fibres) to which the rods are connected. From the observations in this paragraph and the properties of the primary image (Fig. 20.2) it would appear that the number of quanta will be least when the stimulus is a brief flash of such intensity that its action time is less than ·05 second.

To arrange the necessary conditions for measuring the light threshold experimentally is a complicated procedure.

A determination was made in 1942* on the completely dark-adapted eye using light of wavelength 510 $m\mu$; the flash was of a size subtending 10′ at the eye, stimulating the retina at a point 20° from the fovea and of duration ·001 second. Many measurements were made over several months on seven observers. The results were found to vary by nearly 100 per cent between individuals and in the same individual at different times. The mean result obtained for the threshold energy was 4×10^{-10} erg, individual variations ranging from $2{\cdot}1$ to $5{\cdot}7 \times 10^{-10}$ erg. At wavelength 510 $m\mu$, the value of the quantum is $3{\cdot}88 \times 10^{-12}$ erg (§17.3) so that the number of quanta reaching the eye varies approximately from 50 to 150. HECHT calculated that when allowances are made for absorption and reflection of light by the ocular media and for other conditions, the number of quanta reaching the retina is only 5 to 15. Since a retinal area of 10′ angular extent contains about 250 rods, it is extremely unlikely that any rod would receive more than one quantum. Thus the result of the investigation is that the light threshold is given by the stimulation of 5 to 15 rods, each by a single quantum. That is to say, the eye is so extremely sensitive to light that it approaches the limit set by the quantum properties of light.

No matter how carefully an experiment is arranged and controlled there will be variability in the number of quanta delivered to the eye in succeeding flashes; and of those reaching the retina there will be variability in the proportion that is absorbed—a variable proportion will pass through to the choroid and be lost as far as vision is concerned. Therefore some flashes of the above intensity will be seen and some will not be seen—but the former will exceed 50 per cent.

21.3. Upper Intensity Limit. Glare.

It is scarcely possible to assign a numerical value to an upper limit of visibility; this limit is set, not by what the eye can see, but by the disturbing effects of excessive light. For certain very precise visual tasks it is desirable to raise the illumination to high levels (e.g. to 500 ft. candles or more in the case of the operation table in a hospital), provided the distribution of this light and of the surrounding

---

* By HECHT, SHLAER and PIRENNE; see *Vision and the Eye*, by M. H. PIRENNE, Pilot Press, 1948.

illumination is carefully arranged; and some people are called upon to work out-of-doors where the illumination, due to sun and sky, may approach 10,000 ft. candles. However, high illuminations and particularly isolated sources of high luminous intensity may produce a condition called GLARE, which is characterised by discomfort and by impairment of vision. The source of light responsible for the troublesome effect, whether it be small or diffuse, is called the glare source. A short definition of glare sources would be that they are sources which prevent us from seeing what we wish to see.

The extent to which a glare source may interfere with the individual's comfort or vision depends on several factors concerned, as usual, partly with the source—its intensity, size, position and whether steady or fluctuating—and partly with the properties and condition of the eye. At night, when the eye is dark-adapted, a motor headlight causes a blinding glare which may render vision for a time impossible, whereas in daylight it is relatively innocuous. But lights much less intense than this may cause trouble if they are badly placed in relation to the work in hand; and because of the importance of the subject in relation to the comfort and efficiency of operatives in many fields of industrial activity, it has received much systematic study. Because of the difficulty of the subject and of the varied requirements in different occupations the results obtained by investigators have not always been in agreement and it is not easy to generalise; but the following broad conclusions have emerged.

Any marked regional variations in, or any rapid fluctuations of, illumination within the field of view are distracting and should be avoided. "Good light" is always steady and not unduly discontinuous over the field. A naked or intense light in a dark field may be most disturbing.

The many manifestations of glare may be subdivided into (1) *discomfort* and (2) *disability*, or impairment of vision. The discomfort may vary from mild irritation to actual pain in aggravated cases, brought about largely by the strain of undue pupil contraction and accommodation. It makes concentration difficult and leads to errors and accidents; it varies considerably according to the temperament of the individual and is not easy to assess in terms of the characteristics of the glare source. Discomfort glare, provided it is not too serious, and disability glare appear to be quite separate effects and need not occur simultaneously ; impairment of vision is not always accompanied by discomfort and discomfort may be felt without any deterioration in visual performance.

DISCOMFORT GLARE.

This, especially in relation to large glare sources, has not received as much attention as disability glare, but recent investigations show how discomfort glare is affected by the brightness, size and shape of the source, by the brightness of the background and by the position of the source in relation to the line of sight. It is found that in order not to increase the discomfort, if the brightness or area of the source is increased, the brightness of the background must be increased also, in greater proportion in the first case and somewhat smaller proportion in the second case. It is because too little attention has been paid to the background conditions that many lighting installations giving the desired higher illumination on work benches, etc., have proved to be unsuccessful.

With regard to the shape of the source, a long source such as a fluorescent lamp is more disturbing when vertical than when horizontal.

In all cases discomfort is reduced the further the glare source is removed laterally from the line of sight.

DISABILITY GLARE.

Visual efficiency is impaired in two ways : within and around the area covered by the glare source there is a reduction in visual acuity and in the light sense ; both the light threshold and the differential light threshold are raised. It is difficult, for example, to discriminate the expressions on a person's face if he is sitting with his back to the bright window ; the window is a glare source.

These disabilities arise from :

(a) the scattering of light within the ocular media, producing a halo around the glare source ; in consequence the eye cannot recognise such small brightness differences as before, but only differences appropriate to a higher general brightness level.* Because of the position of a lamp standard or of reflection from wet patches on a roadway at night, it may be extremely difficult to detect a person in the road. The amount by which the brightness

* §21.4.

level has been raised by the glare source is said to be given in ft. lamberts by an expression of the form

$$\triangle B = k\frac{E}{\theta^2}$$

where E = illumination in ft. candles produced by the glare source in the plane containing the observer's eye.

θ = angle between line of sight and direction of glare source.

k = a constant, varying from 30 for foveal to 50 for peripheral vision.

(b) the lowering of retinal sensitivity due to spatial and temporal induction ; a powerful glare source may depress all the visual functions.

(c) localised temporal induction effects which produce blind spots and after-images on the retinal areas stimulated by the glare sources.

A type of glare additional to the above two categories and called veiling glare is experienced when a diffusing material such as fog is present in the space between eye and object. When this is illuminated, as by the head-lights of a car in the case of fog, it creates a veil of light and raises the adaptation level of the eye in the same way as a glare source.

The effect of high illumination on visual acuity has been discussed in Chapter II ; some comments on its effect on colour vision will be made later.

Although it has not been investigated, the fact that a localised bright source can sometimes improve visual acuity should be mentioned.

21.4. Sensitivity to Brightness Contrast. The Differential Threshold.

Our efficiency in all kinds of practical visual tasks depends a great deal on our ability to recognise small differences of brightness between one part of the field and another. This is especially true of conditions at night and in dim illuminations generally when our visual acuity is very low and does not help us. WEBER enunciated a law* concerning this sensitivity to contrast, stating that : the increase of stimulus which produces a just perceptible

* §1.4 (B)

increase of sensation bears a constant ratio to the whole stimulus. This law is roughly true, within limits, with respect to all our senses.

To illustrate its importance in vision, consider the simple example of a piece of self-coloured material of brightness 10 m.l. with a patch on it of brightness 11 m.l. If, due to a cloud moving away from the sun or some other cause, the illumination is doubled, the two brightnesses become 20 and 22 m.l. If our increase of sensation were directly proportional to the stimulus, the contrast between the material and the patch would appear to have been doubled

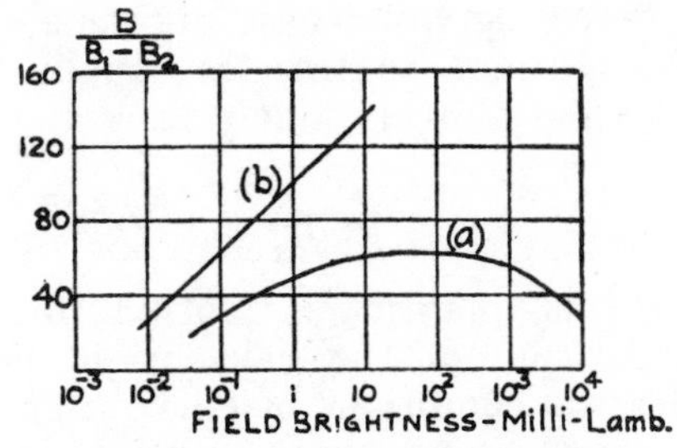

Fig. 21.1—Sensitivity to Brightness Contrast. Reciprocal of Fechner Fraction plotted against Field Brightness; (*a*) Dark surround; (*b*) Light surround. See text.

and so the relative appearance of this and of all objects around us would be continually changing with fluctuations in illumination. But the law tells us that the increase in sensation is proportional to the *ratio* that the increase of stimulus bears to the whole stimulus; this is $\frac{1}{10}$ under both illuminations in the example, and so the general appearance of the scene remains unchanged.

For long, however, there has been argument about the strict truth of the law or at least as to the conditions under which it can be accepted as true. Discrimination of brightness differences varies considerably between individuals; it is affected to an appreciable extent by the size and colour of the object or test patch and the duration of its exposure, by the illumination of the surrounding field and the state of adaptation of the eye. And different experimenters have obtained contradictory results because these conditions have not always been adequately controlled.

Modern work appears to establish results which are illustrated in Fig. 21.1. In the experiments leading to curve (a) the test area is small; it consists of the two spots of light that are to be compared and the surroundings are dark. If B_1 and B_2 represent the brightnesses of the two spots when the difference between them can just be distinguished, then the quantity $(B_1 - B_2)$ is the differential threshold of the stimulus at the brightness level $\frac{1}{2}(B_1 + B_2)$, which we may write simply as B. The ratio $(B_1 - B_2)/B$ is sometimes called the FECHNER fraction; WEBER'S law states that this is constant over a wide range of brightness levels. The smaller this ratio the more acute is the eye in detecting brightness differences; hence the sensitivity to brightness contrast is usually expressed as the reciprocal of the above, namely as

$$\frac{B}{B_1 - B_2}$$

In Fig. 21.1 this quantity is plotted (for white light) against the logarithm of the field brightness, B. It is seen that under the conditions of curve (a) the sensitivity *is* approximately constant over the brightness range 1 to 10^3 m.l., its mean value being about 55. This covers the brightnesses encountered in ordinary daylight and illuminated living and work rooms. Outside the above range the sensitivity is not constant, but decreases rather rapidly. Thus in dim illuminations, under street lighting conditions for example, we do not recognise objects unless they differ appreciably in brightness from one another or from their surroundings; and even then we cannot distinguish their details since our visual acuity is poor under such conditions.

Curve (b) is obtained from experiments in which the whole field is of uniform brightness B_1, the test patch being a small area within it, of brightness B_2. Under these conditions WEBER'S law does not hold; the contrast sensitivity is not constant over any range of brightnesses but progressively increases with field brightness up to 10 m.l. or so, and reaches much higher values than before. Over the range of brightnesses to which both curves apply the eye is much more sensitive to contrast when the whole field is illuminated than when it is dark. Open country and diffusely-lighted interiors are practical examples approximating to these (b) conditions. The variable conditions encountered in everyday life will usually lie somewhere between the extreme cases (a) and (b). If the surrounding field is brighter than the test patch, and especially if there are bright local glare sources, the sensitivity rapidly decreases. If experiments are carried out in monochromatic light, the results show that contrast sensitivity is better for the shorter wavelengths at low values of the field brightness.

FECHNER's name is associated with WEBER's law because of his attempt to express it in mathematical terms. Treating the changes in brightness (B) and sensation (S) as increments, he argued that since $dS \propto \frac{dB}{B}$, the sensation is proportional to the logarithm of the stimulus, i.e. $S = k \log B$; but this is untenable both on mathematical and physiological grounds.

In the above we have been discussing the ability of the eye to compare the brightnesses of two adjacent areas of the field. This is not to be confused with a different kind of performance, namely the ability of the eye to appreciate the difference between two successive stimulations of different intensity on the *same* retinal area. It may be that investigations have been made of this problem.

It will be appreciated that to obtain accuracy in determining the differential threshold and contrast sensitivity experimentally, the conditions which influence them (such as those enumerated) must be carefully controlled, and this requires complicated apparatus. The student can gain a rough idea of their value in the laboratory, however, by using simple apparatus, an example of which is MASSON's disc [Fig. 20.3 (c)]. On a circular disc of white paper are affixed three sectors of black paper or material; sector *a* might be made of angle 20°, *b* of 10° and *c* of 5°. If this disc is fixed to a hand-driven revolving wheel or to a circular plate geared to an electric motor, and rotated at an appropriate speed, three grey rings will be seen corresponding to sectors *a*, *b* and *c*. Between and beyond these will be white rings. The disc is to be illuminated and the brightness of the white portion can be measured by means of an illumination photometer. Assuming for a moment that the black sectors reflect no light and assigning the number 360 as the brightness of the white paper, the brightness of the three grey rings will be 340, 350 and 355; the differences between the grey rings and the white back ground will be 20, 10 and 5 respectively. Rings *a* and *b* will probably be easily distinguished. If ring *c* can only *just* be distinguished, then the differential threshold is $\frac{5}{360}$ of the measured brightness of the white paper and the contrast sensitivity is $360 \div 5$ or 72.

The angular size of sector that can just be distinguished may, of course, have some value other than 5° ; this can be determined by experiment. The illumination can be varied ; the diameters of the sectors can be made large or small ; the white disc itself can be made large or small, so affecting the illumination conditions of the background and the state of adaptation of the eye. In such ways the contrast sensitivity can be roughly determined under various conditions. The black sectors will reflect some light and this must be taken into account in working out results.

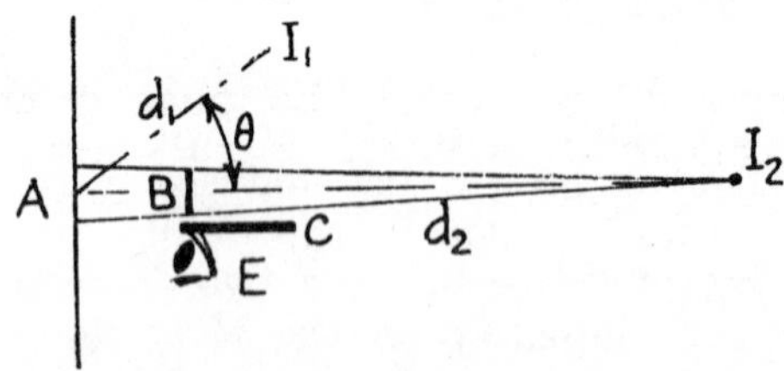

FIG. 21.2—EXPERIMENTAL ARRANGEMENT FOR DETERMINING BRIGHTNESS CONTRAST SENSITIVITY OF EYE.

Another laboratory method is possible with an arrangement similar to the shadow photometer (Fig. 21.2). A shadow is cast at A on a matt white screen by means of an obstacle B and a lamp I_2. A second lamp I_1 illuminates the screen and the shadow. If distances $I_1A = d_1$ and $I_2A = d_2$ and I_1 and I_2 represent the candlepowers, then

illumination on shadow at A $= E_1 = \dfrac{I_1 \cos\theta}{d_1^2}$

illumination on screen near A $= E_2 = \dfrac{I_2}{d_2^2} + \dfrac{I_1 \cos\theta}{d_1^2}$

difference between illuminations $= \dfrac{I_2}{d_2^2}$

The observing eye at E can be shielded from the lamps and the obstacle by means of a screen C. The distance of the lamp I_2 is adjusted until the difference between the shadow A and the screen near to it can just be distinguished ; to increase the accuracy the obstacle B can be in the form of a thick ($\frac{1}{8}''$) wire bent into some geometrical shape—circle, triangle, rectangle, etc.; these can be inserted at random unknown to the observer. We then have

$$\text{differential light threshold} = \frac{I_2}{d_2^2}\rho$$

where ρ = reflection factor of screen.

If CS represents the brightness contrast sensitivity of the eye

$$CS = \frac{\text{brightness of background}}{\text{just perceptible brightness difference}}$$

$$= \frac{\left(\frac{I_2}{d_2^2} + \frac{I_1 \cos\theta}{d_1^2}\right)\rho}{\frac{I_2}{d_2^2}\rho} = 1 + \frac{I_1 d_2^2}{I_2 d_1^2}\cos\theta.$$

The distance d_2 will usually be much greater than d_1 so that, in comparison with the second term on the right of the equation, the first term, 1, can be neglected; or

$$CS = \frac{I_1 d_2^2}{I_2 d_1^2}\cos\theta$$

The FECHNER fraction is the reciprocal of this.

21.5. The Field of Vision.

The normal extent of the visual field in ordinary daylight vision was stated in §2.4. But, as we have seen above, whether an object will be seen in any given region of the retina depends upon the nature of the object and its surroundings and the state of adaptation of the eye. Under photopic conditions a very small object is visible at the fovea but not elsewhere; as the object is increased in size it can be seen at progressively greater distances into the periphery of the retina, the distances depending upon the colour of the object and its brightness.* Moreover, the results obtained also depend on the duration of exposure. Under scotopic conditions, a dim object seen by indirect vision at 20° to 30° from the fovea will not be seen at the fovea nor further out in the periphery. Thus the extent of the visual field cannot be stated in precise terms unless all the characteristics of the stimulus and the conditions of observation are specified.

The manner in which the sensitivity of the eye to light (light sense) varies across the retina is illustrated in Fig. 21.3 under both photopic and scotopic conditions. The

* §2.10.

curves are to be taken as suggesting the general trend of the regional variations, though they accord broadly with the measurements of sensitivity that have been quoted in this chapter. They show that in photopic conditions the fovea is the most sensitive; that if the eye is dark-adapted, all regions become more sensitive to light; to the extent of a hundred-fold or so at the fovea and approaching a million-fold at 20° from the fovea.

The photopic curve shows that the variation of the light sense across the retina is very much less marked than the variation of the form sense.*

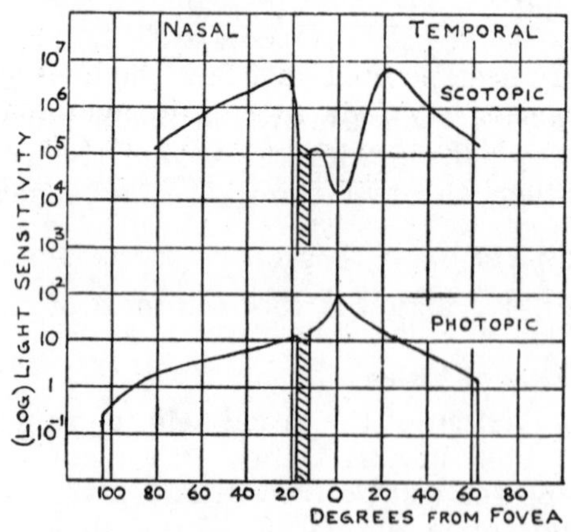

FIG. 21.3—LIGHT SENSITIVITY ACROSS RETINA. THE DATA ARE APPROXIMATE. SENSITIVITY IS EXPRESSED AS RECIPROCAL OF THRESHOLD IN MILLILAMBERTS.

THE COLOUR SENSE.

21.6. Colour Sense. Specific Threshold.

A visual sensation has a quality which we call its colour, i.e. that attribute of it by virtue of which it belongs either to the achromatic series of white-grey-black or to the chromatic series which possesses the more specific quality of hue. The effectiveness with which we appreciate hue and variations of hue under various conditions is determined by the acuteness of our colour sense.

Colour was discussed in Chapter XIX, which the student should recapitulate. There we were concerned mainly

* §2.10

with the stimulus ; but since colour is, after all, a sensation it was necessary to explain some of the capabilities of the visual mechanism in appreciating hue. To summarise, we found that :

All colour sensations are due to mixtures, in varying proportions, of the constituent radiations lying within the visible spectrum.

The same sensation may be evoked by entirely different physical stimuli.

Any colour sensation can be matched by using a suitable mixture of three selected radiations.*

Colour equations are additive.

Further aspects of colour vision must now be considered. It has already been pointed out† how the hues of the visible spectrum successively fade away into achromatic grey as the brightness level is reduced below 10^{-1} ft. lamb. or so until, at about 10^{-3} ft. lamb., all the hues (except a faint blueness) have disappeared. The level at which any particular hue changes to grey is the colour or SPECIFIC THRESHOLD for that hue or wavelength. The brightness has to be reduced still further before the light threshold is reached ; i.e. before the grey sensation completely disappears to darkness. The interval between the two thresholds, during which the sensation is colourless, is the PHOTOCHROMATIC INTERVAL. This varies for different hues, being least for red ; it is doubtful whether there is any photochromatic interval for red beyond λ 670. We are all aware of the blue interval ; blue appears first at dawn and disappears last at evening. During this photochromatic interval the cone mechanism, we believe, is inactive and vision has been taken over by the rods. The faint blue with which grey is tinged is characteristic of the rod mechanism. There does not appear to be any marked photochromatic interval at the fovea for any hue.

21.7. Field of Vision for Colours.

From the manner in which the cone population decreases at increasing distances from the fovea it might be anticipated that there would be a regional variation in the sensitivity to colour ; and this is found to be the case. When, in moderate illumination, a coloured test object is moved outwards from the point of steady fixation, at a certain

* To be more accurate we should add : for foveal vision and a 2° field.
† §20.9.

distance out the hue disappears, the object appearing grey until finally it disappears altogether. The angular distance from the fovea at which the hue disappears is a measure of the field of vision for that hue in the particular meridian explored. With most colours the hue changes before it gives place to grey, passing through a yellow stage in the case of long wavelengths and a blue stage for the shorter wavelengths. This change of hue does not occur, however, in the case of four colours; blue λ 470 and yellow λ 574; blue-green λ 496 and red λ 650; though these wavelengths are probably approximate, it will be observed that they are two complementary pairs. Because of this property

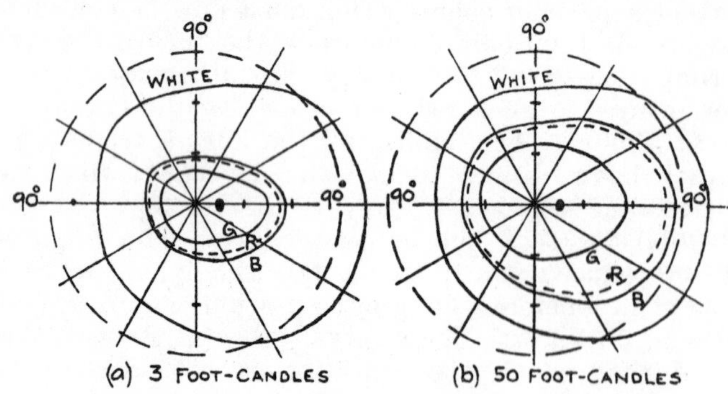

FIG. 21.4—THE COLOUR FIELDS COMPARED WITH EXTREME VISUAL (WHITE) FIELD AT TWO LEVELS OF ILLUMINATION; LIGHT-ADAPTED EYE.

of retaining their hue without changing, these four colours have been called physiologically pure colours.

The field of vision for any selected hue depends upon the degree of saturation of the hue, the size and brightness of the stimulus (test object), the illumination of the surrounding field, size of the pupil and the state of adaptation of the eye; and, in the case of dim illuminations, upon the manner in which the test stimulus is moved into or across the field. The size and brightness of the stimulus are particularly important factors. It may be that slight variations in one or other of these conditions will not seriously affect diagnosis in clinical work, but the evidence on this point is not conclusive.

The normal extents of the colour fields that are usually quoted and illustrated in the literature are probably not reliable as they are based on early work, with the perimeter in which the factors enumerated above were not adequately controlled. Such as they are, however, and pending the publication of more accurate information, they are illustrated in Fig. 21.4 for three spectrum colours: red λ 670, green λ 510 and blue λ 460 at two levels of illumination, namely 50 and 3 ft. candles, the angular size of the stimulus being about 2° and the eye light-adapted. The extreme field for white light is also indicated on each diagram. The field surrounding the test object is grey and illuminated to the same extent as the test object itself. The brightness of a background, and whether it be black or grey or white, influences the recognition of a hue.

The plots show that at moderate intensities of the stimulus (a) the peripheral portions of the retina are insensitive to colour and that as the intensity increases, (b), the fields expand. It is found that if the intensities are raised sufficiently high (requiring varying amounts of energy for the different colours—most for red) all the colour fields, with the possible exception of the green, can be made equal to the maximum white field; and even the green field is only slightly restricted. In other words, all regions of the retina are sensitive to colour if the stimulus intensity is high enough. When, on the other hand, the stimulus intensity is reduced to low levels, the colour fields shrink to a region closely surrounding the fovea; the green field is still the smallest under these conditions. In the light-adapted eye the fovea is the most sensitive region for all colours.

When the eye is dark-adapted, the fields for blue and green do not exceed 30° to 40° at any intensity whereas for red and yellow they extend practically to the whole maximum, as in the light-adapted eye. These limits are reached, however, with stimuli of somewhat lower intensity than under conditions of light adaptation. That is to say, the eye is more sensitive to colour when in the dark-adapted state, though over a restricted field in the case of blue and green; but the increase of sensitivity is very small compared with the hundred-thousandfold increase in the sensitivity to light.*

Whether the hue of a coloured test stimulus will be appreciated depends also upon the size of the stimulus. If the size is reduced the field is restricted unless the intensity

* §21.5.

be increased. Test objects of various sizes are consequently used in clinical perimetry.

The hue will not be appreciated if the duration of exposure of the stimulus is too short; and the needed exposure varies with wavelength; the longer the wavelength the longer the exposure.

It may be that when these colour fields have been explored by more carefully controlled scientific experiments, the above account of them will require modification.

A Clinical Perimeter

In clinical work it is not possible to control all the determining factors relating to the stimulus and the examinee to the extent that is necessary in scientific

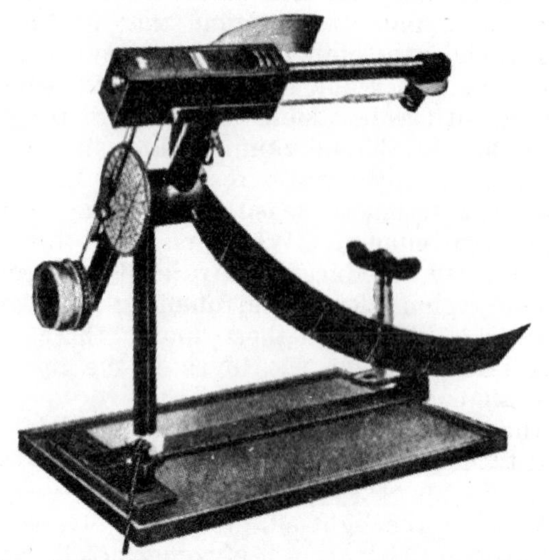

Fig. 21.4a—The Aimark Projection Perimeter.

investigations. An instrument will be described to illustrate how an appreciable measure of control may be achieved in a modern recording perimeter.

Since the introduction of the perimeter by Aubert and Fœrster during the years 1857–69 the technique of perimetry has been improved as a means of detecting the position and severity of lesions in the visual pathway. To obtain the required information with some precision the perimeter should present a stimulus which is under control as to size, brightness and colour in all parts of the field; the stimulus should also be capable of smooth and silent movement so as not to distract the patient and to call for the minimum of effort on the part of the practitioner.

In the instrument illustrated in Fig. 21.4A, the inner surface of the semi-circular arc over which the stimulus moves is grey in colour and the arc has a radius of curvature of one third of a metre. Together with the illuminating system it can be rotated about the horizontal axis through 360° so that measurements can be taken in any meridian. The test stimulus is projected on to the arc by means of a lens and prism system which is contained in the upper horizontal arm of the instrument; the lamp is housed in the box-like compartment at the top of the instrument and is used, not only as the source for the test stimulus, but also to illuminate the fixation cross at the centre of the arc and the chart at the back of the instrument on which the positions of the test stimulus are recorded.

At one end of the box compartment are three rotatable discs; the first of these has four circular apertures of different diameters; by rotating this disc a test stimulus of diameter 1, 3, 5 or 10 mm. can be obtained, for the test stimulus is the image of whichever aperture has been rotated into position. A second disc, alongside the first, also has four apertures one of which is free, the others containing selected filters of red, green and blue. The filters provide coloured test stimuli of relatively high saturation and with dominant hues of approximately 700, 510 and 440 $m\mu$ respectively. The C.I.E. specification of the light transmitted by these filters is given in the Table.*

	Equal energy source			*Illuminant A* (S_A)		
	x	y	z	x	y	z
Red ..	0·709	0·291	0·000	0·712	0·288	0·000
Green ..	0·145	0·467	0·388	0·239	0·507	0·254
Blue ..	0·145	0·051	0·804	0·118	0·073	0·809

In the third disc with four apertures, one is free and the others contain neutral filters of optical densities 0·6, 1·2

* See §19.1 and §19.7.

and 1·8, transmitting therefore $\frac{1}{4}$, $\frac{1}{16}$ and $\frac{1}{64}$ of the incident light respectively. With the free apertures of this and the second disc in position, the brightness of the white test stimulus is about 12 ft. lamberts and consequently 3, 0·75 and 0·19 ft. lamberts respectively when the neutral filters are interposed. The percentage visual transmissions (to tungsten light of colour temperature 3073° K) of the three coloured filters are respectively : red 6·8, green 16·1 and blue 1·2 per cent. Thus the instrument provides means for graduating the test stimulus in size, hue and brightness, to an extent sufficient to detect a small central scotoma.

The patient's head is supported in the headrest which can be adjusted for height and for distance from the arc so that the patient's eye can be placed with some precision at 33⅓ cm. from the arc. He observes the fixation cross at the centre of the arc. For patients with a central scotoma an alternative fixation object is provided in the form of a white annular ring which can be placed in position when required. When the practitioner operates the engraved drum at the back of the instrument, a prism housed in the outer end of the horizontal arm carrying the optical system is rotated and so the test stimulus moves silently along the perimeter arc ; at the same time a pricker marker moves in the appropriate direction and to a proportionate extent over the chart which has been inserted in clips at the back of the instrument. Thus the practitioner can see the pattern the field is taking ; he can remove it from the instrument and study it at leisure when the field plotting is completed and can file it as a permanent record.

21.8. Discrimination of Hue. Differential Colour Threshold.

The hundreds, indeed thousands, of different " colours " that we see around us in nature and in manufactured articles are due partly to differences in hue but also to variations in saturation and in luminosity of each hue. Observation of a continuous spectrum shows that the prominent hues—red, yellow, green, blue, violet—merge gradually into one another ; it is also noticed that the hue changes much more rapidly in the yellow region than it does in the green or red regions ; indeed at the red end there is scarcely any observable change of hue from wavelength 670 $m\mu$ to the extreme end of the spectrum.

That is to say, the least change of wavelength $d\lambda$ that can just be perceived as a change of hue is smaller at λ 590 (yellow) than it is at λ 530 (green) or λ 640 (red).

Values of the smallest detectable change of wavelength at different parts of the spectrum are plotted against wavelength in Fig. 21.5, as determined by WRIGHT and PITT (1934) on five observers. Such a curve is called the *hue discrimination curve.* It does not apply at very low or very high intensities. The observations from which it is plotted are made by exposing light of wavelength λ in one half-field of a colorimeter* and light of wavelength $(\lambda + d\lambda)$ in the other half-field, adjusting $d\lambda$ until the difference between the two hues can be just distinguished.

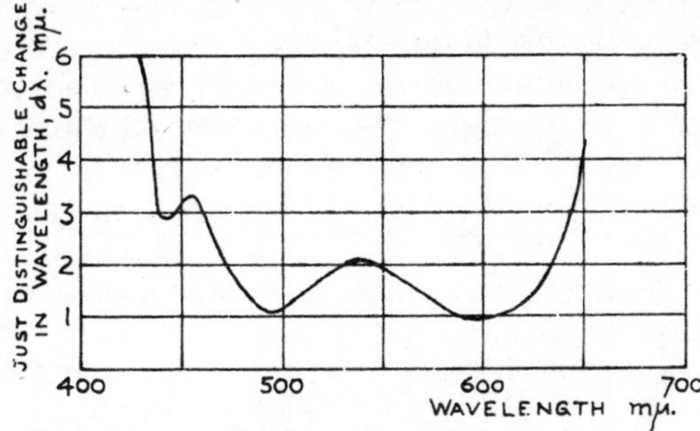

FIG. 21.5—HUE DISCRIMINATION CURVE FOR NORMAL EYE (WRIGHT AND PITT, 1934).

The whole field subtends 2° at the eye; the two half-fields are separated by a fine dividing line. To ensure that we test hue-discrimination alone, the two lights are carefully adjusted to be equal in luminosity. The curve shows that under such conditions the average eye is very sensitive to hue changes in the yellow at λ 590 and in the blue-green at λ 490, its sensitivity being about 1 $m\mu$, which is scarcely twice the separation of the two lines of the sodium spectrum. A trained observer working under favourable conditions will discriminate an even smaller wavelength change than this, probably 0·1 $m\mu$. The rapid rise of the curve towards infinity as it approaches λ 670 bears out the above remark about the constancy of hue at the red end of the spectrum. It can be calculated from the curve that about 150 different hues can be discriminated in the spectrum by the normal

* Fig. 19.3.

observer, provided the stated precautions are observed in the experiment.

If the method of conducting the experiment were to expose restricted widths of the spectrum successively by using a slit of adjustable width and widening the slit until a change of hue can be just detected between its edges, the number of hues that can be distinguished along the spectrum is then very much less than 150—only 20 or 30. But under these conditions it is a different function of the eye that is being investigated; its task here is to compare two hues which are some distance apart (the width of the slit) the hue and the luminosity varying *gradually* from one side of the field to the other.*

21.9. Discrimination of Saturation.

A saturated colour is a pure colour; the more it is diluted with white light the lower is its saturation and

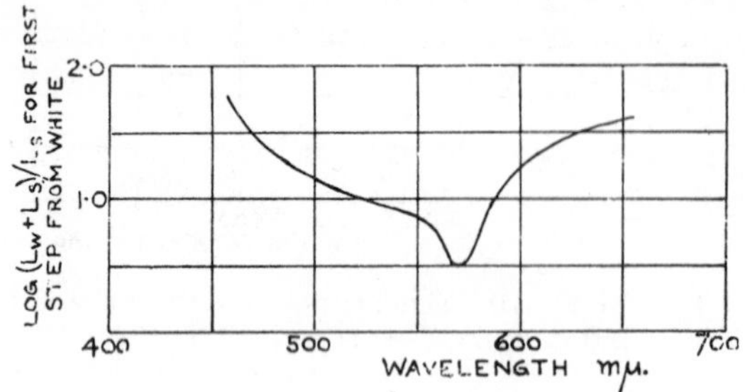

FIG. 21.6—SATURATION DISCRIMINATION CURVE FOR NORMAL EYE.

the paler it appears. If we were to arrange a number of lights of the same hue, say λ 550 light (green), in order of saturation, the first light would appear a green of the purity we obtain in the spectrum and the last light would appear white with no trace of the original hue. If L_s is the luminosity of a given pure spectral hue and it is mixed with a specified white of luminosity L_w, then the saturation may be expressed as $L_s/(L_w + L_s)$.

We can measure the sensitivity of the eye to changes of saturation by using a photometer arrangement. Both half-fields are illuminated with standard white†; monochromatic spectral light of a certain wavelength λ is then

* See also §20.5. † §19.1.

introduced into one half-field (and extra white into the other half to equalise the luminosities) until the difference between the two halves can just be appreciated. The saturation discrimination of the eye for this wavelength may then be expressed as $\log (L_W + L_S)/L_S$. Measurements of this kind have been carefully made on a few individuals* and the mean values of the results are shown plotted against wavelength in Fig. 21.6, giving the *saturation discrimination curve* for the normal observer.

The curve reaches a pronounced minimum at λ 570; this means that for this particular wavelength in the yellow part of the spectrum a relatively large amount L_S is needed to produce a just noticeable difference from white. This is due to the fact that this hue and those nearest to it are already relatively desaturated; this is evident on inspecting the spectrum; for it is seen that though the luminosity is high these colours are pale, not rich and full of colour like the blue or red hues of the spectrum.

It may be worth noting that the wavelength range of highest luminosity appears the least saturated.

21.10. The Luminosity Mixture Curves or Sensation Curves.

Ever since the tristimulus basis of colour sensation was realised† and HELMHOLTZ had elaborated the famous suggestion made by THOMAS YOUNG, there has been a strong belief, supported by much of the experimental evidence acquired since, that some kind of triple mechanism exists in that part of the visual mechanism (cones) that is concerned with colour vision. Some words of HELMHOLTZ, used in a lecture delivered in 1868, are worth repeating:

> " The theory of colours, with all these marvellous and complicated relations, was a riddle which GOETHE in vain attempted to solve; nor were we physicists and physiologists more successful. I include myself in the number; for I long toiled at the task, without getting any nearer my object, until I at last discovered that a wonderfully simple solution had been discovered at the beginning of this century and had been in print ever since for anyone to read who chose. This solution was found and published by the same THOMAS YOUNG who first showed the right method of arriving at the

* By WRIGHT, PITT and NELSON (1937); also by MARTIN, WARBURTON and MORGAN (1933).

† §§ 19.3 to 19.7.

interpretation of Egyptian hieroglyphics. He was one of the most acute men who ever lived, but had the misfortune to be too far in advance of his contemporaries. They looked on him with astonishment but could not follow his bold speculations. . . . Dr. YOUNG supposes that there are in the eye three kinds of nerve-fibres* the first of which, when irritated in any way, produces the sensation of red, the second the sensation of green and the third that of violet. He further assumes that the first are excited most strongly by the waves of ether of greatest length; the second, which are sensitive to green light, by the waves of middle length; while those which convey impressions of violet are acted upon only by the shortest vibrations of ether. . . ."

Over the years, great efforts have been made to discover the nature of these three supposed component mechanisms. It would be extremely useful in this search if we knew to what extent each component responds to the various wavelengths of the spectrum and especially to what wavelength it responds maximally; that is, if we knew the forms of their luminosity or sensation curves. This knowledge might assist in the search that is in progress for light-sensitive substances, other than visual purple, in the retinæ of various creatures. Some such substances have been found and their absorption curves determined; arguing from the similarity between the absorption curve of visual purple and the human scotopic luminosity curve, it would be a great help in exploring these newly found substances if we knew the sensation curves of the assumed three components against which to compare the absorption curves.

Various investigators have selected three lights or stimuli—red, green and blue—and have determined experimentally the quantities of each that are required to produce a sensation which matches the sensation produced by each wavelength of the visible spectrum. The results obtained by WRIGHT, using monochromatic matching stimuli R, G and B of wavelengths 650, 530 and 460 $m\mu$, are given in Table V, and discussed in Chapter XIX. Those figures give the quantities of R, G and B in the so-called trichromatic units; these, it will be remembered, were

* YOUNG did no more than suggest this as a useful working hypothesis.

obtained quite arbitrarily on the basis that the quantities of R, G and B needed to match standard white are considered to be equal when expressed in these units. But although their contributions to colour are thus equal, their contributions to luminosity, i.e. the quantities of *light* that they supply to the mixture, are far from equal. The luminosity curve (Fig. 18.1) tells us that, even from an equal energy source, the luminosity factors of λ 460 and λ 650 radiations are respectively only 0·06 and 0·11 as against 0·86 for λ 530.

If we were to measure the amounts of *light* that R, G and B respectively contribute in matching the successive spectrum radiations, i.e. if the results were expressed in luminosity units instead of the arbitrary trichromatic units, we should obtain a set of curves quite different in shape from those of Fig. 19.4; the ordinates of the blue and red curves would be very much smaller than those for the green curve. And if we were to change to another set of three matching stimuli, again the shapes of the curves would be modified. It would be possible to decide upon a hypothetical set of stimuli such that positive quantities of them would always be needed to arouse any sensation, just as the reference stimuli of §19.7 were chosen for colorimetric purposes. There is an infinite number of such choices and investigators have attempted to discover which one of these choices provides the response curves of the three components of the physiological system —the luminosity mixture curves, fundamental sensation curves, fundamental response curves, etc., as they have been variously described.

By various methods all the known facts of colour vision have been analysed—relating to colour mixture, hue discrimination, adaptation, etc., of both normal and defective individuals—and most of the results of such analysis indicate that whereas there is still much uncertainty, the curves may well be similar to those illustrated in Fig. 21.7 in which the maxima are in the regions: red, 580 to 600 $m\mu$; green, 550 $m\mu$; blue, 460 $m\mu$. They give the proportions based on luminosity units in which the three supposed physiological systems in the eye would respond to the various wavelengths emitted by a certain white light source. It will be observed that the ordinates of the blue curve have been increased a hundred-fold. If the ordinates are added together we obtain the light distribution curve (§18.2) for the particular source. If this were the equal energy source the summation would give the luminosity curve of Fig. 18.1. This is the case in Fig. 21.7 and the summation, shown by the dotted curve, should be compared with Fig. 18.1. The areas under the three curves give the proportions in which the response systems of the eye would be stimulated by white light.

Thus if the eye were stimulated by radiation of wave-length 450 $m\mu$ obtained from an equal-energy source, Fig. 21.7 tells us that all three component mechanisms would respond, in relative proportions: blue component

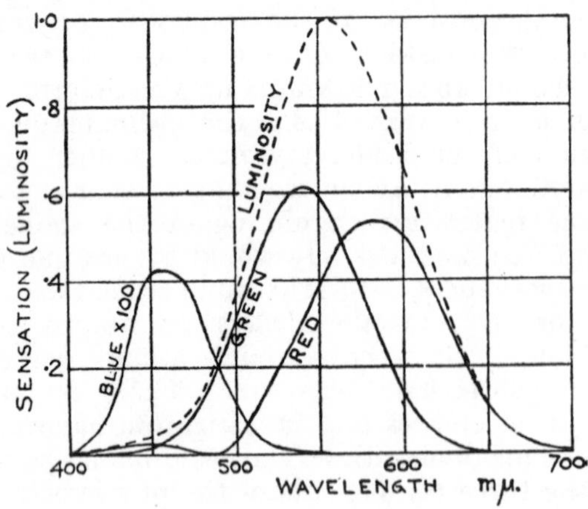

Fig. 21.7—Suggested Luminosity Mixture Curves or Sensation Curves for Equal Energy Spectrum (Wright). Ordinates add up to the Photopic Luminosity Curve.

·004; green component ·02 and red component ·025; the resultant sensation aroused by the transmission of these responses from retina to brain would be of blue-violet quality. (The small subsidiary rise of the red curve in this λ450 region is of some interest.) The responses to λ550 radiation would be in the proportions: blue negligible, green ·59 and red ·39, the resultant sensation being green. Light of wavelengths from 650 $m\mu$ upwards would evoke a response only in the red component.

If we take a pair of complementary colours from the table of §19.2, say λ 580 and λ 482·5, we see from Fig. 21.7 that λ 580 radiation stimulates the green and red components to relative extents ·325 and ·54 (blue negligible);

and that λ 482·5 radiation stimulates the blue and green components to relative extents ·003 and ·15 (red negligible). The two complementaries together are equivalent to a mixture of all three matching stimuli in certain proportions.

The student is reminded that the sensation curves of Fig. 21.7 are only tentative. Further research will quite possibly modify them ; it may even challenge the adequacy of the whole three-components theory ; but that possibility does not deny the usefulness of the theory at the present time (see §23.1).

21.11. Colour Vision in Small Fields.

In numerous instances we have seen how the sensation is dependent on the duration and size of the stimulus (and hence upon the area of the retina stimulated) and on the region of the retina concerned ; for this reason it is necessary in many experiments to restrict the size of the field under examination and to exercise great care in maintaining the observer's fixation in a specified direction. In colour matching it is usual to restrict the field to 2°, partly because this is about the extent of the yellow macular " pigment ", and the results quoted above apply mostly to a field of this size.

It has been found (it was noted by KÖNIG fifty years ago but the observation was neglected) that when the field is reduced to very small dimensions, so small that the retinal image occupies only a part of the rod-free area at the fovea subtending 30′ or less, it becomes much more difficult to recognise colours and below a certain minimum size of field they cannot be recognised at all. A small yellow object on a black background appears white ; a blue object appears black. The same difficulties arise when the field is kept constant but the intensity of stimulus is reduced. Experiments seem to show that, in a normal individual, the colour vision becomes at first dichromatic, lacking the blue mechanism, and then is lost altogether.

This kind of result is obtained with small fields in different parts of the fovea and also in extra-foveal regions. Various hypotheses, based upon the response curves obtained electrically from single nerve fibres of the frog and other animals, have been advanced to account for the phenomenon, but the matter is too controversial to be included here ; it is still under discussion.

ANOMALIES OF THE SENSES

21.12. Anomalies of the Light Sense.

NIGHT BLINDNESS: in this condition vision is normal in ordinary illuminations but is deficient in feeble illumination and the individual does not acquire the normal increase of sensitivity, either to light or to light difference, under dark adaptation. It is usually associated with other conditions and may be divided into categories. The evidence indicates a derangement of the rod mechanism of the retina and one of the various causes is known to be deficiency of vitamin A in the diet, in consequence of which there is reduced formation of visual purple. The dark-adaptation curve for a relatively severe case of night-blindness is indicated in Fig. 20.5; in milder cases the sensitivity proceeds to the normal maximum but does so more slowly than normal.

DAY BLINDNESS or *nyctalopia*: this is the reverse of the above, vision being normal in the dark but poor in daylight.

21.13. Anomalies of the Colour Sense.

In a fair proportion of people, about 8 per cent of males and 0·5 per cent of females, colour vision is defective in some way. In modern industry, especially in connection with navigation and transport, such people would be unable to perform certain occupations and may even be potential sources of danger. It has become a matter of importance to devise tests which will

(a) separate colour defectives from normal people;

(b) classify the colour defectives according to the type and degree of the defect.

The problem would be simplified if we had definite information about the cause of defective colour vision, but this will scarcely be possible until we know more about the manner in which the normal person distinguishes one colour from another.

The famous chemist JOHN DALTON aroused interest in the subject when he described his own defective colour vision in 1794. The considerable volume of experimental work that has been carried out since then, notably by MAXWELL, HELMHOLTZ, KÖNIG and ABNEY, has been continued in recent years in America and Britain with more refined apparatus. Much of the British work has been done at the Imperial College of Science, with the help and encouragement of the Medical Research Council, and it is on the published reports of this work and on the Physical Society's excellent "Report on Defective Colour Vision in Industry" (1946) that the following account is largely based.

The most characteristic disadvantage from which all colour defective people suffer is that they cannot discriminate one colour from another as easily as the normal person. If we suppose that the latter can distinguish, say, 50 hues in the yellow to red region of the spectrum (§21.8), it is found that there are certain people who can distinguish only 25 hues within that range and others who can appreciate only five; in the worst cases no difference of hue is seen at all over the whole range. These defective people may appreciate a difference of *brightness* between one part of the range and another; if a test of this kind were being used, care would be necessary to arrange that the brightness was constant for all the hues, otherwise the colour defective may escape detection. It is on this account that he is so often quite unaware of his defect. It is in attempting to distinguish between red and yellow and between yellow and green, when these hues are of about equal luminosity, that colour defectives find their greatest difficulty; to a less extent they also confuse blue-green, grey and purple.

The above remarks concerning the manner in which the colour defective uses differences in brightness to distinguish one hue from another is but one illustration of the difficulties that are encountered in testing colour vision. It is also to be realised that the colour defective child will learn to associate the names of hues used by normal people with particular objects; the words red, green and blue are used in association with objects like a cherry, grass and the sky, which he will be able to distinguish because of their brightness differences. In many cases he may therefore succeed in naming the hue correctly though it is not hue but a difference of brightness that he appreciates. In more difficult circumstances he will be confused and in a test so devised that incidental aids such as brightness differences and names are absent, he will make detectable errors. Some of the names used by the normal person will mean little or nothing to the defective person and he may therefore describe the same stimulus by different names.

The following classification of colour vision anomalies founded on the trichromatic basis of colour sensation, has been generally agreed :*

I MONOCHROMATIC VISION

also called total colour blindness, achromatic vision or achromatopsia. In this condition there is no colour discrimination, the spectrum is of a uniform grey and all colours can be matched with only one radiation.

II DICHROMATIC VISION

also called red-green blindness (SEEBECK, 1837) and Daltonism. There is reduced colour discrimination, the spectrum is reduced to two colours and all colours can be matched by using only two radiations.

Adopting the terminology introduced by von KRIES, the condition is subdivided into :

II (P) PROTANOPIA : all colours can be matched by mixture of two coloured lights such as blue and yellow or blue and red ; appreciation of brightness in the red and yellow is much below normal.

II (D) DEUTERANOPIA : all colours matched by mixture of two coloured lights such as blue and yellow or blue and red ; appreciation of brightness much the same as normal.

II (T) TRITANOPIA : all colours matched by mixture of red and green lights. This condition is very rare, is usually accompanied by affections of the retina and reliable information is lacking.

III ANOMALOUS TRICHROMATIC VISION

Although, as with normal individuals, three radiations are required for colour matching, colour discrimination is reduced in that the relative quantities of the three radiations differ markedly from the normal. The condition is subdivided into :

III (P) PROTANOMALY : the red end of the spectrum stimulates subnormally ; in mixing red and green

* There have been objections to the terms protanopia, deuteranopia, etc.

lights to produce yellow, more red than normal is needed so that the match appears reddish or red to the normal observer.

III (D) DEUTERANOMALY: in mixing red and green lights to produce yellow, more green than normal is needed so that the match appears greenish or green to the normal observer.

III (T) TRITANOMALY: this condition is very rare and reliable information is lacking.

Defective colour vision can be acquired, as by the excessive use of tobacco or alcohol and it accompanies certain diseases; but in nearly all cases it is congenital. It is largely hereditary. The daughters of a congenitally colour defective father will be carriers of the defect though not defective themselves; none of his sons will be defective or carriers. Half the daughters of a carrier mother will be carriers and half of her sons will be defective. If both parents are defective all daughters will be defective. If the father is defective and the mother a carrier, half the daughters will be defective.

In what follows it is congenital defective colour vision that is under discussion.

21.14. Characteristics of Defective Colour Vision.

The (P) subdivisions differ from the normal to a greater extent than the (D) subdivisions, but they are less numerous.

Detailed examination of a number of colour defectives of groups II and III has shown that their colour mixture curves, luminosity curves and hue discrimination curves differ from the normal. Not enough cases have yet been examined to enable entirely reliable views to be formed but the general tendency is illustrated in Fig. 21.8. In the mixture curves 1, 4 and 7 the matching stimuli are WRIGHT'S.

MONOCHROMATIC VISION

This condition is rare, though in isolated communities where inter-marriage is common, the number increases. It is usually one symptom of a pathological condition which includes: reduced visual acuity, maybe as low as $\frac{6}{60}$; nystagmus; photophobia and discomfort in bright

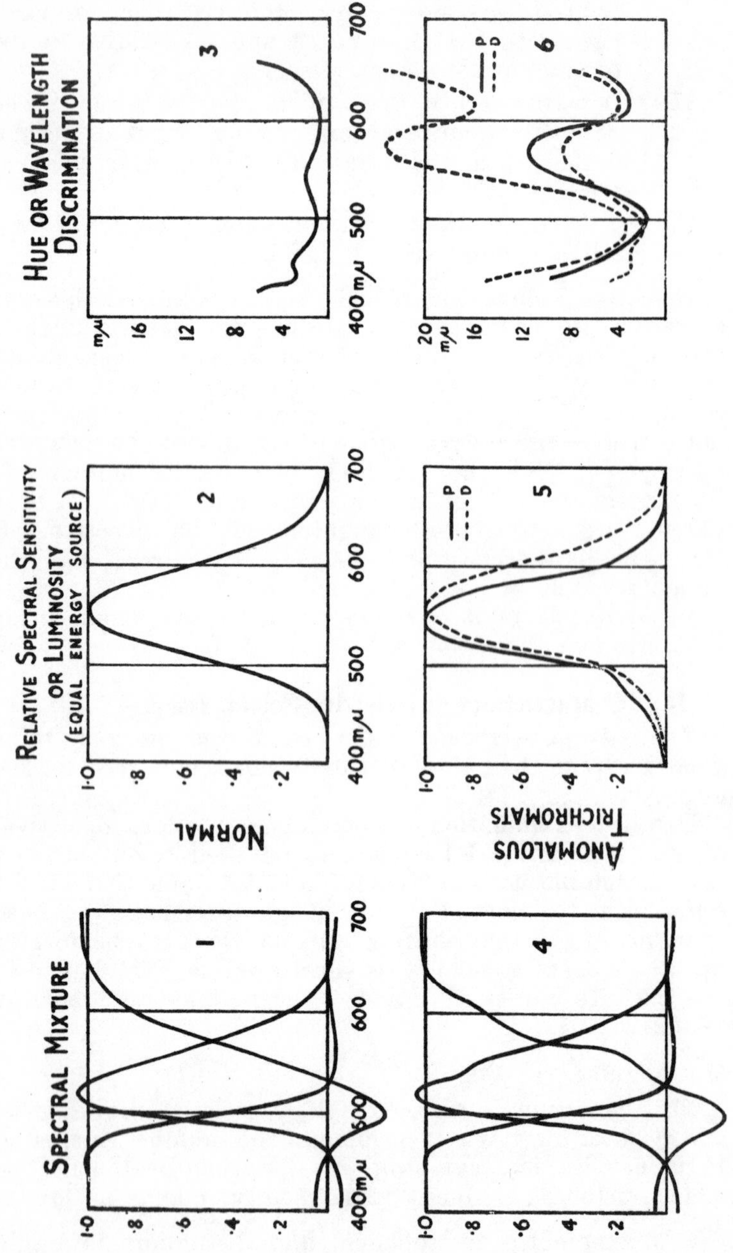
SPECTRAL MIXTURE
RELATIVE SPECTRAL SENSITIVITY OR LUMINOSITY (EQUAL ENERGY SOURCE)
HUE OR WAVELENGTH DISCRIMINATION
NORMAL
ANOMALOUS TRICHROMATS
1
2
3
4
5
6
P
D
1·0 ·8 ·6 ·4 ·2
mμ 16 12 8 4
20 mμ 16 12 8 4
400 mμ 500 600 700

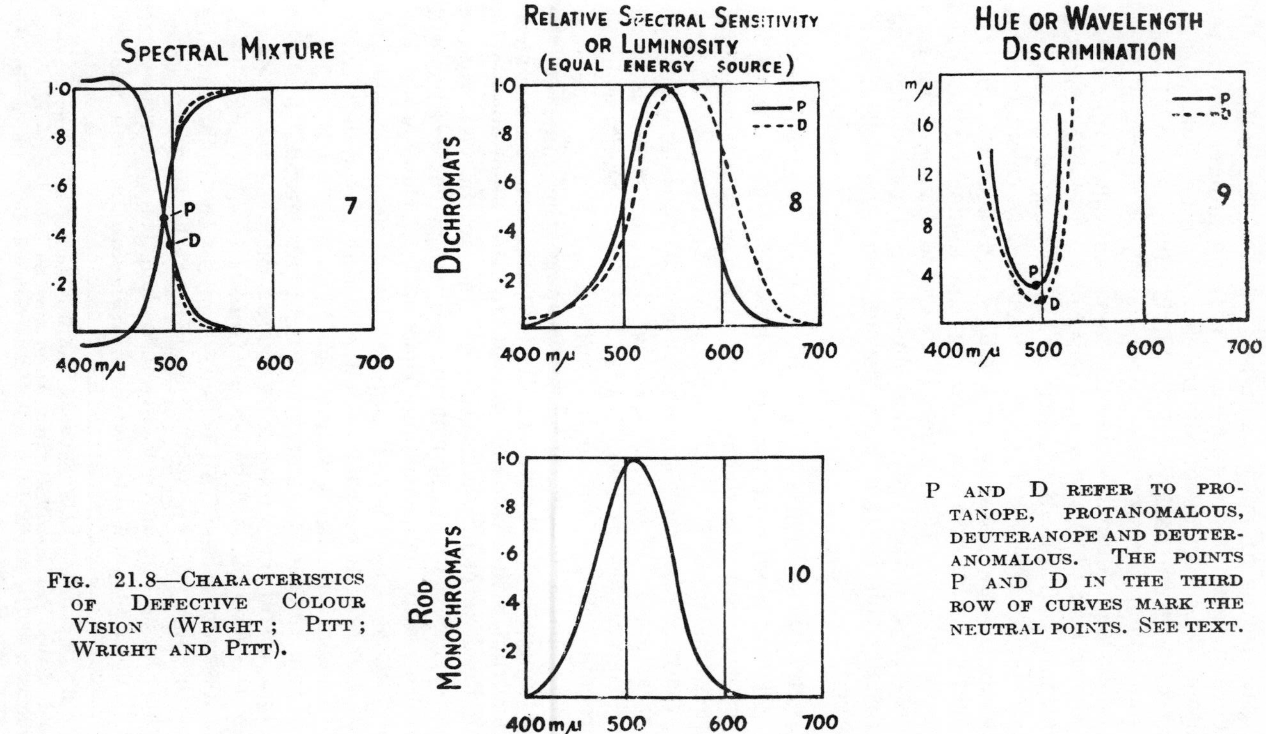

FIG. 21.8—CHARACTERISTICS OF DEFECTIVE COLOUR VISION (WRIGHT; PITT; WRIGHT AND PITT).

P AND D REFER TO PROTANOPE, PROTANOMALOUS, DEUTERANOPE AND DEUTERANOMALOUS. THE POINTS P AND D IN THE THIRD ROW OF CURVES MARK THE NEUTRAL POINTS. SEE TEXT.

light or even ordinary daylight; good vision in dim light. Thus it seems to be something entirely different from the other two categories of colour deficiency. The monochrome grey spectrum varies only in luminosity; as will be seen from the luminosity curve (10), which is very similar to the normal scotopic luminosity curve, the spectrum appears brightest at λ 510 and is shortened at the red end. Spectral mixture and hue discrimination curves are, of course, not possible for this condition. It is found that colour matches made by the normal trichromat and accepted by the dichromat are not accepted by the monochromat. The indications are that vision is mediated through the rods and visual purple only, the cones being inactive for some reason; this has not been conclusively established, however.*

Dichromatic Vision

Of the 8 per cent of colour defective males, about 2·5 per cent are dichromats and 5·5 per cent anomalous trichromats.

Leaving the rare tritanopes out of consideration, the characteristics of the vision of the dichromat are illustrated in diagrams 7, 8 and 9 of Fig. 21.8. If we assume, which is probable though not easily proved, that the blue and yellow parts of the spectrum appear the same to the dichromat as to the normal trichromat, then the complete spectrum will probably appear to the dichromat as a modified spectrum, consisting of blue, white, yellow-green and yellow with orange at the red end. The orange will be especially darkened and shortened in the case of the protanope (P). There is a general weakness of green and red, varying in severity with the extent of the defect, the two main hues being yellow and blue.

From the fact that only two lights are needed to match any spectral hue or white it follows that the colour chart for the dichromat degenerates from a triangle (Fig. 19.5) to a straight line. All colours seen by the dichromat lie on this line and are in the spectrum as he sees it; somewhere along this line and therefore along the spectrum there will be a place where the two lights are in such relative

* It has been suggested that there are two kinds of monochromat; one kind of the type described above, which may be described as rod monochromats, and a second kind, called cone monochromats, whose vision is normal except for their inability to discriminate hue.

proportions as to produce white; this so-called *neutral point* occurs at about λ 495 for the protanope and λ 500 for the deuteranope, in the region which appears blue-green to the normal person. The dichromat's spectrum varies very little in hue from about λ 510 to the long wavelength end, which makes it evident why he confuses green, yellow and red.

Protanopes are differentiated from deuteranopes most characteristically by their luminosity curves (8). For the protanope the curve has a sharper maximum and this occurs at λ 540, nearer to the blue end than the normal; the deuteranope's curve is not very different from the normal luminosity curve (2), its maximum being a little nearer to the red end, at λ 565. The P and D luminosity curves agree with one another more closely at short wavelengths than long wavelengths.

The dichromatic hue discrimination curves (9) are very different from the normal (3); the absence of the curves over the long wavelengths illustrates once again, and strikingly, the difficulty experienced by the dichromat in distinguishing red from yellow and yellow from green. The confusion is always between red and green and not between blue and green, indicating that the relationship between the red and green response systems of the visual mechanism is in some way quite different from the relationship between the red and blue or green and blue response systems. The blue mechanism seems to be dissimilar to the others as if it had a different physiological origin, as was indeed suggested by König many years ago. It can be calculated from the hue discrimination curves that the average protanope can distinguish about 20 hues in the spectrum and the average deuteranope about 30 hues as compared with the 150 hues of the normal trichromat.*

Anomalous Trichromatic Vision

Of the 5·5 per cent of anomalous trichromatic males, about 1 per cent are protanomalous and 4·5 per cent deuteranomalous.

Ignoring the rare tritanomalous group, the characteristics of anomalous trichromatic vision are illustrated in diagrams 4, 5 and 6 of Fig. 21.8. With regard to the spectral mixture curves, the anomalous subjects (more particularly the

* §21.8.

deuteranomalous) who have been exhaustively examined* show some irregularities from the normal and variations amongst themselves, but the general tendency indicated by diagram 4 has been observed.

These defectives, like the normal person, need three radiations for colour matching and so their spectrum does not differ so markedly from the normal; the red end tends towards orange and the green towards yellow-green and, in the case of many of the protanomalous, the red end is dull and shortened as indicated by 5 P. The part of the spectrum which to them appears to be pure yellow, devoid of red or green, is located towards the green side in the protanomalous and towards the red side in the deuteranomalous. It was discovered by RAYLEIGH in 1882 (the Rayleigh equation) that when homogeneous red and green radiations are used to match a homogeneous yellow, some colour defectives require more red than the normal and others more green; the former are the protanomalous and the latter the deuteranomalous. RAYLEIGH used lithium red (λ 671) and thallium green (λ 536). This R/G ratio test is incorporated in the Nagel anomaloscope and provides what is probably the best of all practical tests for detecting anomalous cases and segregating them into the two groups.

The protanomalous are differentiated from the deuteranomalous cases most effectively by their luminosity curves (5) which deviate from the normal in the same direction as with dichromats (8), the protanomalous towards the blue and the deuteranomalous slightly towards the red.

As with the spectral mixture curves, there is much variation between individual deuteranomalous subjects with regard to their hue discrimination curves (6). They all agree in having poorer discrimination than the normal in the yellow and red regions and the minima and maxima of the curves are shifted towards the red, whereas in the blue-green region the departure from normal is much less marked. The lower D curve is typical of some deuteranomalous cases which show a minimum in the violet region.

This poor discrimination in the yellow and red regions together with the dimness of some of the spectral colours results in colour matches made by anomalous trichromats

* By PITT (1935) and NELSON (1938).

not being acceptable to normal trichromats. This suggests that anomalous trichromatism is not due to a uniform reduction of one or more of the three component mechanisms of the eye ; it has been suggested that it may be caused by a distortion or displacement of one or more of the sensation curves (§21.10). Nor is the condition due to abnormal macular pigmentation. Anomalous subjects are more hesitant than normal in making their colour matches ; they need more time and prefer more luminosity and larger test objects.

21.15. Tests for Defective Colour Vision.

All tests for defective colour vision are based upon the difficulty experienced by colour defectives in distinguishing one colour from another. To be satisfactory the test must be so devised as to eliminate the accessory aids of brightness and experience on which the defective person relies in everyday vision ; and to be practical it should be simple and quick to use, relatively inexpensive and reproducible and related to the work the testee is to perform. No one of the available tests completely fulfils these requirements. In the Report on Defective Colour Vision in Industry, tests are divided into five groups :

1. Confusion Chart Tests (pseudo-isochromatic charts).

Introduced by Stilling in 1883, probably the most popular, until recently, have been those devised by Ishihara (1921). The test consists of a series of cards on each of which there is a background of irregularly spaced coloured spots of various sizes ; interspersed amongst these are figures, letters or other shapes also made up of coloured spots. The colours used are those which the colour defectives habitually confuse and they are printed to be of low saturation and so adjusted that brightness discrimination cannot be used by the testee. Whereas the letter or numeral can be easily distinguished against the background by the normal person, it cannot be distinguished, or is mis-read, by the colour defective. On one card, for example, the normal person sees a figure 5, the dichromat sees a 2 and the anomalous trichromat often reads this as a figure 8. These charts are easy to use and form one of the quickest tests of defective colour vision, though they are not infallible. It is important that they be used in daylight or whatever illumination is recommended by the makers.

Needless to say, the charts must be very carefully manufactured in order to present the proper selection of confusion colours—green, yellow, orange, brown, red, pink, etc.—in the correct brightness and saturation; their efficiency depends largely on the care with which they have been printed. Attempts are in hand in U.S.A. to produce a graded series of these confusion charts so that they may be used more effectively for segregating the different categories of colour defectives.

2. Lantern Tests

These were introduced to meet the needs of railway and shipping companies. They are simple to use and will reject people with defective colour vision but will not always enable the latter to be separated into the various groups. They are often preferred to confusion charts as they require less intelligence on the part of the testee. The tests are carried out in a darkened room, the testee having been dark-adapted for about 15 minutes.

Many lanterns have been produced, but they are all similar in presenting coloured apertures, of apparently equal brightness to the normal eye, which have to be recognised and named by the testee. Dimming filters are provided to modify the brightness and to simulate such conditions as fog, etc. It can be seen from the luminosity curves of Fig. 21.8, for example, that red and green lights of equal brightness for the deuteranope will not be adjudged as of equal brightness by the protanope; a dimming filter can be introduced as desired.

3. Wool Tests

These were probably the first colour vision tests to be used. Based upon earlier tests by Seebeck (1837) and Wilson (1855) and following a serious railway accident in Sweden, Holmgren devised his well-known wool test in 1877. The testee is given three specimen skeins of wool—bright green, purple and red; from among about 125 other skeins of various hues and brightnesses he is asked to select just one which he judges to be the nearest match in hue and brightness to each of the three specimens.

Various modifications have been introduced from time to time but these wool tests are now considered to be unreliable and are being superseded.

4. Matching Tests

Under this heading, which includes spectrometers (adapted), colorimeters and specially designed apparatus, are to be found the most accurate tests for detecting and diagnosing defective colour vision. With some of them, e.g. colorimeters, a complete analysis of the colour vision characteristics can be made (Fig. 21.8). For practical purposes, however, they are too elaborate, take too much time and require too much skill on the part of the examiner.

One of them, the *Nagel Anomaloscope*, is less elaborate than most and is sufficiently practical to be considered one of the best of all tests for both detection and diagnosis, being especially useful for anomalous trichromatic cases which frequently cannot be detected and classified by the simpler tests already described. It is designed to determine the red-green ratio of the Raleigh equation (§21.14). By means of a direct vision prism a spectrum is formed of the light from an electric lamp; slits are mounted in the plane of the spectrum at the green, yellow and red positions; the yellow light is directed into the lower half and the red and green together into the upper half of a circular test field. The widths of the slits can be varied by the testee by the manipulation of two drums one of which controls the yellow slit while the other is so connected to the red and green slits that as one opens the other closes. In this way the testee regulates the proportion of red and green lights until the mixture as seen in the upper half-field matches the yellow in both hue and luminosity. If the reading shows that the amount of red is greater than normal, the case is protanomalous; if the green exceeds the normal it is a deuteranomalous case. If difficulty or irregularity is experienced, the testee may be a dichromat, in which case he will be able to match either the full red or the full green by adjusting the intensity of the yellow. To match a bright red a protanope will need little yellow and the deuteranope will use much more yellow.

With this instrument it is thus possible to differentiate between protanopes, deuteranopes, protanomalous and deuteranomalous subjects. The instrument is no test for monochromatism but this is detectable by simpler methods. A drawback of the anomaloscope is that it requires a certain amount of intelligence and practice.

5. Miscellaneous Tests

In general practice it is satisfactory to use one of the reliable sets of confusion charts and in those cases of anomalous trichromatism which are not readily detected by such charts, to confirm on the Nagel anomaloscope. For some special purposes, railways and the fighting services, it is prescribed that an acceptable lantern test must be used.

CHAPTER XXI. *EXERCISES.*

1. Accepting Fabry's value for the illumination produced by a star of the first magnitude as $7 \cdot 7 \times 10^{-8}$ lumens per foot^2, calculate the illumination produced by a star of the sixth magnitude, which is just visible to the eye under ordinary conditions.

2. Describe the factors upon which the value of the light threshold depends in the case of (*a*) a steady source of finite extent; and (*b*) a flash source. For the flash source quote approximate figures for the threshold in terms of the erg and the quantum.

3. Give a definition of glare. Explain how a glare source affects visual efficiency; and describe the general illumination conditions necessary for comfortable and efficient seeing in everyday life.

4. State Weber's psycho-physical law and discuss its importance in relation to everyday vision. Describe a laboratory experiment for investigating the approximate truth of the law.

5. State Weber's law of stimulus-sensation relationship. Discuss the conditions under which it may be accepted as applicable; give explanatory graphs.

6. Explain what is meant by the sensitivity of the eye to brightness contrast. Describe, with the aid of graphs, how this depends upon the brightness of the test patch and its surroundings. Explain the meaning of the Fechner fraction in this connection.

7. In a shadow photometer arrangement for determining the contrast sensitivity of the eye the intensities of the two lamps are respectively 54 and 36 candles. The average of a number of settings gives the distance of the lamps from the screen as one foot and $8 \cdot 75$ feet respectively; the light from the near (54 C.P.) lamp is incident on the screen at 35°. Calculate the contrast sensitivity of the eye. Assuming the reflection factor of the screen to be $0 \cdot 70$, what is the differential light threshold of the eye in the experiment?

8. What is threshold vision? What law connects stimulus and sensation? Draw a diagram showing the relation expressed by the law. How can a disc be made of black and white areas which will appear to shade uniformly from black at the centre to white at the edge, when it is rapidly rotated about its centre? (B.O.A.)

9. With the aid of graphs discuss the variability of the light sense across the retina in photopic and scotopic conditions. Describe also, in the light of these variations, the meaning to be attached to the term "field of vision".

10. Explain how an approximate value for the contrast sensitivity of the eye may be obtained by using a rotating disc. Indicate what measurements are made and how the contrast sensitivity is calculated from these measurements.

11. A bright spectrum is thrown on a screen in an otherwise dark room; this spectrum is very gradually dimmed down so that the room only seems completely dark after about an hour. Describe and explain the changes an observer perceives during this darkening. (B.O.A.)

12. Give a brief description of the apparatus and technique employed in investigating the field (*a*) for white, (*b*) for colours, and give sketches illustrating the general form of the records obtained. (B.O.A.)

13. Explain the meaning of the terms: specific threshold and photochromatic interval. Is there any variation of the photochromatic interval with wavelength or with the region of the retina concerned ?

14. Describe a method for determining the field of vision for colours. Describe the conditions on which the extent of such colour fields depends. Give graphs showing these extents, making clear the conditions under which they apply.

15. Describe how observations may be made in order to determine the hue discrimination curve of the eye. Give such a curve for the normal eye. What are the approximate values of the sensitivity of the eye in discriminating hue at wavelengths 430, 490, 590 and 650 $m\mu$?

16. Explain the terms: hue discrimination and saturation discrimination. Describe a method for measuring the latter capability of the eye and show on a graph how it varies with wavelength.

17. Differentiate between the trichromatic coefficient curves and the so-called fundamental sensation curves. Explain what each of these sets of curves is intended to express and the units used in plotting them.

18. Write a short essay on the so-called fundamental sensation curves, making clear their meaning and their significance in connection with visual theory.

19. Explain the importance, when investigating the various capabilities of the eye, of careful control of the intensity, wavelength, size and duration of the stimulus, of the region of the retina stimulated and of the state of adaptation of the eye.

20. Explain briefly the Young-Helmholtz theory of vision. What is a colour equation ? What is a colour triangle ? Give an example to show the connection between these. (B.O.A.)

21. Give a brief account of the symptoms of the condition called night blindness. Draw dark adaptation curves for a normal person, a severe case of night blindness and a mild case of night blindness. Assume that in all three cases the pre-adaptation level was high. What indication do the curves give as to a possible contributory cause of night blindness ?

22. What is the most characteristic way in which the vision of the colour defective person differs from the normal person ? Why is the colour defective often unaware of his defect ? What precautions must be observed in testing colour defectives ?

23. Give a classification of colour vision anomalies and describe briefly, with the aid of appropriate graphs, the characteristics of the vision of each class.

24. Differentiate between dichromatic and anomalous trichromatic vision. How does the spectrum appear to each of these classes? What is meant by the neutral point and where in the spectrum does it appear?

25. Show on a diagram the hue discrimination curves of (*a*) a normal person, (*b*) a dichromat, (*c*) an anomalous trichromat. With the aid of these curves discuss the difficulties experienced by (*b*) and (*c*) in distinguishing certain colours from one another.

26. Describe how the spectrum as seen by (*a*) the protanomalous and (*b*) the deuteranomalous person differs from the spectrum as seen by the normal person. What test can be used to distinguish between (*a*) and (*b*) cases? Give a diagram showing the luminosity curves for these two types of colour defective.

27. Explain the essential differences between normal and defective colour vision. Describe three types of test that can be used to distinguish the normal from the defective observer. (B.O.A.)

28. Give an account of the experimental factors underlying the Young-Helmholtz theory of colour vision. How are they applied to the specification of a colour on the trichromatic system? (B.O.A.)

29. Give an account of the experimental work underlying Weber's law as it applies to vision. Under what conditions does the law break down? To what extent does visual acuity depend on brightness discrimination? (B.O.A.)

30. What do you know concerning visual thresholds for light and colour (*a*) for large areas, (*b*) for small areas?

What flux of light enters an eye whose entrance pupil diameter is 8 mm. from a source of area one square millimetre with a brightness of one candle per square centimetre and placed ten metres away? (S.M.C.)

31. Write an essay on the classification of colour vision tests. (S.M.C.)

32. Describe the requirements that should be met by a satisfactory colour vision test. Explain the basis upon which confusion chart tests (or pseudo-isochromatic charts) and wool tests are constructed. Describe briefly one other type of test which is considered to be more comprehensive than these.

33. Enunciate Fechner's Law of sensation and describe any group of experiments on light difference sensitivity which aims at testing the law over a wide range of intensity. Give a rough graph to indicate the variation of the Fechner fraction with intensity. (S.M.C.)

34. Write an account of the influence of time, size and brightness factors on the recognition of illuminated areas (rough values at least of the magnitudes should be given). Apply the information to discuss visibility of light signals and of faintly visible objects at night time. (S.M.C.)

35. Distinguish between visibility of point sources of light, contact setting of discs and the resolving power of the eye. What physical and physiological factors influence visibility and acuity? (S.M.C.)

36. Write an essay on the adaptation of the eye to darkness and to light, including an account of the thresholds of vision for light and colour. Has the information any clinical or practical value ? (S.M.C.)

37. Give an account of the chief phenomena associated with normal colour vision. Comment briefly on their possible theoretical explanation. (B.O.A.)

38. Give an account of the phenomena associated with defective colour perception, indicating the relation between the vision of normal trichromats, anomalous trichromats, dichromats and monochromats. (B.O.A.)

39. Compare and contrast foveal vision and peripheral vision. (B.O.A.)

40. In what way does the sensitivity of the retina vary over its surface ? Describe experiments to illustrate your answer. (B.O.A.)

41. Describe the chief peculiarities and difficulties of vision of those commonly described as " red-green colour blind " and comment on the appropriateness of that description.

Explain the meanings of the terms " deuteranopia " and " deuter anomaly ". (B.O.A.)

42. What do you understand by complementary colours ? Why, on current theories, is there no spectral complementary to pure green ? Explain why a red-green colour blind subject sees a colourless region in the spectrum. (B.O.A.)

43. Give an account of the method of determining the sensation produced by various spectral colours in terms of the three primary colours or matching stimuli. Make a sketch of a form of the necessary apparatus. How do you account for the existence of complementary colours ?

44. Give a description of the type of instrument employed for measuring the limits of the field of vision and for accurately locating blind areas within the field. What difficulties are experienced in making these measurements ? Can you suggest any alterations in the design of most instruments of this type which would overcome the difficulties ?

45. Describe (*a*) a perimeter and (*b*) a keratometer, giving reasons for the selection of the forms you describe. Explain briefly their uses and importance in eye examinations. (B.O.A.)

46. Write a short essay on glare. (B.O.A.)

CHAPTER XXII

PHYSICO-PHYSIOLOGICAL PROCESSES

22.1. Changes in the Retina on Stimulation.

The previous few chapters have been concerned with facts and experimental observations concerning the relationships between the physical stimulus and the sensation that ultimately arises in consciousness. No *explanation* of such relationships is possible until the intermediate physiological stage* of the visual process is thoroughly understood; until we can say what it is that happens in and behind the retina when it is stimulated by light. It is not surprising, therefore, that great efforts have been made to penetrate the secrets of the physico-physiological exchanges that occur; to find out how radiant energy is converted into neural energy, to discover any evidences there may be of the triple response system to which reference has been made in earlier chapters†; or, failing this, to determine what *is* the nature of the mechanism that enables us to appreciate light and colour.

The problem is partly a chemical or physico-chemical one and partly electrical, for there is little doubt that an initial photo-chemical action in the retina is the trigger, as it were, which starts the discharge of electrical action currents or impulses along the nerve fibres. Just how the impulses arise from the chemical action we do not yet know.

Early investigations into the chemistry of the process commenced by SCHULTZE (1866) and KÜHNE (1878), have been continued by many workers up to the recent researches of LYTHGOE (visual purple) and in the electro-physiological field by GRANIT (retinal potentials), ADRIAN, HECHT and HARTLINE (nerve impulses) and others. Research in this field is difficult since the structures concerned are so delicate and the effects to be measured are so very small.

Of all the radiant energy that falls on the eye, the infra-red and ultra-violet ranges have frequencies which correspond respectively with the periodicities of the atoms and

* §§ 1.2 and 1.7. † §§ 1.7, 19.3, 19.7 and 21.10.

sub-atomic particles of the various ocular media and so are absorbed by these tissues* and may, if of sufficient intensity and duration, produce thermal and chemical (abiotic) lesions in them. It is not with these radiations and their effects that we are here concerned, but with the radiations lying within the visible spectrum (light) and which are responsible for visual sensations. This light disturbs the equilibrium of the retina by causing structural, chemical and electrical changes in it.

Most of the information that has been gradually obtained is the result of experiments on fishes, birds, insects and animals and must be used with appropriate caution when applying it to or comparing it with the subjective visual sensations of human beings. The effects observed in, say, frogs and cold-blooded animals may not be observed or may be observed to a different extent in mammals; the eyes of vertebrates are more highly developed than those of invertebrates; some eyes, e.g. the cat's, contain chiefly rods whereas others, e.g. the snake, are mainly cone eyes and others, like our own, are "mixed".

STRUCTURAL CHANGES

When the eyes of frogs, fishes, birds and certain reptiles are exposed to light there is a movement inwards of pigment from the retinal pigment epithelium; at the same time there occurs an elongation of the rods and a contraction of the cones, so that the pigment envelops the rods and the outer tips of the cones. Reverse movements occur when the eye is dark-adapted; the pigment slowly returns to the cells of the epithelium, the rods contract and the cones elongate so that only the outer tips of the rods as well as of the cones extend into the pigment. These phenomena have not been observed in man nor generally in mammals; their significance is not clear.

22.2. Chemical Changes.

The most important chemical change occuring in the retina when it is stimulated by light appears to be the bleaching of the VISUAL PURPLE.† This important substance (sometimes called rhodopsin) absorbs light selectively so that it is purple or pink in colour. Its chemical nature is a protein with attached chromophore groups of carotenoid

---

* §17.8. † §20.7.

substances related to vitamin A; it is to the absorption by these substances that it owes its colour. By chemical operations visual purple has been extracted from the rods of several creatures, particularly from frogs, and the action of light on it has been most carefully studied; it is said to be found also in the rods of the higher animals. It is found that, after a latent period, the incident light is rapidly absorbed, the attached coloured molecules being destroyed or radically altered in the process. This bleaching corresponds very closely with the quantity of radiation absorbed when this is expressed in energy units, e.g. quanta.* The amount of absorption, and therefore of bleaching, varies with wavelength in the manner illustrated (by the full line curve) in Fig. 22.1. This absorption curve is found to bear a striking resemblance to the human scotopic

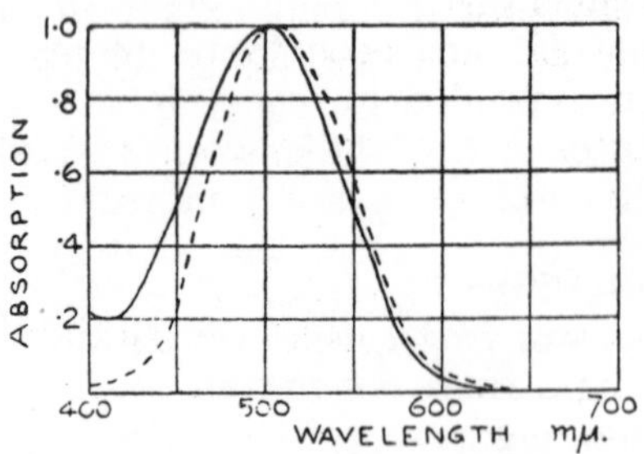

Fig. 22.1—Absorption by Visual Purple. Full Line, Visual Purple; Broken Line, Scotopic Luminosity Curve.

(rod) luminosity curve—curve S in Fig. 20.6 and the broken line curve in Fig. 22.1—except possibly, for reasons not yet fully explained, at the far violet end of the spectrum. Its maximum falls at about λ 504, which is practically coincident with the maximum of the scotopic luminosity curve when this has been corrected for quantum considerations.†

The quantity of energy absorbed in producing the effects is also found to agree with that required subjectively to produce the light threshold (§21.2). When experiments are carried out on complete animal eyes so that contact is maintained with the pigment epithelium and hence to the supply of fresh raw material to complete the physiological cycle, the removal of the stimulating light is followed by a

* §17.3. † §18.10.

process of regeneration, slower than the bleaching process; just as the recovery of sensitivity in dark-adaptation is a slower process than adaptation to light. Indeed all the evidence accumulated points to the fundamental character of the photo-chemical properties of visual purple.

There is recent evidence that the bleaching of visual purple by light sets free a number of intermediate coloured products the first of which is orange-coloured and has been called "transient orange"; this quickly decomposes to "indicator yellow" and then gradually to "visual white". These breakdown processes have, however, not yet been elucidated. A substance which has been called retinine has also been obtained from the chemical breakdown of visual purple; the relation between retinine and indicator yellow is not clear, though it has been suggested that they are the same substance.

Visual purple has not been found in any cones. Much effort has been expended in trying to find in the cones of various creatures some substance with an absorption curve bearing the same kind of correlation with the photopic luminosity curve as that already found to exist between the absorption of visual purple and the scotopic luminosity curve; even, maybe, substances which would reveal properties showing some connection with the colour perception mechanism. Some light-sensitive substances have indeed been found in different retinæ; substances with absorption curves having maxima at different wavelengths in the region 520–545 $m\mu$ have been extracted from the retinæ of sea fishes. WALD (1937) has isolated a substance which he calls iodopsin from the chicken, which has a cone retina; the maximum occurs at λ 575. These substances have not yet been sufficiently analysed for a claim to be made that we know anything very reliable about the photo-chemical system of the cones, but it is quite possible that a substance or substances with the necessary properties will be discovered in the cones, or that the above-mentioned breakdown products of visual purple will have properties suitable for cone, including colour, vision. GRANIT has found differences between the scotopic and photopic curves of certain fishes and the corresponding curves of the eel and a similar difference between their retinal substances; which lends support to the view that the cone (photopic) substances are related to the rod (scotopic) substances, and that they may indeed be transformed from one to the other.

22.3. Electrical Changes. Electro-physiology.

It has been known for a long time that electrical changes accompany, indeed are almost certainly initiated by, the chemical changes just described; that is, the breakdown of the visual purple in the rod mechanism, and of some light-sensitive substance or substances in the cone mechanism, immediately disturb the electrical equilibrium of the retina and initiate trains of electrical impulses which travel inwards across the neurones of the retina and thence along the optic nerve fibres to the brain. These electrical actions are very minute and their investigation has been made possible only comparatively recently by the use of amplifiers and delicate recording instruments such as the string galvanometer of EINTHOVEN and the oscillograph. It is now possible to isolate a single nerve fibre and measure and record the electrical changes that arise in it when it is disturbed. Indeed it has become essential to operate on single fibres because the latest work has shown that there are different kinds of fibres which behave in different ways under a given set of conditions; and there is little chance of resolving the complexities of the electrical events except by dealing with individual fibres. All the information we receive about the outside world through our visual sense derives from these electrical impulses passing to the brain.

A. Changes in the Retina

Between the cornea and the posterior pole of an eye, or the cornea and the severed optic nerve of a still surviving excised eye, there is a potential difference of a few millivolts, depending upon the animal; the pole or optic nerve is negative with respect to the cornea. There is a similar P.D. between the rod-cone layer and the nerve-fibre layer of the retina, the rod-cone layer being negative. If, with the eye in the dark, one electrode of the recording apparatus is applied to the cornea and the other electrode to the optic nerve, a steady " current of rest " is indicated by the instrument, flowing in the direction: cornea—instrument —optic nerve—cornea. If now a flash of light is directed into the eye there is at first a latent period lasting up to 0·05 second, being shorter as the intensity of the stimulating light is greater; then a small negative change in the current, i.e. in the opposite direction to the current of rest; this is shown at *a*, Fig. 22.2. This negative dip is followed by a much larger positive change which rises rapidly to a maximum at *b*, called the *b* wave; and then, maybe with some fluctuations, the current begins to subside to a steady value or a steadily rising value, *c*, for the duration of the stimulation. In some cases, immediately after removal of the stimulation a further abrupt positive rise, *d*, occurs before the current finally subsides to its original rest value; this is the off-effect. The sequence of events, illustrated in Fig. 22.2, should be compared with Fig. 20.2 depicting the growth and decay of sensation.

The experiment has been performed in various ways, sometimes without removing the eye, and although the results do not agree in every detail, there can be no doubt that the sequence of events is due to activity in the retina following its stimulation by light. It has been shown that

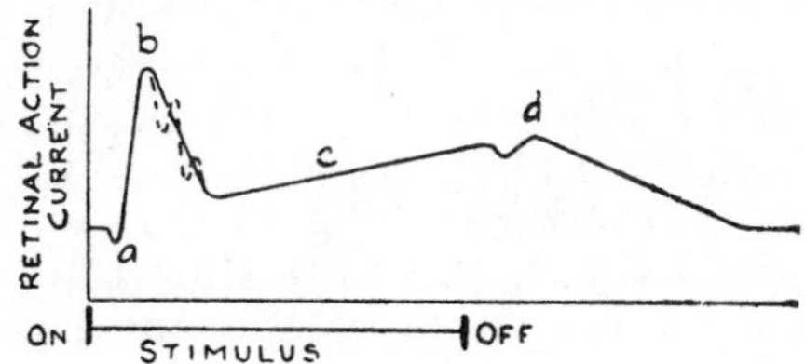

FIG. 22.2—RETINAL ACTION CURRENT PRODUCED BY LIGHT. THE ELECTRORETINOGRAM (E.R.G.).

the *magnitude* of these action currents varies with the wavelength of the light in the same way that the response of a photographic plate varies with wavelength (§17.8); the same *kind* of effect is produced by all wavelengths. There seems to be no differentiation here to account for the quality or colour variation of our sensations.

When the eye under test is kept in the dark the maximum response is produced by green light at λ 505 or so and in the light-adapted eye by yellow light around λ 560, which correspond to the scotopic and photopic luminosity curves and the Purkinje effect. It will be observed that the latent period is somewhat shorter than the latent period for sensation to develop (§20.3); the time to reach the initial positive maximum current at b, Fig. 22.2, is also somewhat shorter than the time needed for the primary image of sensation to reach its maximum, M_1 or M_2 of Fig. 20.2. It is found that the minimum quantity of energy needed to produce the action current also agrees with that necessary to initiate a sensation (§21.2). Thus there are undoubted resemblances between the electrical activity in the stimulated retina and the development of sensation in the human eye.

Again, when the eye under test is subjected to intermittent light stimuli, the electro-retinogram, or E.R.G., as the curve of Fig. 22.2 is sometimes called, exhibits a series of undulations corresponding in frequency with the frequency of the stimuli; and when the latter frequency is raised beyond a certain point, the undulations are smoothed out; results which correspond with the subjective sensation of flicker and its critical frequency (§20.11).

Further progress has been made recently by GRANIT (1936) who has shown that the retinal action-potential curve of Fig. 22.2 can be analysed into three components two of which are positive and one negative, representing an inhibitory reaction. That is to say, this negative component shows that one effect of stimulation by light may be not to elicit excitation but to inhibit it—to prevent the discharge of impulses along the optic nerve. This is a most significant discovery in relation to the phenomena of induction. This negative component has been found to be more marked in cone retinæ (pigeon, light-adapted frog) than in rod retinæ (rat, cat). He has also recorded the spectral sensitivity of individual elements in various retinæ and finds different cones responding maximally to widely different wavelengths. Whilst, in the frog's retina, most of the elements have a sensitivity with a maximum at 560 $m\mu$, there are three other groups with maxima around 580–600 $m\mu$, 520–540 $m\mu$ and 450–470 $m\mu$; which are most suggestive results from the point of view of a triple response system. GRANIT suggests that the majority of the elements, with maximum sensitivity at λ 560, are concerned with the sensation of luminosity and he calls them *dominators*; the other three groups, not so numerous, he calls *modulators* since he considers that their function is to modulate the response in some way to give the sensation of colour.

B. CHANGES IN THE OPTIC NERVE. OPTIC NERVE CURRENTS.

The rapid rise of the *b* wave of the retinal action current is accompanied by the discharge of a train of electrical impulses along the optic nerve fibres. Investigation into nerve currents of this kind was initiated by ADRIAN and his colleagues in 1926 and has been continued, with particular reference to the nerves subserving the sense of vision in various creatures, by HARTLINE in America.

The arrangement of the type of apparatus employed is suggested diagrammatically in Fig. 22.3. The eye of the particular creature being investigated, with a centimetre or more of nerve attached, is mounted in a moist chamber which is so supported that it can be moved with precision in the vertical and two horizontal directions. In this way it can be carefully positioned in relation to the optical system which focuses the stimulating light on the eye. This system includes a shutter and variable diaphragm

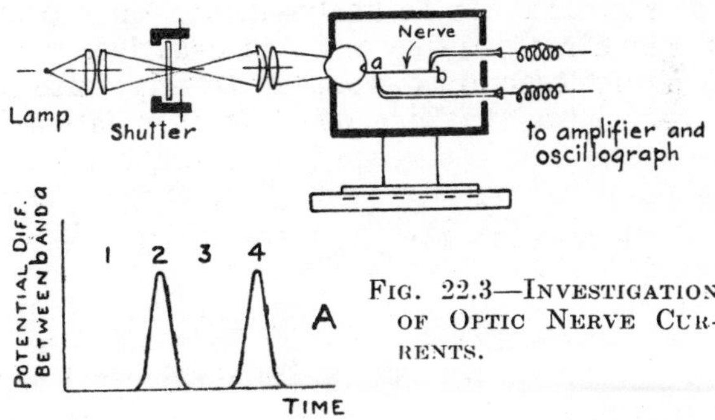

FIG. 22.3—INVESTIGATION OF OPTIC NERVE CURRENTS.

so that the duration, size and intensity of the stimulus can be controlled. Applied to the nerve at *a* and *b* are two non-polarizable electrodes which are connected to an amplifier and thence to an oscillograph which records the changes of electrical potential in the fibre between a and b. The amplification can be made sufficient for the impulses to work a loud speaker or a recording pen if required.

In an unstimulated condition of rest there is a steady P.D. between a and b and the instrument records an undisturbed straight line. On stimulating the fibre, as by illuminating the eye and so starting off the chemical and electrical reactions in the retina already described, a train of impulses begins to travel along it, after a latent period of about 0·1 second. When the first impulse passes over the point a, this point becomes momentarily electrically negative in relation to point b. The instrument records a jump as at 2 in diagram A. This pulse of electro-negativity passes on towards b and the oscillograph reading returns to the original value, as at 3. Presently the second impulse of the train reaches a and a second jump 4 is recorded; and so on.

The duration of these individual jumps is of the order of one or two thousandths of a second and so they appear as short vertical lines or spikes on the oscillogram. Hence the appearance of the latter during a period of steady illumination of the eye is as shown at A, Fig. 22.4. With

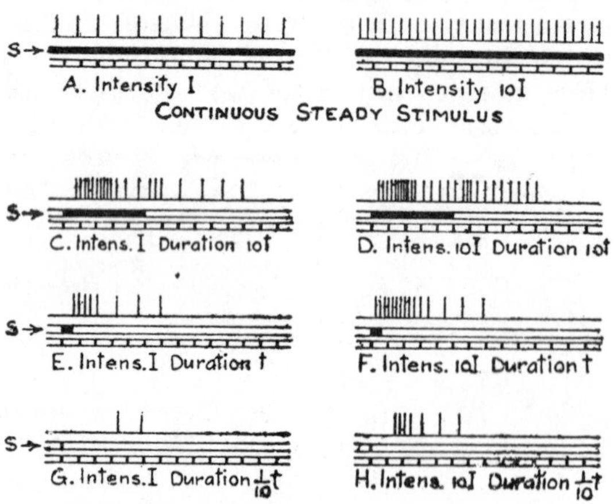

FIG. 22.4—TYPICAL OSCILLOGRAMS SHOWING ACTION CURRENTS IN A SINGLE FIBRE AT DIFFERENT STIMULUS INTENSITIES AND DURATIONS. TIME MARKED OFF IN $\frac{1}{5}$ SECONDS AT BASE OF EACH DIAGRAM. DURATION OF STIMULUS SHOWN IN SPACE S.

a steady stimulus of higher intensity the record will appear as at B; in this, it is to be noted, the spikes are of the same height as before, but their frequency (the number of spikes per second) has increased. This is in conformity with the all-or-none law described in §1.4.

If the wavelength of the stimulating light is changed, the result is of just the same character; the same kind of spikes are obtained in the oscillogram and their frequency will be just the same for one wavelength as another when the intensities are suitably adjusted. There is no qualitative difference between the two trains of impulses, so that here again there is no evidence of the manner in which we are able to discriminate one hue from another.

When, with the eye and fibre at rest, the stimulating light is first admitted to the eye, there commences, after the latent period mentioned, a rapid sequence of events which is of the type represented graphically in Fig. 22.5 and which corresponds very closely with the rise and fall of sensation experienced by humans, discussed in §20.3 and Fig. 20.2. Following the latent period there is a rush of impulses which rapidly attain a maximum frequency; the frequency then falls, sharply at first, and subsides to a steady value so long as the stimulation continues with its starting intensity. Immediately after the light is cut off there is a short period of decline and then a renewed positive effect; i.e. another rush of impulses, the "off-effect", which fairly rapidly declines to zero. The actual shape of the curve depends upon the stimulus intensity and adaptation of the eye, etc. The corresponding oscillogram is shown beneath the graph.

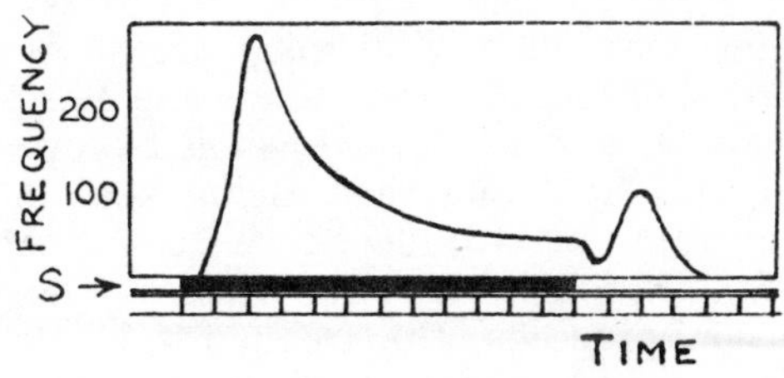

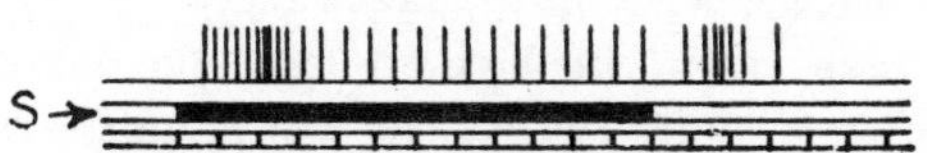

FIG. 22.5—FREQUENCY OF IMPULSES IN CURRENT IN OPTIC NERVE OF CONGER EEL (FROM ADRIAN). BELOW: CORRESPONDING OSCILLOGRAM. DURATION OF STIMULUS SHOWN IN SPACE S; TIME MARKED OFF IN $\frac{1}{5}$ SECONDS, AT BASE OF EACH DIAGRAM.

The diagrams C to H of Fig. 22.4 are typical of the oscillograms obtained from a single fibre of the primitive eye of such a specimen as the King Crab (limulus polyphemus) under different conditions of stimulus intensity and duration. A study of these diagrams reveals, in addition to the characteristics already mentioned, that the frequency of the impulses increases with the intensity though not in the same proportion; roughly, the frequency varies with the logarithm of the intensity; also that (for stimuli of short duration) the intensity and duration are inter-dependent, the effect depending upon the total quantity of light. Thus diagrams C and F are similar; so are E and H. Note that when the stimulus is a flash of very short duration, as in G and H, the sequence of events in the fibre does not commence until the flash has ended.

It is also the case, in vertebrate retinæ, that the intensity and area of stimulation are, within certain limits of area, similarly interconnected, showing that processes initiated in a localised area spread to adjacent areas. The latent period shortens with an increase either of intensity or of area.

The range of stimulus intensity over which a fibre will conduct impulses is found to be of the same order as that to which the human eye responds (§§ 20.7, 21.2). The energy needed to produce a threshold effect in a fibre is of the same order as that requred to arouse sensation; different fibres may have different thresholds, however, especially as between rod fibres and cone fibres.

If the eye under test is first subjected to a pre-adapting stimulus of bright light and then, being kept in the dark, is exposed at intervals to successive stimuli of constant intensity and duration, it is found that as the process of dark adaptation proceeds, the frequency of the impulses in the fibre continuously increases; i.e. the electrical response increases with dark adaptation as the sensational response increases in the human eye (§20.7).

Thus we see that there are very close resemblances between the electrical response to stimulation in the retina and optic nerve fibres of many species and the sensational response to stimulation in the human visual mechanism; the electroretinogram and the oscillogram exhibit the same features as the curve illustrating the growth and decay of visual sensation. Useful as this information is in providing us with clues concerning the manner in which the physiological sources of sensation begin to develop, it contains little evidence as to how *colour* vision arises. In the above account the only references that may have a bearing on this important and difficult problem are those relating to the breakdown products of visual purple; the discovery of certain light-sensitive substances in cone retinæ; and of groups of cones in the frog's retina possessing different absorption maxima (GRANIT'S modulators).

Strenuous attempts are being made to improve electro-physiological technique so that these clues concerning colour vision can be further analysed.

Although the sequence of events illustrated by Fig. 22.5 is initiated by the commencing of the photo-chemical decomposition process in the retina, this latter process is too slow to account for the shape of the curve, which is probably due largely to the combination of excitation and inhibition mentioned in §22.3A.

It is probable that complex events occur within the body of a nerve fibre during the building up of the conditions necessary for the discharge of impulses along it. Further refinements in the experimental technique may elucidate these fundamental nerve processes.

22.4. Nerve Fibres in the Vertebrate Eye.

" On " and " Off " Fibres

A most interesting field for speculation has been opened up by recent electrical investigations on the above lines* on individual fibres of vertebrates such as the frog; for it is revealed that there are surprising differences of behaviour in different fibres of the same eye. Some fibres show the type of response described above for the more primitive eye of *Limulus*. Others give a short burst of impulses when first exposed to the stimulus and another short burst when the light is switched off but give no response during the intervening period of steady illumination; these may be called " on-and-off " fibres—about half of the total fibres are of this kind. More surprising is the type of fibre that remains quiescent when the light is switched on and while it continues to stimulate the eye, and then gives a brisk discharge of impulses when the stimulus is removed; these are " off-fibres ".

The on-and-off fibres respond in the manner described not only when the stimulation is switched on and then off completely, but also when it is increased or decreased or when a spot of light, or a shadow, is moved across the retina. It may be that these fibres are specially concerned with intensity discrimination.

The character and extent of the " off " effect depends upon the properties of the stimulus and the condition of the eye. It is obtained only with a fairly intense stimulus;

* By Hartline and by Granit, using different techniques.

it rises more abruptly and reaches a higher magnitude as the duration of previous exposure is lengthened. In eyes previously light-adapted it is large and fast; with previous dark-adaptation it is small. The retina thus appears to have developed a mechanism for discharging impulses when a stimulus ceases; the effect arises only after previous stimulation—there is no question of a response to absence of stimulation, or darkness. The off-effect would appear to have a connection with the after-images described in §20.6.

Apparently the off-fibres are not found in primitive eyes such as that of *Limulus*, in which there is direct connection between the fibres and the percipient elements; but only in eyes which contain a more or less complicated system of nervous connections, corresponding to the bipolar and ganglion cells in our own eyes. It appears, therefore, that the bipolars are not just simple relay stations, but that they mediate complex processes. These variations of behaviour in " on " and " off " fibres occur whatever may be the wavelength of the stimulus; they do not provide a basis for explaining the mechanism of colour vision.

Receptive Field of a Nerve Fibre

By manipulating the optical system of the apparatus illustrated in Fig. 22.3 the area of stimulation on the retina can be varied and made to cover a large area or a small spot. By using the latter it is possible to explore the extent of the retina that is effective in exciting the individual fibre, i.e. the receptive field of the fibre. In vertebrate eyes this field has a definite location and may extend up to 1 mm. in diameter, or larger than this with very high stimulus intensities. In the central part of the receptive field of a given fibre the stimulus intensity needed to produce a discharge in the fibre is less than in peripheral portions of the field; and when the whole receptive field is stimulated the effects add together, the final result depending upon the total quantity of light falling on the field. It is found that the receptive fields of different fibres may overlap one another.

Here is unmistakable evidence of the lateral interconnection between retinal receptors, referred to in §1.5. It appears that not only are large numbers of rods or cones (except within the fovea) connected to one fibre, but a given receptor element, though more closely connected to one certain fibre, may be connected to several; thus relatively large areas of the synaptic layers of the retina may operate together as a whole.

Inter-action can occur between areas that are not adjacent to one another in the retina; unstimulated elements may be left between them.

How is this inter-connection between adjacent, and separated, areas of the retina to be reconciled with the ability of the eye to distinguish fine detail? This latter capability would seem to require a distinct separation between different receptors and yet the evidence of inter-action between them is unmistakable. This is one of many questions concerning the visual processes to which there is at present no answer.

CHAPTER XXII. *EXERCISES.*

1. Give a general account of the structural, chemical and electrical changes that occur in the retina of various species when stimulated by light.

2. Describe the resemblances that have been found between (*a*) the chemical and (*b*) the electrical changes that occur in the retinæ of various creatures and the subjective response of the human eye to light. Give appropriate curves.

3. Describe what is believed to be the chemical nature of visual purple. Give an account of the action on it of light and the resemblance between such action and human scotopic vision.

4. Show on a diagram the curve, sometimes called the electro-retinogram or E.R.G., which illustrates the electrical events that occur in certain retinæ when stimulated by light. Discuss this curve and the ways in which it shows resemblances to the sensational response of the human visual mechanism to light.

5. Give a brief account of the results of investigations into optic nerve currents with a sketch of the kind of apparatus used. Give examples of the diagrams (oscillograms) that are obtained from such investigations, for different intensities and durations of the stimulus.

6. What changes are supposed to take place in the retina when it is illuminated? What appearances are observed if two adjacent areas of the retina receive white and coloured light respectively, and what suggestions have been made to account for these appearances? (B.O.A.)

7. Give a detailed account of the probable changes which occur in the retina under the influence of light. (B.O.A.)

8. Give an account of the photo-chemistry of the retina as understood at the present time. To what extent are both the rods and cones capable of light and dark adaptation? (B.O.A.)

9. It is commonly stated that the eye is similar to the camera. Discuss this statement, showing in what important respects the eye differs from the camera. (B.O.A.)

10. Give a summary of the main results that have been obtained from investigations into the electrical events occurring in the light-stimulated retinæ of various creatures. Have any results been obtained which might be related to human vision with respect to (*a*) induction effects and (*b*) colour vision ?

11. Electrical investigations on nerve fibres of the frog's eye have shown that different kinds of effects are revealed by different fibres. Give a description of these effects and of any significance they may have.

12. Write a short account of the following:
(*a*) the receptive field of a nerve fibre ;
(*b*) differences between the cat's retina and the pigeon's retina ;
(*c*) differences between the eyes of the crab and the frog.

13. Describe what happens in a sensory nerve when the appropriate end-organ is stimulated. (B.O.A.)

14. What manifest changes occur in the retina under the action of light ? Describe the relations between the reaction of the visual purple, the electrical currents in the optic nerve and the visual sensation. How do the experimental results on optic nerve currents support the all-or-none theory of nerve impulse ?

CHAPTER XXIII

THEORIES OF VISION. PERCEPTION.

23.1. Theories.

The preceding chapters have dealt with a selection of the experimental observations that have been made over the years by many investigators; observations concerning the relationships found to exist between light stimulus and visual sensation and also about the intermediate physico-physiological processes that occur in the retina and in the nervous connections leading from the retina. These observations have been gradually accumulated by experiment and reasoning with the object of increasing our knowledge of visual processes and thus contributing to our ability to control the environment in which we find ourselves. Some of the observations have been repeated by very many individuals and are accepted as true experiences common to all normal persons; such are called *facts*. Others, however, are not sufficiently well substantiated to be accepted as facts; they may have been observed in good faith by a certain scientist but are meanwhile considered as no more than provisional. It may be that other scientists are not quite satisfied with the conditions under which the experiment was conducted or that the observations are contradictory to others on the same subject, and so on. Not until the same results have been experienced by a substantial number of normal individuals can they be accepted as facts. They may ultimately prove to be true facts or they may be disproved, or at least qualified.

Even those observations which prove to be facts are not of much use until they are gathered together, classified and brought into relationship with one another and with the general body of knowledge; i.e. until they are correlated. It is not until this has been done, especially, where possible, in the form of mathematical equations or graphs, that the significance of the facts, or a group of them, can be properly appreciated; it is not until this stage has been reached that we can say that the facts have been "explained"; so that we can decide more clearly what are the next steps to be taken in order to probe the subject further. It is this process of classification and correlation that constitutes the formulation of a theory. A theory should "explain", i.e. should be reconcilable with, the facts already established and should point the way towards further advancement. If it does so it is a good, a useful, theory at the particular time, even though it may be extended or modified or even rejected as further facts are acquired. There is no finality in any theory. So long as the known facts, and new facts as they are established, fit in with the theory, we are able to say that the phenomena concerned are understood, are explained by the theory.

Sometimes progress is made by proposing a hypothesis, which is merely a supposition made perhaps without reference to any facts, to see what consequences will follow from it. If the hypothesis has been made by someone with the qualities of inventiveness and resource, the consequences inferred from it may be found to agree with many of the known facts. In that case it is a good hypothesis and may, after certain corrections, be developed into a theory.

23.2. The Main Problem. Colour Vision.

The student, reviewing the foregoing chapters and his knowledge of the anatomy and physiology of the eye, will agree that many of the observations described are sufficiently well founded to be acceptable as facts and that these provide us with a good general picture of the manner in which the eyes function. It should be mentioned in passing, however, that in some cases the general acceptance of the observations as facts rests on indirect evidence only; and that in these, or in other cases, there are people who dissent from the general belief.

For example: it has never been directly proved that the rods and cones are the receptor or percipient elements where the physical energy of the light beam is transformed into energy of a type that can be conducted along nerve fibres; but our belief that the rods and cones *are* the site of this energy exchange rests on a most imposing array of indirect evidence. Again, although there is an overwhelming body of factual evidence in support of the duplicity theory concerning the rod and cone duplex mechanisms in the retina, the theory will probably have to be modified or extended before all observed facts can be reconciled with it.

There are certain characteristics of vision, well established by repeated observations, for which we have as yet no adequate explanation ; to account for which no-one has succeeded in formulating a satisfactory theory. It is not clear, for example, just why visual acuity improves with increase of illumination on the target and on the surrounding field, even when an artificial pupil is used ; nor is it an easy matter to explain the high performance of the eye in the discrimination of detail and contours in view of the fact that it is in continual movement, even when the gaze is concentrated as steadily as possible on one particular point ; added to which are the defects of the retinal image caused by diffraction and aberrations of the optical system. Many phenomena associated with adaptation, temporal and spatial induction, after-images, flicker, etc., though well established by repeated observations, are incapable of satisfactory explanation at the present time. Indeed there are few functions concerned with vision (and this probably applies to other senses) about which we can claim to be reasonably clear. Consider the accommodation of the eye, which is a fundamental act of vision : if a distant object is presented to an emmetropic eye it is seen clearly ; if a negative lens is placed before the eye, the latter immediately accommodates ; and when the lens is removed the eye relaxes at once. If a positive lens is placed before the eye, it makes no attempt to change its refractive state. Why ? The image is blurred just as much in the second case as in the first. The pencils of light reaching the retina are convergent in the first case and divergent in the second, but how does the brain know that ? The discussion can be carried further, but it is very difficult, if not impossible at present, to give a satisfactory explanation.

When attempts are made to probe more deeply into these phenomena—and research is continuous in many parts of the world—it is usually found that further progress cannot be made until more information is obtained about the photo-chemical and electrical events occuring in the retina ; about visual purple and its products and the functioning of the rods in relation to that of the cones. And of all the problems associated with these retinal reactions, the most puzzling of all is the problem of colour vision. It is understandable why a pencil of light of wavelength 555 $m\mu$ and intensity I should produce an effect on the retina which differs in magnitude from a pencil of wavelength, say, 650 $m\mu$ of the same intensity so that the two sensations differ markedly in luminosity. Other selective detectors exhibit this kind of spectral variation,* which is due to the relations that exist between the frequencies of the radiations and the natural periodicities of the atoms and sub-atomic particles of which the sensitive receiving surface is composed. But why is it, in the case of the eye, that one sensation has a quality of yellowish-green and the other a quality of red? How does this differentiation in quality of sensation arise?

This problem has fascinated scientists for a very long time and is still the one that engages the most attention, probably because it is generally agreed that it is fundamental and its solution would provide a key with which many of the other difficulties could be removed or considerably simplified.

Innumerable hypotheses and theories of colour vision have been propounded since the time of THOMAS YOUNG. There would be no point in attempting to review them here. They have followed two main lines which may be described respectively as the physical and the psychological. Following the lead of NEWTON, YOUNG and HELMHOLTZ, the physicists base their reasoning on the most striking and fundamental physical fact of colour vision that any colour can be produced by mixing three lights in suitable proportions. They argue that the visual mechanism or that part of it concerned with colour vision must therefore contain, in some form or other, three component response systems which are stimulated in certain relative proportions by any light whatever that impinges on the retina. A general idea of this view will have been gathered by the student from the repeated references to it in previous pages.† It is admitted that there are several well-substantiated facts of colour vision that cannot be reconciled with the YOUNG-HELMHOLTZ three-components theory in the simple form in which it has been usually stated, particularly phenomena concerned with induction and with the dependence of colour perception on the duration and area of the stimulus‡; but these

---

* §§ 17.8 and 18.1. † §§ 19.3, 19.7 and 21.10. ‡ §21.11.

difficulties do not invalidate the main triplicity basis of the theory. It is likely that the three response systems are not completely independent of one another and that the theory will have to be modified or extended in other ways.

To the psychologists, on the other hand, the true facts of colour vision are the sensations themselves, not the physical events leading up to them. They argue with GOETHE, who strenuously opposed the ideas of NEWTON and YOUNG, that the spectrum contains not three but unmistakably *four* " primary " hues: red, yellow, green and blue; the intermediate regions of the spectrum are blends of these. For reasons that emerge in their arguments these four principal hues are subdivided into the two pairs: red-green and yellow-blue. (When we include the achromatic sensations (§19.1) we may say there are six pure or primary sensations: red, yellow, green, blue, black and white.) The psychologists will not admit that the yellow sensation is less " primary " than the others or that it is a mixture of red and green; nor that the simple and primitive sensation of white is a mixture of red, green and blue. They maintain that psychologically such views are completely inadmissible; their approach to the problem is fundamentally different from that of the physicist.

The trichromatic character of colour mixing is, however, as firmly based today as in the early days of the YOUNG-HELMHOLTZ theory and so the psychologists, in general, perforce accept it and try to harmonise it with their conviction of four primary sensations of hue. In doing so they have proposed various modifications such as the subdivision of one or more of the three component systems or, accepting the triplicity as far as the initial stages of the retinal activity are concerned, they introduce subdivision or modulation at a later stage in the visual process.* A theory of this kind was proposed by DONDERS but the most prominent exponent of the psychologists' position has been HERING and no discussion of colour vision would be complete without at least an outline of his theory.

23.3. Colour Vision. Psychological Theories. Hering.

HERING proposed (1876) that there are three mechanisms or substances in the retina or visual pathway which, in common with living tissue generally, are continually

---

* See also §19.3, footnote.

undergoing a two-way process of regeneration or assimilation (A effect) in one direction and of breakdown or dissimilation (B effect) in the other direction. The three substances are the white-black, the yellow-blue and the red-green; the first deals with achromatic and the other two with chromatic sensations. In the absence of any stimulation the two opposing metabolic changes autonomously neutralise

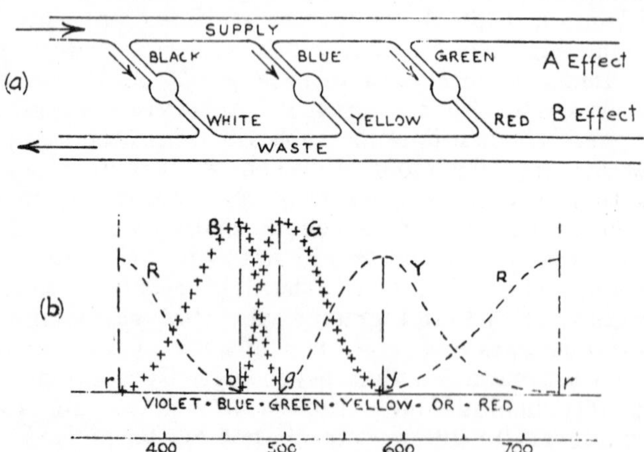

FIG. 23.1—ILLUSTRATING HERING'S THEORY OF COLOUR VISION. THE CURVES SHOW HOW THE THREE SUPPOSED SUBSTANCES ARE AFFECTED BY THE WAVELENGTHS OF THE VISIBLE SPECTRUM: THEY MAY BE CONSIDERED AS SENSATION CURVES ON THIS THEORY.

one another so that each mechanism is in a state of equilibrium; they will always tend towards this state after stimulation ceases. Fig. 23.1 (a) is intended to suggest the arrangement diagrammatically.

When the eye is stimulated by luminous radiation of any wavelength or combination of wavelengths, the red-green and yellow-blue mechanisms are actuated in one direction or the other. The effects of stimulation by the various wavelengths in the spectrum are illustrated in Fig. 23.1 (b), which may be considered as the sensation curves on this theory. The four primary colour sensations suggested by HERING are those evoked by the wavelengths marked r, y, g and b; at each of these points one curve reaches a maximum and two of the others have zero value or nearly so, the sensation being a pure one of red, yellow, green or blue respectively. Except that HERING'S pure red is situated in the red-violet gap (§19.6), these are the physiologically pure colours mentioned in §21.7. The red-green mechanism suffers a breakdown effect under stimulation by the light of the spectral regions ry and br and evokes a red sensation; stimulation by the yb region regenerates it (A effect) and evokes a green sensation. In the yellow-blue mechanism a B effect and a yellow sensation follow stimulation by the rg region and an A effect with blue sensation from the gr region. The white-black mechanism breaks down (B effect) under stimulation by any wavelength and evokes a white sensation; the magnitude of the effect varies with the wavelength, reaching a maximum in the yellow region; the curve representing this effect corresponds to the luminosity curve of §18.1. The reverse (A) effect occurs during the absence of stimulation with an accompanying sensation of darkness.

This opponent-colours theory of HERING'S affords a reasonably satisfactory explanation of induction and after-images, but does not account for some of the facts of defective colour vision, especially anomalous trichromatic vision, and is on the whole less successful than the YOUNG-HELMHOLTZ theory. Of other psychological theories, the one proposed by MRS. LADD-FRANKLING (1892 and later) is in some respects more successful than HERING'S.

No theory, physical or psychological, has so far proved really satisfactory. Recent discoveries, particularly in the photo-chemistry and electro-physiology of the retina, have shown that our knowledge of the visual process is as yet too meagre for theory making; and that the exertions of investigators should be directed to further experiment in the attempt to formulate a common principle to embrace both the physicist's and the psychologist's point of view.

23.4. The Triple Response System.*

Although there are differences between the physicist and psychologist viewpoints, it is generally agreed by all to adopt the hypothesis that, in addition to the duplicity of the rod mechanism and the cone mechanism, there is

---

* An excellent general account of the physicist's view of the problems associated with colour vision and existing knowledge concerning them is to be found in W. D. WRIGHT'S Ettles Memorial Lecture entitled "A Survey of Modern Researches on Colour Vision" and published in *The Refractionist*, Vol. 31, 1942.

also a further sub-division into three component systems of some kind; related, directly or indirectly, with three fundamental response curves.

There is no direct physiological evidence of the existence of these three response systems. Despite the great range of the information we possess about so many physiological and sensory aspects of vision, no one has yet succeeded in discovering three kinds of cones, or a triple structure in individual cones, or three kinds of substances in or around the cones, or three kinds of nerve impulses in the fibres leading from the cones.* But some of the observations described in the last chapter are promising since they have revealed the existence, in the eyes of certain fishes, birds and animals, of different light-sensitive substances in various retinæ, of cones differing from one another in that they respond maximally to widely separated parts of the spectrum and of nerve fibres which differ, not in the type of individual impulse they transmit, but in the manner in which these are transmitted. Though promising, such information is at present too scanty and too disconnected to permit of the laying down of a firm foundation on which to build a satisfactory theory of colour vision.

Let us, however, suppose that (neglecting the rods entirely) three kinds of receptor have been found in the human retina and, further, that they take the form of three different kinds of cone. There would still remain the very difficult problem of discovering how each response is transmitted to the brain, there to give rise to our sensations of luminosity and hue. Do the cones operate in conjunction with one photo-chemical substance or are three substances required? If one, is it the visual purple or some other substance? If three, are these the breakdown products of visual purple or different substances? What is the exact nature of the photo-chemical cycle of breakdown and regeneration? Where, within the exceedingly small volume of the cone, is the substance (or substances) secreted? Both LYTHGOE and GRANIT have suggested that, in the case of the rods, the visual purple might exist on their surfaces. On the other hand, the Stiles-Crawford effect

* The lateral geniculate body contains six laminæ, three of which make connection, through the fibres of the optic tract, with one eye and three with the other eye. It may be significant that a retinal lesion leads to atrophy in all three laminæ related to the eye concerned, as if there exists some kind of triple connection from all parts of the retina; whether this may have any bearing on the triple response system remains indefinite.

(§2.15) would appear to require that a greater photo-chemical action would result if the light travels straight down into the interior of the cone, suggesting that the sensitive substance or substances lie within the cones. Also, the result of the photo-chemical reaction is the production of a train of impulses and these must presumably emerge through the base from the interior of the cone since they are to travel inwards through the retina at the start of their journey to the higher centres. And what is the relationship between the photo-chemical process and the discharge of the electrical impulses ? The former appear to be too slow to account for certain sensory phenomena associated, for example, with the initial stages of adaptation.

Let us suppose further that the above problems have been solved so that we know how the retina, the end-organ of vision, transforms the innumerable wavelengths of the incident light into three forms of nervous energy ready for transmission to the brain. How is this transmission carried out ? Two alternatives seem possible. First, the "red" cones may be supposed to have a straight-through connection to specialised "red" sensation cells in the brain, the "green" cones to "green" cells and the "blue" cones to "blue" cells ; but, considering the great number of cones and all the intervening neurones and nerve tissue in the considerable length of path from retina to brain, such unique connection from individual cone to individual cell would appear to be unbelievable. And in any case, we have much evidence of inter-connection within the retina and of the comparatively large area of receptive field of individual fibres, which cannot be ignored in any theory.

The other alternative is this : does the "red" cone originate a "red" type of impulses in its nerve fibre which differs from the green impulses and blue impulses despatched respectively by the green and blue cones ? In other words, is there difference in quality (specificity) of nerve impulses ?

Recent investigations have failed to reveal any such specificity in nerve currents. MÜLLER'S law of specific nerve energies still appears to stand ; the individual impulses appear to be of the same character in all nerve fibres whatever sense they subserve ; they do not appear to be specific. It is true that when the impulses are derived from the eye, we see ; when they are derived from the ear, we hear ; but the distinction is due to the end-organ and the brain. The sensations are specific because the optic nerve fibres and the auditory nerve fibres lead to different areas of the brain. The end-organs, the eye and the ear, are specific since they select the particular kind of stimulus to which they will respond—electro-magnetic waves in the one case and sound waves in the other. Electro-physiological research has so far shown that when light of wavelength, say, 650 $m\mu$ enters the light-adapted eye in such intensity that the electro-retinogram is equal in magnitude to that obtained with light of wavelength, say, 555 $m\mu$ at some lower intensity, the two electroretinograms are equal in every other respect; they exhibit no difference between one wavelength and the other.

Thus neither of the two alternatives would appear to be acceptable. It is the case, however, that the optic nerve fibres have been shown to vary in diameter; and in certain nerve fibres serving muscles and other senses it is known that fibres of larger diameter transmit bigger impulses.* But as to whether it may be found possible to associate fibres of different diameters with different wavelengths in the spectrum there is no information.

Thus we see that, even making the large assumption that there are three kinds of cone, the difficulties in the way of formulating a satisfactory theory are still formidable. A great deal of patient and highly technical experimental work still remains to be done. And if these difficulties are overcome so that we obtain a reasonably clear picture of the manner in which our assumed triple-cone retina and the brain operate together in evoking colour sensations, the picture must be correlated with the many well-founded subjective facts of vision described in Chapters XX and XXI. Belief in the existence of some kind of triple response system is based mainly upon the one important fact that any colour sensation can be produced by mixing three coloured lights in suitable proportions; but there are many other sensory phenomena—concerned with after-images, adaptation, spatial induction, regional variations over the retina (e.g. colour fields), visual acuity, defective colour vision, colour vision in small areas, etc.—with which the triple physiological model would have to be reconciled.

As an example consider visual acuity. It has been advanced as a reason against the three-cone hypothesis

---

* W. D. Wright and Ragnar Granit, *On the Correlation of Some Sensory and Physiological Phenomena of Vision*; Monograph published by the British Journal of Ophthalmology, 1938.

that with a retina thus constituted visual acuity could not be so good as we know it to be. "Red" light entering the eye from a "red" object would stimulate only "red" cones and so only a third of the total number of cones would be available for building up the details of the retinal image. This would surely result in a worsening of visual acuity if the retina were immobile like a photographic plate. Because of the continual quivering movements of the eye about the mean fixation position, however, the image is, as it were, being scanned by a vibrating pattern of cones. The sensation must be averaged out of a succession of impressions differing from one another to some extent; so long as the cones are individually small it would not matter if they were fewer in number. If this argument is sound, visual acuity would maintain its known value with the triple-coned retina.

PERCEPTION

23.5. What is Mind?

In §§ 1.2, 1.4 (D) and 20.1 brief references were made to the complex character of the processes called co-ordination and perception whereby the central nervous system of the body makes the necessary adjustments between the incoming messages from the sense organs and the outgoing messages to the muscles and glands to enable the individual to survive and to understand and, in part, to control his environment. Apart from these references the treatment in the book has been restricted to the physical and physiological stages of the visual process; these can be, and are, examined by the methods of physics and physiology. This takes us no further than the production of a complicated pattern of disturbances in the nerve cells of the brain, still at the physiological level; it does not explain the sensation and perception which follow at the higher level of consciousness. Even in Chapters XX and XXI we were not concerned with the *nature* of sensation but only with the relations existing between sensations (which were simple sensations of light and hue) and the physical events or stimuli giving rise to them.

Sensation was defined as a state or a change of consciousness. But what is consciousness? The answer may be made that it is a becoming aware of the conditions of the environment, assumed to have a real existence, through the mediation of the sense organs and their physiological messages; but who or what is it that becomes aware? If it is said to be the mind which becomes aware, or conscious, what is this mind and what is the relationship between it and the brain? To such questions, in spite of continuous controversy amongst great philosophers, there seems to be no answer.*

There has to be some agency to co-ordinate all the impressions received from the organs of the body, first into elementary sensations of hunger, pain, taste, smell, light and colour, etc., and then into perceptual patterns which give unity and meaning to the environment from which the stimuli originated; and that agency is usually called the "mind". If a familiar object, say a red rubber ball, is supported in a homogeneous field by an invisible support and I observe it binocularly from a distance of a few feet, my only sensory impression of it consists of two circular images on my two mobile retinæ, which are receiving a flow (flux) of electromagnetic radiations of a certain combination of wavelengths. Within a fraction of a second, however, my mind "recognises" the object as a ball, not as two coloured circles. Although the back of the ball cannot be seen, my mind fills in the information that the back is there, that there is but one ball, that the ball is spherical, that it is smooth or rough in texture, that it is light in weight, that it will bounce, and so on. These extra attributes of the percept, which are superimposed upon the simple visual sensations derived from the two eyes, have come from the stored memories of the mind; their presence in the mind is the result of characteristics that I have inherited and experience that I have previously gained through all my senses. Without such memories I could not "perceive". The adding together of all these attributes to form the final percept is a psychological summation, quite different from a mathematical summation restricted to things all of the same kind.

To an infant with no experience of a ball, the percept would scarcely differ from the simple visual sensation; he has still to learn how to "see" in the full sense.

---

* It does not lie within the scope of a class book such as this to attempt to describe the theories of extra-sensory perception propounded by certain psychologists: according to such theories visual perception does not depend essentially on the eyes at all.

Most people have had experience of the remarkable feats of memory; of the recognition of the face of a person who has not been seen for thirty years or more; of the way in which a certain smell or a tune will immediately awake a memory of a scene of years ago.

On occasion the mind may make a mistake in that part of the percept which it imposes on the sensory impression and so we have miscalculations, illusions and hallucinations. It would be possible, for example, to present a flat picture of the ball (or two pictures, one to each eye, in a stereoscopic device) under such conditions that the mind would be deceived into interpreting the presentation as a real three-dimensional ball. If, in the original experiment with the real ball, I were suffering from jaundice, the ball would appear yellow or orange in colour. If I press one eyeball at the side with my finger, or if I imbibe too much alcohol, there appear to be two balls. The ball will not appear red to certain colour defectives.

If the interest of the mind is concentrated on other matters, its attention to the ball percept will wane and the whole percept may be inhibited and relegated to the outer fringe of consciousness even though the sensory images have not changed in any respect.

We see how profoundly the neural images presented to the brain in consequence of physiological activity derived from the stimuli may be influenced by the mind when forming the final percept at the higher level. No account of vision which is restricted to the physical and physiological levels can be complete, even though these processes are sufficiently complicated, as we learned in the previous chapters. But when we come to contemplate the far more abstruse phenomena concerned with the manner in which, on the higher psychological plane, these events become elaborated and sublimated into a percept in consciousness, the immensity of the process is such as almost to stagger the imagination. We can use our higher mental (perceptual) faculties to examine and analyse physical experiments and even to interpret our sensations, but to analyse and "explain" our mental faculties would require equipment at a still higher level; and this we do not possess. It does not seem possible, therefore, that we can ever know all that consciousness is and does.

This does not mean, however, that it necessarily operates entirely at a super-physiological level. Modern research into the anatomy and physiology of the nervous system, especially the brain; into the characteristics of unconditioned reflexes and the acquirement of conditioned reflexes; into the effects of lesions in various parts of the visual mechanism and into heredity have shown that at least a foundation for the processes concerned with the mind and perception is incorporated in the cells and pathways of the brain. For example: it has been shown that the crouching of young chicks in response to the appearance of a hawk is not due to an instinct or inherited *idea* of fear of a hawk. Experiments with wooden and cardboard models of various shapes and sizes show that, within certain limits of size, any object of shape similar to the hawk and moving rapidly overhead elicits the same reaction. The chick has inherited, not an idea, but a mechanism of nerve cells on the sensory side of the nervous system which responds to a particular form of visual stimulus; when the effect of this response reaches the central nervous system a further mechanism is released on the motor side which produces the muscular movements of crouching. From experiments of this kind it appears that some aspect at least of that which is called mind consists of, or is tied to, the physiological mechanism; and that this works automatically in certain ways according to the pattern of the external stimulus and is incapable of working in any other way in response to that stimulus (§1.2). And yet, in man, the mind can check this automatic process and substitute spontaneously some other pattern of interpretation and behaviour.

A study of perception would necessitate a classification of the subject into subdivisions such as:

- perception of light and colour; monocular and binocular; lustre;
- perception of form and contour; monocular and binocular;
- perception of space; monocular and binocular: position, direction, size, depth, distinctness, motion, etc.;

Such a study lies outside the scope of this book; but a few random examples will be briefly described in order to illustrate the effect, always important and often paramount, of the psychological (perceptual) stage of the visual process in normal everyday vision; and of the consequent necessity to eliminate all accessory perceptual aids when drawing conclusions from experiments on the physiology of vision and, conversely, to refrain from attributing to processes at the perceptual level those effects which arise physiologically in the retina.

The examples to be quoted could be considerably extended: many of them are commonly described as optical illusions and there has been much controversy concerning their explanation. Sometimes the disagreements have been due to ascribing to the mind effects, e.g. induction, for which there is, at least partially, a physiological basis. In those cases, and these are the most numerous, in which the incongruity *is* due to faulty interpretation at the perceptual level, the cause seems to arise from the upsetting of the normal standards by which the mind assesses its visual experiences. As with after-images (§20.6), these illusions do not intrude unduly on the attention in daily life. But the effects may nevertheless be present.

23.6. The Perception of Colour.

When using an instrument such as a colorimeter the field of view is restricted to 2° or so and all the usual surrounding aids which operate in normal vision are eliminated; as far as the stimulus is concerned the sensation derived from the left (test) field is determined solely by the intensity and spectral composition of the light reaching it from the specimen under test and by the inductive effect of the light in the right (matching) field. There results a simple sensation of a certain luminosity and hue. If the test specimen is a piece of paper containing a dye which absorbs light of all the short wavelengths up to, say, 560 $m\mu$ and reflects the remaining wavelengths of the spectrum, and if the paper is illuminated with white light, then light entering the eye from the left field will evoke a sensation of unsaturated orange (we will ignore the inductive effect of the other half of the field which will in any case be small as a match is approached). If the paper is illuminated with blue light, there will be no reflection except the small amount of surface reflection and the field will appear a very dark blue. The percept differs scarcely at all from the simple sensation; there is no opportunity for the mind to elaborate the sensation since there are no factors of experience and memory to enter into the observation of such an unfamiliar scene.

If, on the other hand, a familiar object such as snow is observed, it always appears white however it is illuminated. If illuminated by blue light, the mind will not hesitate to recognise it as snow, which memory says is normally white and so the mental percept will be " snow, white, but illuminated in an unusual manner ". Some agency at the perceptual level over-rides the blue of the sensation. In the case of all objects with which we are familiar, the colour we " perceive " belongs to the object and is not determined by the spectral composition of the retinal stimulation.

The colour that we normally associate with a given object, that is the colour it appears to have when viewed by the normal light-adapted eye in diffuse daylight, is called its *true colour*. After considerable experience this colour becomes stored in the memory in association with that object, and then becomes the *memory colour*. When the object is presented to the eye under such conditions that all its usual associations are eliminated, the colour in which it appears is determined solely by the physical stimulus on the retina and is called the *plane colour*. In the colorimeter experiment described above, the colour of the field is a plane colour. If the snow, illuminated by blue light, were observed through a narrow tube so that it is seen isolated and robbed of its usual associations, it would appear blue—the plane colour.

If a somewhat overcast sky be observed through a yellow filter, the quantity of light entering the eye is reduced by the filter and yet, to most people, the sky appears definitely brighter.

If, in a dark room, a black disc is illuminated with white light from a projector lamp, the disc appears black. If the disc is rapidly rotated it will appear grey. If a strip of white paper is held in the light beam close to the rotating disc, the disc will immediately appear black. The stimulus has remained unchanged ; the white strip will have introduced some effect of induction on the physiological level, but the major reason for the striking changes in the percept is psychological.

23.7. The Perception of Form.

Of all the factors that are combined in the formation of a percept the strongest is the *meaning* that the mind attaches to it. When once this meaning has been grasped by the mind, it persists even though the usual conditions of presentation may be altered; as, for example, in the case of snow illuminated by blue light. If a square be drawn on a piece of paper, it is still interpreted as a square when the paper is viewed obliquely so that in the perspective the angles are not right angles and the upper and lower sides are not parallel.

If very little meaning can be attached to a presentation, or if it be of such a nature that more than one meaning

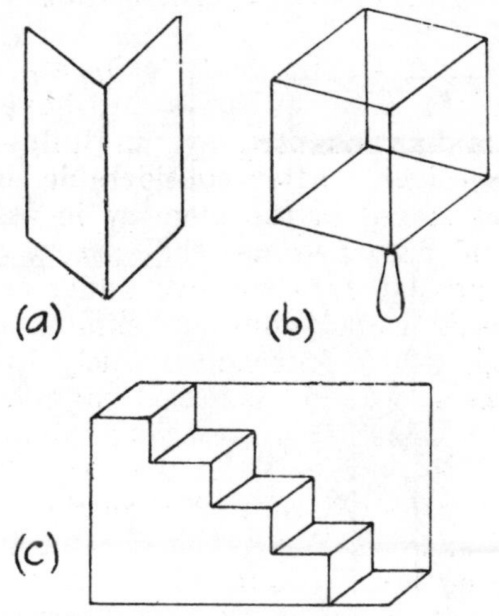

FIG. 23.2—PERCEPTION OF FORM. INADEQUATE PRESENTATION.

can be attached to it (inadequacy of presentation), the mind will interpret it in different ways at different times. If each of the diagrams in Fig. 23.2 be observed intently for many seconds, the percept will change from one meaning to another. With continued fixed observation, the rhythm of the fluctuation from one meaning to the other will vary with different observers.

The cube of example (b) may be made of wire with, say, one inch sides and held by means of a small handle, as indicated. If viewed with one eye from a distance of two feet or so and, when the apparently farthest corner appears as the nearest corner, it is rotated about a horizontal or a vertical axis, it will appear to turn in the opposite direction.

23.8. The Perception of Space.

The above are but a few simple examples of the operation of psychological factors in seeing, but they are sufficient to give some idea of the complexity of such factors during our perception of objects in three-dimensional space and of our own relation to them. The manner in which the mind appraises a given object or group of objects lying within the scene is affected by the interplay between the factors of size, distance, direction, clearness, colour, the

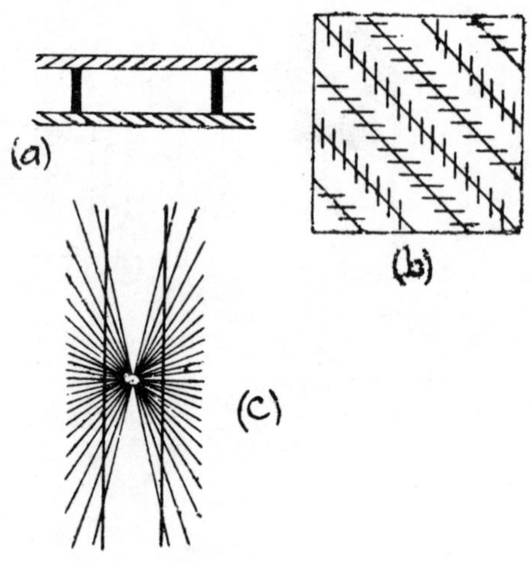

Fig. 23.3—Perception of Relative Directions.

presence of surrounding objects, their relative movements and by inequalities between the two eyes. The subject was discussed in its binocular aspects in Chapters XII and XV. A few further examples are given below.

Perception of Shape and Size.

In Fig. 23.3 (a) the upper and lower horizontal bars are strictly parallel; in (b) the long diagonal lines are strictly parallel; in (c) the two vertical lines are parallel.

The effect of neighbouring or surrounding objects or contours on our appreciation of size is well illustrated in Fig. 23.4. In (a) the two centre circles are strictly equal in size. The three vertical pillars in example (b) are equal in height, but the slanting lines induce the impression of depth so that the pillars, being conceived as lying at increasing distances, are judged to be gaining correspondingly in size. The two horizontal lines in (c) are equal in length. Example (d) illustrates the common error of judging a distance which is subdivided into steps to be greater than an equal distance not so divided; the left-hand half of the diagram appears larger than the right-hand half though in fact they are equal; reference was

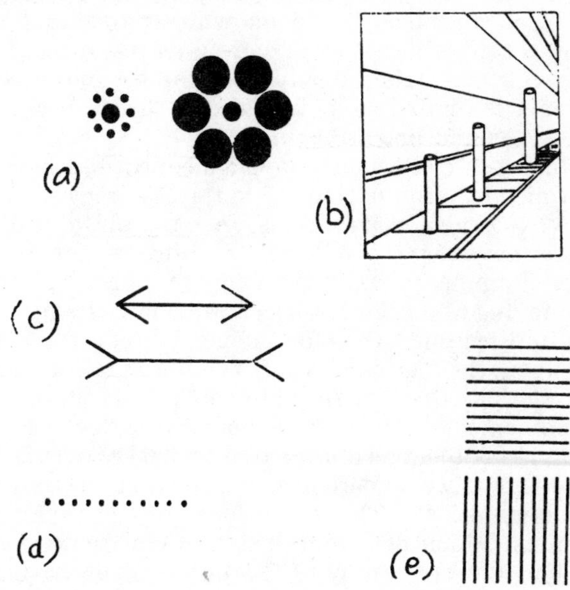

Fig. 23.4—Perception of Size.

made to this when discussing errors of space perception in §15.2. The same kind of illusion is illustrated in (e) for of the two squares the one below appears longer horizontally and the upper one longer vertically.

The Perception of Movement

When an object changes its position in the field of view the physical basis for our perception of its movement is provided by the shift of the retinal image over the mosaic of retinal receptors (§22.4); the manner in which the movement is apprehended in consciousness depends upon the speed of the object and other factors and will not be discussed here. There are various ways, however, in which the illusion of movement of a stationary object is created. If the gaze is fixed for some time on an object or objects moving steadily in one direction, then when the gaze is shifted to stationary objects they appear to be moving in the opposite direction. After gazing at a waterfall, for example, stationary objects appear at first to be moving upwards. This phenomenon of motion after-images provides a striking demonstration for an audience. A bold black spiral is drawn on white paper and this is pasted on a card which is steadily and slowly rotated about its centre; after gazing steadily at this for many seconds the audience is invited to look at the lecturer's head, which appears to expand or shrink in size.

The illusion of continuous movement may also be created by intermittent stimulation of adjacent regions of the retina; *stroboscopic movement* is an example of this type of illusory movement. A moving object which is intermittently illuminated may be made to appear stationary or to be moving at a different speed or to have its movement reversed in direction; the effect depends upon the relationship between the periodicity of the illumination and the speed of the object. By suitable control of these factors the phenomenon can be put to many practical uses. We know that if an object be illuminated by flashes of sufficiently high frequency, we experience a sensation of continuous uniform luminosity. The conditions, of the eye and of the stimulus, which determine this critical frequency were discussed in §20.11. Suppose the object is a circular disc carrying a mark of some kind, say X, near its edge. If the disc is rotated at a speed exceeding the critical frequency and is illuminated by intermittent flashes of the same frequency, the mark X will occupy the same position at every flash and will consequently appear to be stationary. In this way objects such as rotating and reciprocating parts of machinery can be examined as if they were at rest and, granted that the frequency of illumination can be controlled to known values, the speed of rotation or movement of a part can be measured.

If the speed of rotation of the disc in the above example is slightly greater or less than the frequency of illumination, the mark X will appear to drift slowly forwards or backwards respectively. This effect is often observed in the cinema; the wheels of a carriage appear to rotate backwards because of a lack of phase between the speed of rotation of the wheels and the frequency of exposure of the camera when the scene was filmed. The flicker shown by discharge lamps when run on low-frequency alternating current is occasionally responsible for stroboscopic effects with rotating machinery.

Various forms of stroboscope are manufactured in which the intermittent illumination is secured by using low-pressure mercury vapour tubes or neon lamps the frequency of the flashes of which is controlled by the electrical circuit to any value between certain limits; in the B.T.H. stroboscopic tube, for example, the duration of the individual flashes is of the order of 10^{-5} second and the frequency is variable from 250 to 500 flashes per second.

It is interesting to observe that when the gaze is rapidly shifted, in ordinary vision, from one part of a scene to another, we experience no impression of movement although the images of the objects present in the scene travel across the retina. This is presumably due to the fixing of the mind's attention upon the object that is to be observed when the movement is terminated, intermediate objects being psychologically ignored. If, however, the movement is continued in an unaccustomed manner, as when the whole body is whirled around several times, the intermediate stages are not obliterated and dizziness ensues; the ballet dancer learns to prevent this by resting the head momentarily at each 180° of the rotation and regaining fixation.

Physical Space and Visual Space

Through the mediation of all our senses but mainly our visual sense, through our sensations of luminosity, colour, form and location, elaborated and conditioned by inherited tendencies and by the factors of interest and memory in the mind, we perceive in ourselves a certain mental picture of the changing world around us; this we might call "visual space". In so far as there exists a real physical world of objects and space which is distinct from our inner perception of it and which we might call "physical space", what kind of relationship exists between the two? Physical space consists of length, mass, time, of luminous flux, brightness, reflection and transmission factors, wavelengths, etc., all of which we can measure in terms of units that we have set up for ourselves. In what units are we to assess the ingredients of visual space existing in the mind; how are we to set up units of perception?

Physical space and visual space are not identical. In the former the lines of a railway track are parallel; in the latter they meet in a distant point; a so-called frontal plane is flat in physical space whereas it is curved, sometimes convex and sometimes concave to the observer according to the distance, in visual space; a star is thousands of light-years distant in physical space but we can attach no meaning to its distance perceptually. Our senses tell us about the outside world in relation to us rather than about the outside world itself.

Such considerations lead to problems that are too advanced for a text of this kind, but until we discover more about the relationships referred to, our progress will be retarded in many practical matters in the domain of ophthalmics: binocular vision and its anomalies (e.g. aniseikonia), the training of personnel for operating visual, especially binocular, instruments, and so on.

CHAPTER XXIII. *EXERCISES.*

1. Give a summary of the evidence upon which is based the belief (*a*) that the rods and cones are the elements in the retina where the physical energy of the incident light is transformed; (*b*) in the duplicity theory concerning the distinction between the rod mechanism and the cone mechanism.

2. Can you propose an explanation to account for the fact that visual acuity improves when there is a certain balance between the illumination of the test object and of its surroundings?

3. Write an essay on the physicist's and the psychologist's points of view in relation to a theory of colour vision.

4. Give a short account of Hering's theory of colour vision. Make an attempt to reconcile this theory with the known facts of anomalous trichromatic vision.

5. Many physicists and psychologists are agreed to adopt as a working hypothesis the view that the visual mechanism contains some kind of triple response system. Describe the evidence on which this view rests and some of the problems that would still remain to be solved before an adequate theory of colour vision could be formulated, even if the triple response basis were established.

6. Describe two ways in which the physiological phenomena of flicker can be used in optical instruments. (B.O.A.)

7. Write an essay on the perception of colour, describing how the percept as to the colour of an object may be affected by familiarity with such objects and by the surrounding field; and including definitions of the terms true colour, memory and plane colour.

8. Describe examples of objects which exhibit "inadequacy of presentation" so that, with the gaze fixed intently upon them, the perceptual interpretation of their meaning changes from one form to another.

9. Give an account of our perception of space, including examples of illusions as to the shape or size of objects which arise because of the presence of other objects or patterns of lines in the field.

10. Explain what is meant by stroboscopic movement. Give an example illustrating the manner in which the phenomenon arises. Can it be put to any practical uses?

11. Write short notes on:
(*a*) the importance of pupil centres as reference points in the study of blurred image formation in the eye;
(*b*) visibility curves;
(*c*) classification of kinds of glare;
(*d*) stroboscopy. (S.M.C.)

12. Write short notes on:
(*a*) available colour vision tests;
(*b*) the recognition of night blindness;
(*c*) the measurement of stereoscopic acuity. (S.M.C.—part question.)

13. The legibility for a given individual of a page of print depends on many factors. Enumerate and discuss the most important of these. (B.O.A.)

14. It has been stated that the eyesight of the general population at the present time is a matter for much concern. What do you consider are the factors which lead to the development of refractive errors under modern conditions? Outline a programme of research and development which might be undertaken to remedy this state of affairs. (B.O.A.)

15. What are the visual functions involved in the recognition of the texture of a surface? Why is it more difficult to recognise the nature of a piece of land (*a*) when the land is viewed from a distance—e.g. from an aeroplane; and (*b*) when the illumination is low—e.g. in the twilight? (B.O.A.)

16. How do you explain the fact that the image upon the retina is inverted and yet we see things the right way up and are quite unaware of the inversion on the retina from our subjective sensations? Has any twist in the optic nerve (which it may or may not have) any bearing upon the problem? (B.O.A.)

17. Explain clearly in what respects the following statements are untrue or only partly true:
(*a*) A sheet of red glass converts white light into red.
(*b*) The hypermetrope is unable to focus objects clearly.
(*c*) It is difficult to see clearly if one goes from bright daylight into a dimly lighted room, and equally so on coming out into full daylight again.
(*d*) Yellow is a primary colour. (B.O.A.)

APPENDIX

SOME USEFUL REFERENCES

The following list of textbooks and Reports dealing with cognate subjects, may prove useful to more advanced students and to teachers. It is not intended to be exhaustive.

Optics. W. H. A. Fincham; Hatton Press, London, 1950.

Principles of Optics. Hardy and Perrin; McGraw-Hill, New York and London, 1932.

Anatomy of Eye and Orbit. E. Wolff; H. K. Lewis, London, 1948.

Visual Optics (Volume I). H. H. Emsley; Hatton Press, London, 1952.

Physiology of the Eye. H. Davson; J. & A. Churchill, London, 1948.

Measurement of Colour. W. D. Wright; Adam Hilger Ltd., London, 1944.

Researches on Normal and Defective Colour Vision. W. D. Wright; Kimpton, London, 1946.

Photometry and the Eye. W. D. Wright; Hatton Press, London, 1949.

Report of Discussion on Vision. Physical and Optical Societies, London, 1932.

"Survey of Modern Developments in Colorimetry." J. Guild; *Proc. Opt. Convention*, London, 1926.

Report on Defective Colour Vision in Industry. Physical Society, London, 1946.

Report on Colour Terminology. Physical Society, London, 1948.

THE GREEK ALPHABET

A	α	alpha	I	ι	iota	P	ρ	rho
B	β	beta	K	κ	kappa	Σ	σ ς	sigma
Γ	γ	gamma	Λ	λ	lambda	T	τ	tau
Δ	δ	delta	M	μ	mu	Υ	υ	upsilon
E	ε	epsilon	N	ν	nu	Φ	φ	phi
Z	ζ	zeta	Ξ	ξ	xi	X	χ	chi
H	η	eta	O	ο	omicrons	Ψ	ψ	psi
Θ	θ	theta	Π	π	pi	Ω	ω	omega

SOME UNITS AND USEFUL RELATIONS

$\pi = 3\cdot 1416$ $\log \pi = \cdot 4971$

1 metre = 39·371 inches 1 inch = 25·40 mm.

1 square metre = 10·76 square feet

1 μ = 1 micron = 10^{-3} mm. = $3\cdot 937 \times 10^{-5}$ inch

1 $m\mu$ = 1 millimicron = 10^{-6} mm. = $3\cdot 937 \times 10^{-8}$ inch

1 radian = $\dfrac{180^\circ}{\pi} = 57\cdot 3^\circ$ = 3438 minutes = 206,300 seconds

1 centrad = $1\nabla = \dfrac{1}{100}$ radian

1 prism dioptre = $1\Delta = \tan^{-1}\dfrac{1}{100} = 1\nabla$ very nearly

If $ax^2 + bx + c = 0$ then $x = \dfrac{-b \pm \sqrt{b^2 - 4ac}}{2a}$

sine = $\dfrac{\text{perp.}}{\text{hypot.}}$ cosine = $\dfrac{\text{base}}{\text{hypot.}}$ tangent = $\dfrac{\text{perp.}}{\text{base}}$

$\tan A = \dfrac{\sin A}{\cos A}$ $\sin^2 A + \cos^2 A = 1$

$\sin 2A = 2 \sin A \cos A$; $\cos 2A = 2\cos^2 A - 1 = 1 - 2\sin^2 A$

$\tan 2A = \dfrac{2 \tan A}{1 - \tan^2 A}$

Triangles : a, b, c are the sides; A, B, C the opposite angles

$\dfrac{a}{\sin A} = \dfrac{b}{\sin B} = \dfrac{c}{\sin C}$; $a^2 = b^2 + c^2 - 2bc \cos A$

Area = $\frac{1}{2} bc \sin A$

1 quantum = $\dfrac{1979 \times 10^{-12}}{\lambda}$ erg where λ is expressed in $m\mu$

$= 4\cdot 95 \times 10^{-12}$ erg ($\lambda = 400\ m\mu$)

$= 2\cdot 83 \times 10^{-12}$ erg ($\lambda = 700\ m\mu$)

UNITS AND DIMENSIONS

To express the magnitude of any physical quantity we must state it as a number of units of its kind. In stating that the length of a rod is 60·96 centimetres we are using the centimetre as our UNIT of length; and the number 60·96 is the MEASURE of the quantity in that unit. The same rod is 2 feet long; i.e. the measure is 2 when the unit of length is the foot.

In any science there are many *different* kinds of quantities and they bear certain relations to one another. All mechanical quantities can be derived from three which are arbitrarily chosen as fundamental. For scientific purposes these three are: length [L], mass [M] and time [T]. For engineering purposes they are: length, force (F) and time, the unit of force being that with which the earth attracts a mass of one pound at a particular place (London); i.e. one pound weight. Units of different sizes may be used for the same quantity, the guiding principle being to avoid writing unnecessarily large or small powers of 10. Thus the spectroscopist measures lengths in millimicrons ($1\ m\mu = 10^{-6}$ mm.), whilst the astronomer needs a very much larger unit and measures distances in light-years; 1 light-year is the distance travelled by light in empty space in one year. The physicist measures work or energy in ergs (1 erg = work done by a force of 1 dyne acting through a distance of 1 cm.); the engineer measures energy, in this country, in foot-pounds; the householder buys electrical energy in terms of Board of Trade Units (1 B.T.U. = $3 \cdot 6 \times 10^{13}$ ergs).

In the centimetre-gramme-second or C.G.S. system of units, largely used in science, the units in which the fundamental quantities are expressed are the centimetre, the gramme and the second. A *volume* is (a length) × (a length) × (a length); we say that a volume has three DIMENSIONS in length or [volume] = [L] × [L] × [L] = $[L]^3$. The unit of volume on the C.G.S. system is the cubic centimetre; it varies as the cube of the unit of length. Unit *velocity* is 1 cm. in 1 second; the dimensions of velocity are $\frac{L}{T}$ or LT^{-1} cm. per second. Unit *momentum* or quantity of motion in a body, is that of 1 gramme moving with unit velocity of 1 cm. per second; or the dimensions of momentum are MLT^{-1}. *Force* is change of momentum per second, hence its dimensions are $\frac{MLT^{-1}}{T}$ or MLT^{-2}, the unit on the C.G.S. system being called the dyne.

Quantities like angle, which is a ratio between two lengths, and refractive index, which is a ratio between two velocities, are mere numbers and have zero dimensions. Dimensions are useful for checking equations, since the terms on the two sides of an algebraic equation relating to physical quantities must necessarily have the same dimensions.

For convenience of reference a number of useful quantities with their units and dimensions are collected together in the accompanying table. Definitions and explanations of those having particular reference to the subject of this book have appeared in the text.

Quantities such as the velocity of light, refractive indices of substances, the dimensions and mass of the electron, and its electric charge, the constants in the radiation formulæ, etc., have to be determined, directly or indirectly, by experiment. It will be understood, therefore, that their accepted values suffer slight modifications from time to time as experimental methods become more precise. For example, the value $4 \cdot 80 \times 10^{-10}$ E.S.U. for the electronic charge e quoted in the footnote to §17.2 is a recent value; MILLIKAN's value is $4 \cdot 77 \times 10^{-10}$ E.S.U.

TABLE I. UNITS AND DIMENSIONS

antity	*Symbol*	*Dimensions*	*Unit*	*Magnitudes and Comparisons*
th		L	centi-metre	1 foot = 30·479 cm.; 1 metre = 39·37 inches
		M	gramme	1 pound = 453·59 gm. = 7000 grains
		T	second	
city	v	cm. per second; LT^{-1}		1 mile per hour = 88 feet per minute
leration	f	cm. per sec. per sec.; LT^{-2}		
ılar ocity	ω		radian per sec.	
entum		mass × velocity; MLT^{-1}		
e		mass × acceleration; MLT^{-2}	dyne	1 gm. = 981 dynes; 1 pound = 444,974 dynes
k or rgy		force × length; ML^2T^{-2}	erg joule	1 joule = 10^7 ergs 1 foot-pound = $13 \cdot 5626 \times 10^6$ ergs = 1·35626 joule
er		work or energy per sec.; ML^2T^{-3}	watt	1 watt = 1 joule per sec. 1 H.P. = 550 ft. lb. per sec. = 746 watts 1 Kilowatt-hour = 1·34 H.P.-hour = 1 B. of T. unit
;		ML^2T^{-2}	calorie	1 calorie = heat to raise 1 gm. water through 1° C. 1 calorie ≡ 4·18 joules = 3·087 ft.-pounds 1 B.Th.U. = 252 cal. = 778 ft.-pounds 1 therm = 10^5 B.Th.U. = 29·312 B. of T. units
inous ux	F	lumen	lumen	1 lumen ≡ 0·00154 watt for λ = 555 $m\mu$
nsity	I	lumen per unit solid angle	candle	1 candle ≡ 4π lumens when emission uniform in all directions
htness	B	lumen per unit solid angle per unit area	candle per unit area	See Table II for comparisons
		or lumen per unit area	lambert	
nination	E	lumen per unit area	lumen per metre²	Also called metre-candle or lux
			lumen per foot²	Also called foot-candle.

TABLE II. LIGHT: CONVERSION FACTORS.

LUMINANCE (BRIGHTNESS)

	Candle / cm.²	Candle / metre²	Candle / foot²	Lambert	Milli-lambert	Fo lam
Candle per cm.² (stilb) ..	1	10^4	929	π	3142	29
Candle per metre² (nit) ..	10^{-4}	1	0·0929	$\pi \times 10^{-4}$	0·3142	0·2
Candle per foot² ..	$10\cdot76 \times 10^{-4}$	10·76	1	$3\cdot382 \times 10^{-3}$	3·382	
Lambert (Lum. per cm.²) ..	$\frac{1}{\pi}$	3183	295·7	1	1000	92
Millilambert	$\frac{1}{\pi} \times 10^{-3}$	3·183	0·296	10^{-3}	1	0·9
Foot-lambert	$3\cdot427 \times 10^{-4}$	3·427	$\frac{1}{\pi}$	$10\cdot76 \times 10^{-4}$	1·076	
Lum. per metre² (apostilb)	$3\cdot183 \times 10^{-5}$	0·3183	0·0296			0·0

ILLUMINATION

	Lumen / metre²	Lumen / cm.²	Milliphot	Lum foo
Lumen per metre² (metre-candle; lux)	1	10^{-4}	10^{-1}	0·09
Lumen per cm.² (phot)	10^4	1	10^3	92
Milliphot	10	10^{-3}	1	0·92
Lumen per foot² (foot-candle) ..	10·76	$10\cdot76 \times 10^{-4}$	1·076	1

Multiply unit in vertical column by conversion factor to obtain unit in horizontal col e.g. 1 candle/foot² equals 10·76 candles/metre² or 3·382 millilamberts; 1 lumen/cm.² e 10^4 lumens/metre² or 929 lumens/foot.²

For perfect diffuser: Luminance (brightness) in ft. lamb. = Illumination in lum./ft.² x l

TABLE III. BRIGHTNESS OF LIGHT SOURCES in Candles per cm.² (stilb).

(Note: the following are to be taken as round figures. Precise values for lamps depend upon wattage, shape of filament, gas pressure, conditions of operation, etc.)

Sun: reduced by atmospheric absorption to about ..	165,000
Sky: clear fine day	0·7 to 0·8
Full Moon:	0·25
Candle flame:	0·5
Carbon arc: depending on current density ..	20,000 to 80,000
Mercury vapour discharge lamp: high pressure ..	120 to 48,000
Tungsten lamps, gas-filled: maximum of filament	450 to 2,650
Projection lamps: equivalent brightness of filament shape	100 to 3,000
Glow-worm	0·005

TABLE IV. ILLUMINATIONS in Lumens per foot^2 (foot-candles)

At earth's surface due to sun and sky; maximum ..	..	10,000
Indoors on fine day: depending on window area	..	10–25
Recommended minima for: precise visual tasks ..	..	25–50
average visual tasks (e.g. reading)		10–15
rough shop work ..	..	2–4
ophthalmic test chart	..	8–15
special tasks (e.g. operating table)		100–500

TABLE V. LUMINOSITY FACTORS (PHOTOPIC) AND TRICHROMATIC COEFFICIENTS (W. D. WRIGHT, 1927).

Wavelength $m\mu$	*Luminosity Factor*	*Trichromatic Coefficients*		
		Red : λ 650	*Green* : λ 530	*Blue* : λ 460
400	·0004			
10	·0012	·051	– ·047	·996
20	·0040			
30	·0116	·045	– ·043	·998
40	·023			
450	·038	·021	– ·024	1·003
60	·060	·000	·000	1·000
70	·091	– ·031	·057	·974
80	·139	– ·094	·182	·912
90	·208	– ·170	·420	·750
500	·323	– ·233	·772	·461
10	·503	– ·207	1·002	·205
20	·710	– ·111	1·049	·062
30	·862	·000	1·000	·000
40	·954	·123	·901	– ·024
550	·995	·232	·797	– ·029
60	·995	·354	·676	– ·030
70	·952	·480	·543	– ·023
80	·870	·604	·414	– ·018
90	·757	·720	·290	– ·010
600	·631	·811	·196	– ·007
10	·503	·881	·124	– ·005
20	·381	·929	·075	– ·004
30	·265	·966	·037	– ·003
40	·175	·988	·014	– ·002
650	·107	1·000	·000	·000
60	·061			
70	·032			
80	·017	1·011	– ·011	
90	·0082			
700	·0041	1·015	– ·015	
10	·0021			
20	·0010			
Standard White (4800° K)		·333	·333	·333

ANSWERS TO EXERCISES

CHAPTER XII. Page 60.

7. 225 and 275 metres. Each 0·000404 mm. nasalward from fovea.
43. 8·2 seconds ; 1635 metres.
44. 15△ each eye ; 4·77 D.
45. Convergence of R.E. 27·27△.
47. 18 metres approx.
48. 10·39 per cent.

CHAPTER XIII. Page 114.

6. (*a*) R. projection 48 cm. below and 30 cm. to left of L. projection.
   (*b*) R. proj. 48 cm. below and 54 cm. to left of L. proj.
   (*c*) 5△ base in.
7. R. projection 72 cm. to right of and 24 cm. above L. projection; i.e. diplopia is uncrossed R. superior.
8. (*a*) R. proj. 72 cm. to right of L. proj ; (*b*) single vision.
   (*c*) single vision ; (*d*) R. proj. 72 cm. below L. proj. ; (*e*) R. proj. 72 cm. below and 30 cm. to left of L. proj.
9. R. proj. 48 cm. above and 24 cm. to right of L. proj. ; (*a*) R. proj. 48 cm. above and 24 cm. to left of L. proj ; (*b*) single vision.
   With long line object, fusion and single vision in all cases.
11. To *test* whether phoria or tropia see Chapter XII.
17. Conditions at 5 metres :
    (*a*) Eso 2△; (*b*) Exo 1·2△; (*c*) L. Hyper 0·3△.
18. At 10 metres : (*a*) Hor. streak through source ; (*b*) R. Hyper ; horizontal streak below source ; (*c*) very slight R. Hyper is simulated ; streak slightly below source.
    At 1 metre : (*a*) Hor. streak through source ; (*b*) for same upward tilt as before, appearance same as for 10 metres ; (*c*) same as (*c*) for 10 metres but more pronounced.
19. Exo 7△; 7△ base in; 16° 58′.
20. Exo 10△.
21. Yes. Exo 6△. (If forward position of – 10 D lenses were taken into account, phoria shown with centred lenses would be approximately Exo 5·5△, the effect of the lenses on the eye being 2·5△ base in).
22. Exo 9¼△.
28. Exophoria ; left hyperphoria ; incyclophoria.
29. (*a*) Eso 4 △ at 6 metres ; (*b*) R. Hyper 1·6△ at 5 m. ; (*c*) Excyclo at near ; (*d*) Exo 2·5△ with R. Hyper 3△, at 6 m. (*e*) Excyclo 10° at distance. Raise front of left carrier or front of right carrier, or both.
45. Indications are that convergence exercises might be of value.
52. 3·43△.

CHAPTER XIV. Page 162.

24. About 15° to 20°, depending on the angle alpha.
28. Approx. $41\frac{1}{2}$°.

CHAPTER XVI. Page 192.

8. R. supravergence (or artificial R. hyperphoria) and R. retinal image larger than L. (assuming axial ametropia).
9. 7·25△ divergent.
10. Each eye $3\frac{1}{3}$△ in direction of frame displacement. Points $4\frac{1}{6}$ mm. from O.C.; 0·107△ in opposite direction to first rotation.
11. 2·22△; or 74 M.A.
12. R. No convergence; 2·59 D accommodation;
    L. 13·5△; 1·94 D accommodation; L. supravergence.
13. R. image 2·65 per cent larger than L. image.

CHAPTER XVII. Page 214.

3. Equation 17.3; 434·1 $m\mu$ (one of violet lines).
5. 376·2 watts/cm.^{2}; 1013° K. At 4000° K total energy increases to about 1460 watts/cm.^{2} and λ_m moves to lower wavelengths, to about 720 $m\mu$.
8. (*a*) has continuous spectrum and energy distribution curve is of type shown in lower part of Fig. 17.6 or similar to tungsten curve of Fig. 17.7; much of energy lies in infra-red; (*b*) has line spectrum and energy dist. curve as in upper part of Fig. 17.6. Much of energy is invisible and u.v. and latter can be made visible by fluorescent coating; thus luminous efficiency higher than (*a*).
10. Student learns about HERTZ and RÖNTGEN in subject of Optics.

CHAPTER XVIII. Page 237.

2. (*a*) 50 candles; (*b*) 25 candles; 0·0628 lumen.
3. 97·3 candles.
4. §18.8; 30 cm.
5. Assuming eye can detect one per cent difference, distance is about 0·5 cm.
6. Intensity of source = 147·8 can.; total flux = 1857 lumens.
7. 0·929 foot-can.; 90·25 per cent.
8. Scale diagram gives distance from source to front edge = 6 ft. and angle of incidence of light as 46°; calculation from these gives $I = \frac{36 \times 2}{\cdot 72} = 100$ can.

   More accurately, $I = 100\cdot 25$ can.

9 At $\theta°$ from vertical, illumination $E = I_\theta \cos^3\theta/625$ ft. can. $\therefore I_\theta = 125/\cos^3\theta$ can.

$\theta°$	10	20	30	40	50	60	70
I_θ	130·9	150·6	192·5	278	470·5	1000	3123

10. 2860 can./foot^2 or 9000 ft. lamb.; 0·746 ft.
11. 2 seconds.
15. §1·6; luminosity curve, Fig. 18.1.
17. 4 ft. and 40 ft.; intensity = 1600 can.; output = 6400π lumens.
19. §18.8.

CHAPTER XIX. Page 268.

11. (*a*) 571, (*b*) 591, (*c*) 492 $m\mu$; §19.2; roughly luminosities in ratio (*a*) 30 : 1; (*b*) 2 : 1.
14. Y = 1·778 R + 1·222 G − 0·222 B; the coeffts. here are not equal on the two sides of the equation nor equal to unity. Presumably there was not a match in hue and luminosity.
15. C = ·261 R + ·826 G − ·087 W.
16. (*a*) Table V for coefficients; (*b*) blue-green; desaturated with 40 per cent white; λ 501 (*c*) Yellow; almost pure; λ 589 (Wright's matching stimuli); (*d*) yellow-green; desaturated with 62 per cent white; λ 562; (*e*) standard white.
17. (*a*) 0, ·3, 1·0, 1·3, 2·0, 5·0; (*b*) 2·62.
18. 0·699; transp. = 4 per cent; density = 1·398.
19. (*b*) right eye, a plain red surface; left eye, black lines on green surface.
25. (*a*) Green-yellow; desaturated about 35 per cent white; λ 553; (*b*) blue-green; desaturated about 32 per cent white; λ 499; (*c*) yellow; desaturated about 90 per cent white (very pale); λ 572.

CHAPTER XXI. Page 344.

1. $7·7 \times 10^{-10}$ lumens per foot^2.
7. 0·94; 0·329 foot-lambert.
15. 6, 1, 1, 4 $m\mu$.
30. 5×10^{-9} lumen.

INDEX